54027000285419

Medicines Library

AF606595

Controlled Drug Bioavailability

Controlled Drug Bioavailability

VOLUME 2
BIOAVAILABILITY METHODOLOGY AND REGULATION

Edited by

VICTOR F. SMOLEN
PharmaControl Corporation
Englewood Cliffs, New Jersey

LUANN BALL
Ciba-Geigy Corporation
Summit, New Jersey

A Wiley-Interscience Publication

JOHN WILEY & SONS

New York • Chichester • Brisbane • Toronto • Singapore

Library of Congress Cataloging in Publication Data:

Main entry under title:

Bioavailability methodology and regulation.

(Controlled drug bioavailability; v. 2)
"A Wiley-Interscience publication."
Includes bibliographical references and index.
1. Drugs—Bioavailability. 2. Chemistry, Pharmaceutical. I. Smolen, Victor F. II. Ball, LuAnn.
RM301.6.B56 1984 615.5'8 83-16679
ISBN 0-471-88200-3

Printed in the United States of America

10 9 8 7 6 5 4 3 2 1

Contributors

LuAnn Ball, Ciba-Geigy Corporation, Summit, New Jersey

Bernard E. Cabana, Division of Biopharmaceutics, Food and Drug Administration, Rockville, Maryland

R. M. J. Ings, Hoechst UK, Ltd., Bucks, England

Goetz Leopold, Human Pharmacology Centre, E. Merck, Darmstadt, Federal Republic of Germany

Keith Rotenberg, Pennwalt Corporation, Rochester, New York

Jerome Skelly, Pharmacokinetics Branch, Division of Biopharmaceutics, Food and Drug Administration, Rockville, Maryland

Victor F. Smolen, PharmaControl Corporation, Englewood Cliffs, New Jersey

Daniel B. Tuey, PharmaControl Corporation, Englewood Cliffs, New Jersey

Series Preface

The purpose of this newly established continuing series of monographs is to provide a forum to disseminate current knowledge that contributes to expediting the design, development, evaluation, manufacture, control, marketing, and clinical use of increasingly safer and more effective drug products at lower costs. A critical problem with the entire health care industry is the high and rapidly escalating costs. A significant contribution to this problem is the cost of drugs. Not only is the research for the development of drug products expensive, but so is the process for the establishment of their quality, safety, effectiveness, and manner of use. It has been estimated that it presently takes an average of seven years and in excess of $50 million to gain approval of a single new drug in the United States by the Food and Drug Administration (FDA). Briefly, a promising new drug must first be tested in up to thousands of animals to assess its possible toxicity. That done, it must then be used in multiphasic tests before the dosage form(s) and dose levels, safety, effectiveness, and possible side effects can be determined. These human subjects must be under the almost constant surveillance of high-priced specialists, and the results of all these studies must be analyzed by statisticians and reported. Finally, this mass of data must be reviewed and approved by drug regulatory agencies such as the FDA before permission to market the drug can be given. It is obviously imperative that the most current knowledge be effectively applied to reduce the costs of drug product development and accelerate the availability of new therapies and improved products to the patients needing them.

In all approaches to drug development it cannot be overlooked that drugs are never used as the pure chemical substances whose molecular structures are responsible for their intrinsic pharmacological activities. Drugs are always put into delivery systems, such as liquids to be injected by mechanical or electromechanical devices, or are formulated into dosage forms such as tablets, capsules, suppositories, and so on, and recently even into patches placed on the skin's surface; such dosage forms become the marketed drug products themselves. In practice, the dynamics of the manner by which a dosage form releases its drug to become available to its site(s) of action in the body is equally as important in determining the safety and effectiveness of the course of drug therapy as is the intrinsic pharmacological activity of the chemical substance that the drug product contains.

The formulation and manufacture of drug dosage forms, as well as how drug delivery devices are designed and operated, has a profound influence on the manner in which drugs access their site(s) of action. In recent years it has become widely recognized among pharmaceutical scientists, clinicians, and government regulatory agencies that drug bioavailability, defined as the time course of the rates and extents of drug entrance into the body or release to its sites of absorption prior to entering into the body, is of the most fundamental importance to the design, development, evaluation, and clinical use of drug products. This importance becomes apparent from simply considering that once a drug enters into the body (i.e., becomes bioavailable), the course of its therapeutic and toxic effects becomes entirely determined by the intrinsic dynamics of the drug's disposition and actions in the body. Since targeting of drug molecules to specific sites of action is not yet achieved, there is presently virtually nothing that can be routinely and effectively done to alter the course of these effects. Therefore, selection of or otherwise affecting the manner in which the drug is allowed to enter the body in the first place (i.e., the bioavailability input of the drug) provides the only practical means to control, or inadvertently alter, the safety and effectiveness of drug products. A potential basis for drug product design and development must, therefore, always consider the relationship between the drug bioavailability inputs that a product will deliver and the resulting time course of pharmacological effects and body fluid drug levels that ensue. Products having the same bioavailability inputs can be considered bioequivalent. Pharmacokinetics, defined as what the body does to the drug (i.e., absorb, distribute, metabolize, and eliminate it), and pharmacodynamics, defined as what the drug does to the body (i.e., elicit pharmacological effects), provide the theoretical and computationally practical means of relating drug bioavailability inputs to the drug level and pharmacological responses that underlie the safety and clinical effectiveness of a drug's usage.

Even though the development of new clinical drug entities—which was incipient and flourished after World War II—continues to produce new and exciting progress, there is presently a rapidly increasing awareness that the drug industry has entered a new era of even greater precision in drug therapy based on controlled drug bioavailability. As is the case with all trends in our society, circumstances of politics, law, and economics, in addition to developments in science and pharmaceutical technology, are providing a strong impetus to the growth of precisely controlled bioavailability. This can be understood from considering the regulatory law requirements and economics of new drug entity development relative to the inordinately lower costs of developing and marketing better drug delivery systems for generic drugs whose intrinsic safety and effectiveness have already been well established.

Generic drugs are those for which patent protection has expired, allowing them to be sold by other manufacturers in competition with the original patenting pharmaceutical company. In 1979 the U.S. market in generic drugs was an estimated $4.37 billion, representing 43% of the total pharmaceutical drug market in that year. A recent Frost and Sullivan report on the generic drugs market forecasts generic drug sales to reach nearly $10 billion by 1989 in the United States alone. Others forecast $10 billion generic sales to be reached by 1985. Significant factors in this growth are the expiration of patents of 48 of the major pharmaceuticals (which had combined sales in the United States of $2.2 billion in 1979) and the time, difficulty, and expense of developing new ethical, patented drugs. Therefore, the competition by both ethical and generic drug companies to retain and capture market shares can be projected to become increasingly fierce. Successful competitors can be expected to offer superior drug products that provide therapeutic advantages. The leveling of competition between multisource suppliers of the same generic drug entity should provide the economic impetus to develop drug products that are not merely satisfactory but have a therapeutically optimal, controlled drug bioavailability. The development of such products would contribute to even more rapidly advancing the pharmaceutical sciences as well as being of obvious benefit to drug-consuming patients. It is to these objectives that this series of monographs is dedicated, through presenting current information relating to the theory and practice of controlled drug bioavailability.

The present and subsequent volumes are devoted primarily to those topical areas whose interaction is requisite to the development of drug products of optimal therapeutic benefit. Most broadly, these topics include (1) pharmacokinetics and pharmacodynamics that provide the theoretical and computational means necessary to relate the dynamic manner in which a drug must be allowed to enter the body to elicit optimally sought pharmacological effects (the performance criteria, on which to design the drug release dynamics of drug products to achieve optimal therapeutic benefits can be determined); (2) methodologies and drug regulatory considerations for the bioavailability–bioequivalency requirements and the evaluation of drug delivery systems; (3) the specific design, development, properties, manufacture, control, and factors that affect the bioavailability of particular types of drug delivery system that most broadly are chemical, mechanical, or electromechanical devices; and (4) the marketing and promotion of drug products. The projected market success of a controlled-release drug product is of course the initiating factor for its development. The manner of promoting a uniquely new product will include a need to educate the physician, pharmacist, nurse, and patient in order to gain its acceptance; therefore, the promotion of a new and novel drug delivery system is even more important than the otherwise unrealized potential therapeutic benefits such products can provide. For example, there is clearly a need for controlled-release drug products that allow for a once-a-day dosing schedule to always be maintained for all the drugs a patient is taking in order to achieve maximum patient compliance and therapeutic benefits. This must be done while permitting the dosage for many of the most important drugs to be readily adjusted to a patient's individualized needs. These objectives would necessitate that the drugs be supplied in unconventional forms. The marketing and promotion of new drug product forms would require the application of both a clinical pharmacokinetic and educational support program to ensure the proper and most successful usage of such products. This example serves to illustrate the need for the integration of all the relevant topics and themes of this series to deliver a maximum therapeutic benefit to patients in what is envisaged to continue to be an era of increasing improvements in controlled drug bioavailability.

VICTOR F. SMOLEN
LUANN BALL

Englewood Cliffs, New Jersey
Summit, New Jersey
August 1983

Preface

In the development of a new drug product, an immense amount of time and money is spent testing for safety, effectiveness, and reliability. The abundance of results obtained must be reported to and approved by the Food and Drug Administration (FDA) before the drug product can be marketed. To minimize the overall effort, it is important to use effective in-vitro and in-vivo testing methods in animals and in humans. Volume 2 in this continuing series on controlled drug bioavailability is of particular value to the pharmacokineticist who designs effective testing methods and reports the results to the FDA. Chapter 1 is concerned with factors that influence the results of a bioavailability/ bioequivalence study performed in humans. Bioavailability testing in animals is the topic of Chapter 2. Chapters 3 through 5 address in-vitro methods for assessing drug product bioavailabilities. Chapter 3 discusses the correlation of in-vitro dissolution test results with in-vivo bioavailability parameters. A method for computationally converting in-vitro dissolution results into a time course of in-vivo response is reported in Chapter 4. Chapter 5 looks at various dissolution testing methodologies, including a computer-controlled dissolution testing apparatus that can, when programmed with in-vivo results from a pilot study, substitute for a panel of human subjects in the determination of drug product bioavailability/bioequivalence. Chapter 6 suggests an approach to effectively reporting in-vitro and in-vivo results and conclusions to the FDA. Poorly written reports can prolong the drug product review process and delay its subsequent approval for marketing. A method for obtaining pharmacokinetic data by computer resolution of recorded physiological signals is discussed in Chapter 7, and an example is shown for organic nitrates.

VICTOR F. SMOLEN
LUANN BALL

Englewood Cliffs, New Jersey
Summit, New Jersey
November 1983

Contents

Controlled Drug Bioavailability

CHAPTER 1

Experimental Factors Influencing the Results of Drug Product Bioavailability/Bioequivalency Studies in Humans

GOETZ LEOPOLD

Human Pharmacology Centre, E. Merck, Darmstadt, Federal Republic of Germany

CONTENTS

To determine relative bioavailability or bioequivalence, various formulations of two or more preparations are compared under identical trial conditions. These conditions are particularly suitable if they permit clinically relevant statements to be assessed economically. We can select suitable experimental conditions and factors only if we know how these factors influence the bioavailability of drugs.

The knowledge and consideration of all experimental factors that can modify the bioavailability of drugs is also important for a safe and effective drug therapy. Experimental factors are those that may affect drug bioavailability and can be influenced by the investigator planning a study with a given substance and formulation. They include the *external trial conditions* and the *physiological and biochemical characteristics* of normal subjects or patients. The second point is especially important when a trial design with independent groups of volunteers or patients is used.

Many relevant factors have been identified and their importance documented and reviewed during the last 15 years (1–17), although some had already been identified in the "Old German Literature" (18). Tappeiner (19) wrote in 1899:

> The common route which is chosen for the application of drugs is that through the mouth. The digestive canal is perfectly equipped for the nutrition business but it has many disadvantages for the use in therapy. First of all, the stomach is not at all an excellent absorption organ. In this respect the stomach is by far inferior to the gut. Secondly, the state of filling often implies a great delay in absorption and in any case uncertainty with respect to its beginning. Thirdly, many substances are decomposed in the digestive canal and thus rendered ineffective, others will not at all be absorbed, and at the end fourthly, even after the uptake into the blood the drug must pass through the liver which is—as is well known—able to chemically convert or retain many substances. All these conditions imply great uncertainty. To this adds, that even in the most favorable cases presumably the first molecules will be already absorbed after 5 minutes and even pass into the secretion, but the main portion will arrive after 10–15 minutes and the last remainder will arrive only at a time when the first have been already excreted a long while ago. Therefore the administered dose will never be entirely present in the blood at the same time to be active in the organs. The effect, therefore, only reaches a certain extent which will gradually be gained and just so gradually abandoned again. [author's translation].

The aim of this chapter is to review concisely all possible influences of experimental factors on the results of bioavailability/bioequivalency studies, including a compilation of relevant references.

A pragmatic *classification of the experimental factors* can be established as follows:

1. External trial conditions.

a. Subject related.

i. Intake of food: time relative to intake of drug, quality, quantity, temperature, and spices (20).

ii. Intake of fluid: time relative to intake of drug, quality, quantity, and temperature.

iii. Social drugs: coffee, tea, tobacco, and ethanol.

iv. Posture and physical activity: supine, rest, and exercise.

v. Psychic stress: specific, necessary inconveniences of the protocol (e.g., duration and physical inconvenience) and situations producing tension or anxiety.

b. Environment related.

i. Climatic variations: temperature, atmospheric pressure, weather condition, and humidity.

ii. Chronobiologic factors: circadian and seasonal variations and chronopharmacokinetics.

iii. Atmosphere of the clinical environment: the surroundings, recreational facilities, contact with the staff, and conflict and tension-producing situations independent of the protocol.

2. Characteristics of volunteers.

a. Somatic characteristics.

i. Anthropometric data: race, sex (pregnancy), age, height, weight, and ponderal-index (height-weight-relation).

ii. Physical state: physical examination (nutritional and physical state) and laboratory data (clinical chemistry, hematology, urinalysis, and hemostaseology).

iii. Special physiological functions: liver, stomach, thyroid, kidney, and GI-tract (genetic constitution, pharmacogenetics, and ethnopharmacokinetics).

b. Psychic characteristics.

i. Personality traits: level of neuroticism and anticipation anxiety.

ii. Tolerance for stress, personal trial experience.

iii. Attitude toward the trial: motivation, cooperation, and compliance.

c. Habits and conditions of living (not the *external* trial conditions *during* a study, but individual habits and conditions of living and environment that have *persistently* affected the *internal* milieu of a subject *before* a study).

   i. Dietary factors: feeding habits, meal times, quantity and composition of food, and fluid intake and volume.
   ii. Social drugs: tobacco, alcohol, and coffee or tea (type and quantity).
   iii. Drugs (common self-medication): contraceptives, laxatives, antacids, vitamins, analgesics, and sedatives.
   iv. Micturition: deliberate control.
   v. Defecation: normal frequency.
   vi. Physical activity: state of training.
   vii. Employment: occupational exposure.

3. Special characteristics of patients.

   a. Pathophysiologic conditions (disease): of stomach, GI-tract, liver, kidney, thyroid, GI-flora, plasma proteins, body temperature, and cardiovascular system.
   b. Interaction with other drugs: antacids, anticholinergics, etc.

1. EXTERNAL TRIAL CONDITIONS

The external trial conditions listed above usually modify bioavailability because they influence one or more *physiological factors* such as (3, 5–7, 12, 21–40): hydrogen ion concentration in the GI-tract (secretion and buffering), gastric juice (volume and viscosity), gastrointestinal motility (pyloric passage and GI-transit time), blood flow rate (mesenterium and liver), GI-endocrine system, flow rate of bile and pancreatic juice, and microflora of the GI-tract.

1.1 Subject Related

1.1.1 *Intake of Food*

The influence of food on the bioavailability of drugs has often been described (41–48), but it is not yet possible to make many general statements. Therefore, the individual results are listed pragmatically in Tables 1–4, as proposed by Welling (14, 49, 50) and Toothaker and Welling (51), who reviewed this topic. The data are supplemented by the results of Weber (52), Melander (53), Beerman (54), Leopold (55, 56),* and others.

Food influences the bioavailability of drugs by modulating physiologic functions of the GI-tract, except in cases exhibiting a direct interaction with food constituents (e.g., formation of poorly soluble salts, chelation, adsorption, etc.). Because of its large surface, drugs are better absorbed in the small intestine than in the stomach (6). Therefore, the moment of passage through the pyloric sphincter is especially important for the enteric absorption of drugs. A delay in gastric emptying often implies a delay of absorption. The rate of gastric emptying can be raised by increasing intragastric pressure; the relevant baroreceptors are located in the gastric wall (57, 58). A delay of gastric emptying can be effected by the impulses of three types of receptors in the duodenal mucosa and by the action of hormones. The receptors exhibit a selective sensitivity to hydrogen ions, fatty acids, or osmotic changes. When ingested food or fluid of low pH, high fatty acid content, or high osmolarity reaches the duodenum, a reflex inhibition of gastric emptying occurs. The inhibition of gastric motility by hormones (gastric inhibitory peptide [GIP], enterogastrin, cholecystokinin-pancreozymin, and motilin) is also triggered by low pH and fatty acids in the duodenum. These inhibitory mechanisms protect the epithelium of the small intestine (59, 60). Furthermore, the higher the temperature of an ingested meal or drink, the more solid a meal, and the more viscous the gastric contents, the stronger the inhibition of gastric emptying will be (61–64).

The regulation of gastric motility is tightly connected with the gastric secretion. Psychic-neural as well as gastric and intestinal influences play a role. Gastric secretion is mainly stimulated by gastrin liberated by distension- and chemo-receptors (e.g., those sensitive to protein fragments). Gastric secretion is inhibited by secretin, cholecystokinin-pancreozymin, and GIP, which are liberated in the duodenum by fatty acids and hydrogen ions. The secretion of pancreatic juice is regulated by secretin and cholecystokinin-pancreozymin.

The production of bile is enhanced by secretin; the contraction of the gall bladder is triggered by reflex or by cholecystokinin-pancreozymin (36, 59, 60).

The blood flow rate in the splanchnic region is increased during a meal and postprandially; the extent depends on the type of food. After a high-protein meal the blood flow rate increases significantly and normalizes only gradually,

*These projects were supported by grants of the German Federal Department for Research and Technology (BMFT) No. MT 417 and BAM 07. Responsibility for the content lies with the author. The publications concerned are references 55, 56, 146, 147, 156, 173, 174, 230, and 309–311.

whereas after a high carbohydrate meal the blood flow rate initially decreases somewhat and then quickly returns to normal (21). In enteral absorption, the diffusion rate of a drug from the lumen of the GI-tract to the blood of the splanchnic capillaries is also determined by the concentration gradient in the membrane to be crossed. Therefore, a modification of the blood flow rate by food intake can be clinically significant for the enteral absorption of drugs, especially those that undergo a pronounced first pass effect and exhibit a high hepatic extraction rate (65, 66). Thus, gastrointestinal motility, blood flow rate, and GI-secretion are the major physiologic functions that modify the bioavailability of drugs.

The reported effects of concomitant food intake on bioavailability can be divided into four groups: reduced, delayed, unaffected, and increased drug absorption (Tables 1–4). Because the trial methods, the documentation, and the validity of the results of many studies exhibit vast differences, it is not possible to discuss in detail the clinical relevance of the individual data. Conflicting data might be the result of dissimilarities in the formulations or experimental factors.

Table 1. Drugs Whose Absorption May Be Reduced by Food

Drug	Reference	Drug	Reference
Acetylsalicylic acid	(67–71)	Levothyroxine	(103)
Amiloride	(72)	Lincomycin	(104)
Amoxicillin	(73)	Methacycline	(105)
Ampicillin	(74–78)	Nafcillin	(106)
Atenolol	(79)	Oxytetracycline	(105, 107)
Benzilonium-bromide	(80)	Penicillin G	(108–110)
Bretylium tosylate	(81)	Penicillin V	(108, 111)
Cephalexin	(82)	Phenethicillin	(108, 112)
Demethylchlortetracycline	(83–85)	Pivampicillin	(75, 76, 113)
Doxycycline (slightly reduced)	(85, 86)	Propantheline	(114, 115)
Emepronium-bromide	(87)	Rifampicin	(116)
Erythromycin	(88, 89)	Sodium-fluoride	(117)
Erythromycin stearate	(89–94)	Sotalol	(118)
Ethanol	(95–97)	Sulfadiazine-sodium	(119)
Fenoprofen	(98)	Sulfalene	(120)
5-Fluoracil	(99)	Tetracycline	(85, 86, 105)
Isoniazid	(101)	Trithiozine	(121)
Levodopa	(102)	Zinc ions	(122–124)

Table 2. Drugs Whose Absorption May Be Delayed by Food

Drug	Reference	Drug	Reference
Acetaminophen	(125–127)	Nitrofurantoin	(55, 56)
Acetylsalicylic acid	(70, 128, 129)	Oxacillin	(161)
Alclofenac	(130)	Penbutolol	(161a)
Amoxicillin	(73, 77, 78, 131)	Pentobarbital	(162)
Ampicillin	(132)	Pindolol	(163)
Bumetanide	(133)	Piroxicam	(164)
Capuride	(134)	Potassium ions	(165)
Cefaclor	(135)	Prednisone	(166)
Cephalexin	(136–138)	Procainamide	(167)
Cephradine	(137, 139)	Quinidine	(168)
Cimetidine	(140–142)	Rifampicin	(169)
Clindamycin	(143)	Sodium salicylate	(52, 170)
Clofibrate	(55, 56)	Sulfacarbamide	(52, 170)
Diazepam	(144)	Sulfadiazine	(119)
Dicloxacillin	(145)	Sulfamethoxine	(171)
Digitoxin	(56, 146, 147)	Sulfamethoxypyridazine	(171)
Doxycycline	(152)	Sulfanilamide	(119)
Erythromycin base	(153)	Sulfasymazine	(171)
Furosemide	(154)	Sulfaisomidine	(52, 170)
Glipizide	(155)	Sulfioxazole	(171)
Indobufen	(157)	Thiopenthal	(172)
Indomethacin	(55, 100, 156)	Tolbutamide	(52, 170)
Indoprofen (capsules)	(158)	Valproic acid	(173a)
Lincomycin	(159)	Vitamin C	(174)
Metronidazole	(160)	Warfarin	(175)

The question of whether a drug should be ingested in the fasting state or concomitant with food does not differentiate enough. Ingestion in the fasting state needs additional statements concerning type, volume, and temperature of the fluid with which the drug is swallowed (14, 63). Ingestion concomitant with food raises questions about its type, amount, composition, and temperature. The influence of a light breakfast on the enteral absorption of a drug must not be the same as that of a heavy meal; and even a breakfast does not look the same everywhere (e.g., Continental vs. English).

Table 3. Drugs Whose Absorption May Be Unaffected by Food[a]

Drug	Reference	Drug	Reference
Acetylsalicylic acid	(70, 176)	Oxazepam	(188)
Ampicillin	(110, 177, 178)	Oxprenolol	(190)
Bendroflumethiazide	(179)	Penicillin V (acid)	(191)
Chlorpropamide	(180)	Phenazone	(176)
Digoxin (elixir)	(150)	Pindolol	(192)
Doxycycline	(181, 182)	Pivmecillinam	(193)
Erythromycin estolate	(90, 110, 183)	Prazosine	(194)
Erythromycin ethylcarbonate	(184)	Prednisolone	(195)
Erythromycin ethylsuccinate (suspension)	(153)	Prednisone	(195a)
		Propoxyphene	(176)
Glibenclamide	(185)	Propylthiouracil	(196)
1-Hyoscyamine	(80, 115)	Spiramycin	(197)
Melperone	(186)	Sulfisodimidine	(198)
Metaproterenol	(187)	Theophylline	(199)
Minocycline	(181)	Tolbutamide	(180)
Nitrazepam	(188)	Triacetyloleandomycin	(91)

[a]With a liquid Lundh meal, the GI-absorption of Amoxicillin, Ampicillin, Cephalexin, Pivampicillin, and Pivpenicillinam is essentially uninfluenced (200, 201).

Table 4. Drugs Whose Absorption May Be Increased by Food

Drug	Reference	Drug	Reference
Carbamazepine	(202)	Lithium ions	(215)
Diazepam	(144)	8-Methoxypsoralen	(216)
Dicoumarol	(203)	Metoprolol	(217, 218)
Diftalone	(204)	Nitrofurantoin	(55, 56, 219–222)
Erythromycin estolate	(93, 153)	Phenytoin	(223)
Erythromycin ethylsuccinate	(110)	Propoxyphene	(224, 225)
Erythromycin stearate	(205)	Propranolol	(66, 217)
Fluproquazone	(206)	Proquazone	(226)
Griseofulvin	(207–209)	Riboflavin	(227)
Hetacillin	(210)	Riboflavin 5′phosphate	(228)
Hydralazine	(211)	Spironolactone	(229)
Hydrochlorothiazide	(212, 213)	Sulfaperine	(55, 230)
Indoprofen (tablets)	(158)	Theophylline	(199)
Labetalol	(214)		

Table 5. Influence of Diet on the Bioavailability of Drugs[a]

Drug	Bioavailability Relative to Intake in the Fasting State						Reference
	Carbohydrate Rich		Protein Rich		Lipid Rich		
	(Rate)	(Extent)	(Rate)	(Extent)	(Rate)	(Extent)	
Acetaminophen	–	Ø	(–)	Ø	/	/	(231)
Acetylsalicylic acid	– –	Ø	–	%	–	+	(232)
Amoxicillin	–	–	–	–	–	–	(73)
Ampicillin	–	–	–	–	–	–	(73)
Clofibrate	+	Ø	+ +	Ø	Ø	Ø	(55, 56)
Digitoxin	–	Ø	–	Ø	–	Ø	(146)
Doxycycline	Ø	Ø	Ø	Ø	(–)	Ø	(86)
Erythromycin stearate	(Ø)	–	(Ø)	–	(Ø)	–	(94)
Ethanol	(Ø)	– –	(Ø)	–	(Ø)	–	(96)
Griseofulvin	/	/	(+)	(+)	+ +	+ +	(207, 208)
Indomethacin	–	Ø	(–)	Ø	–	Ø	(156)
Nitrofurantoin	(–)	Ø	Ø	Ø	(+)	Ø	(55, 174)
Propoxyphene	–	(+)	–	Ø	(–)	Ø	(224)
Sodium salicylate	–	Ø	/	/	–	(Ø)	(52, 170)
Sulfacarbamide	–	Ø	/	/	–	Ø	(52, 170)
Sulfaisomidine	–	Ø	/	/	–	Ø	(52, 170)
Sulfaperine	(+)	Ø	(+)	Ø	+	+ +	(55, 174)
Tetracycline	Ø	–	Ø	–	Ø	–	(86)
Theophylline	Ø	Ø	+ +	+	Ø	Ø	(199)
Tolbutamide	–	(Ø)	/	/	–	(Ø)	(52, 170)
Warfarin	–	Ø	–	Ø	–	Ø	(197)

[a]The following symbols are used in the table: – = reduced; + = increased; Ø = unaffected; ( ) = influence questionable; / = not investigated; reduplication of symbols = increased influence.

The influence of *different diets* on the bioavailability of drugs is listed in Table 5. The rate and the extent of absorption might be influenced alone or together, in a negative or positive manner. Griseofulvin was the first example of a lipid rich diet enhancing GI-absorption (207); other drugs behave similarly (Figure 1).

Whether a modification of the bioavailability of a drug by concomitant ingestion of food is of clinical significance depends on the specific thera-

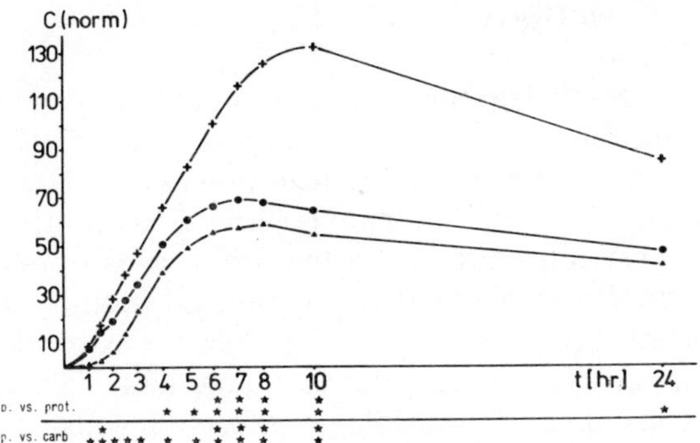

Figure 1. Influence of various diets on the enteral absorption of 2.0 g sulfaperine (55, 173, 174). Serum concentration time curves [C(norm)] after oral administration of 4×0.5 g Pallidin®-tablets immediately after a high lipid, a high protein, and a high carbohydrate standard breakfast. $\bar{x}$: $n=6$ healthy volunteers, three-way-crossover. *: $p \leqslant 0.05$. ⁑: $p \leqslant 0.01$. +——+ High lipid, ●——● high protein, ▲——▲ high carbohydrate breakfast. C(norm) = [(serum concentration) (mg/1)/(dose per kg) (mg kg)] $\times$ 100

peutic use. In an acute indication, for example, when after oral administration of a drug rapid and sufficient GI-absorption is therapeutically desirable, a delay of absorption may be clinically relevant. For an efficient chronic drug therapy, the extent of absorption is usually more critical than the rate of absorption. In some cases it might be necessary to make special recommendations about the time interval between drug and food intake to assure an optimal therapeutic result. Melander et al. (155) demonstrated that glipizide promoted a more optimal insulin profile and improved glucose disposition when it was ingested 30 minutes before a meal.

1.1.2 *Intake of Fluid*

Many drug substances do not readily dissolve in water; hence, the amount of water ingested with the drug may be a critical factor for quick absorption. Welling and his coworkers (94, 199) demonstrated that after ingestion of different compounds with small and large accompanying fluid volumes, a large water volume was necessary for an efficient absorption of erythromycin stearate, which is poorly soluble in water. This was not essential for the absorption of the more water soluble theophylline.

Drugs should always be ingested with at least 100–250 ml of water. In bioavailability studies, not only the volume of the fluid ingested with the drug should be controlled to reduce variability, but also its temperature, since the gastric emptying rate decreases with the rising temperature of gastric contents (61, 233).

1.1.3 *Social Drugs*

Coffee and Tea. Methylxanthines have a number of acute pharmacologic actions significant for the enteral absorption of drugs. Caffeine moderately stimulates the production of gastric acid; this effect is not mediated by gastrin (234–236). The acid production is stimulated far more by coffee than tea, and the gastrin concentration in the serum rises simultaneously (234, 237). The influence of coffee and caffeine on GI-motility described in the literature is somewhat contradictory (238), since the external trial conditions are seldom comparable (different dosages, amounts of fluid, modes of administration, etc.). The pharmacologic effects can also rapidly change; thus, the results depend on which time points have been chosen for measurement. For example, an initially enhanced peristalsis can be followed by a delay of the pyloric passage. Because of the likewise stimulated gastric acid secretion the pH in the duodenum falls. Thus, the initial enhancement of motility converts to an inhibition. The mesenteric blood flow rate is significantly raised by caffeine (239).

The bile flow is especially stimulated by phenolic carbon acids (chlorogenic, neochloric, isochlorogenic, coffee-, *p*-cumaric, and ferulic acid) and other roasting products (furfurol, oxymethyl-furfurol) (240, 241). The plasma concentration of epinephrine, norepinephrine, and renin clearly rises under the influence of caffeine (242). The combination of these effects shows great intra- and interindividual variations, which depend on the type and amount of coffee ingested, and exhibits altering effects during the observation period.

Therefore, it is not surprising that the investigations documented in the literature do not show a systematic influence of coffee and caffeine on the bioavailability of drugs (Table 6).

Tobacco and Nicotine. The acute pharmacologic effects of smoking are numerous. Nicotine stimulates salivation (246, 247). The tone of the cardiac sphincter (248), the pyloric sphincter (249), and the sphincter Oddi (241) is reduced. Contractions in the fasting state will be diminished (246, 247). The influence of nicotine on gastric motility is described variably; it may be unchanged or strongly inhibited. Moreover, after initial hypermotility, normal or subnormal motility is observed (247). The data on the influence of nicotine on gastric emptying are also not uniform. Besides enhanced gastric emptying, a moderate delay is often reported (247). Under the influence of cigarette smoking, liquid food leaves the stomach faster, whereas the pyloric passage for solid food is not enhanced (250). The motility of the colon is promoted (241). Although the volume of the gastric juice seems to be increased by nicotine, the secretion of acid and pepsin is not raised (251–253). The plasma concentration of gastrin is unaffected by cigarette

Table 6. Influence of Coffee and Caffeine on the Bioavailability of Drugs[a]

Drug	Bioavailability		Reference
	Rate	Extent	
Acetaminophen	Ø	+	(243)
Dihydroergotamine	(+)[b]	+	(244)
Ergotamine	(+)[b]	+	(245)
Nitrofurantoin	(+)[b]	(+)	(55, 174)
Phenacetin	Ø	+	(243)
Sulfaperine	Ø	Ø	(55, 174)
Zinc ions	Ø	−	(124)

[a]The following symbols are used in the table: − = reduced; + = improved; Ø = not affected; ( ) = questionable;
[b]Reduced lag-time.

smoking (254). The blood flow rate in the gastric mucosa diminishes significantly during smoking, which is demonstrated easily by gastroscopy (255).

The influence of cigarette smoking on GI-absorption of sulfaperine was examined in smokers and nonsmokers (55, 174). Volunteers who either smoked (S) or did not smoke (N) were studied while smoking (s) and not smoking (n). Figure 2 demonstrates that the absorption of sulfaperine in smokers who smoke is the same as in nonsmokers who do not smoke. When the habit does not match the condition, however, sulfaperine is absorbed faster and more completely. This correlated with qualitative measurements by an endoradiopill indicating that GI-motility was enhanced in "smokers who had to restrain from smoking" as well as in "nonsmokers who were forced to smoke." It is likely that enhanced peristalsis, especially rhythmic segmentation and mixing motions of the small intestine, may enhance dissolution and intensify the contact with the absorptive surface. This in turn may lead to a better absorption of sulfaperine, whose bioavailability is dissolution limited. In cases where habit and condition match, the physiologic function of the GI-tract is normal. Habitual smokers are adapted to nicotine exposure. This could mean that in "smokers who have to restrain from smoking" GI-motility is enhanced because the abstinence from nicotine leads to a relative dominance of the vagal tone in the splanchnic region under additional situation-specific and emotionally negatively colored influences. In "nonsmokers who are forced to smoke" the GI-tract stimulating effect of

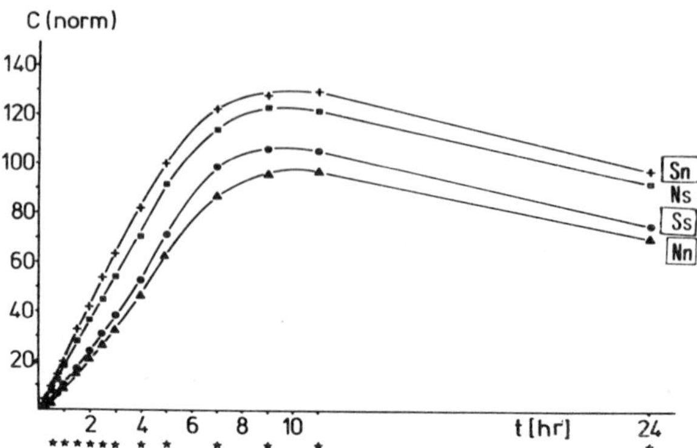

Figure 2. Influence of cigarette smoking on GI-absorption of 2.0 g sulfaperine. Mean serum concentration time curves after oral administration of 4×0.5 g Pallidin®-tablets a half-hour after a standard breakfast to smokers (S) and nonsmokers (N), under smoking (s) and not smoking (n) conditions. C(norm) = see Figure 1. Smoking: six cigarettes, in $\frac{1}{2}$-hour intervals starting after the administraton of sulfaperine. Smokers: $n=6$; nonsmokers: $n=6$. Ss ●——●, Sn +——+, crossover. Nn ▲——▲, Ns ■——■, crossover. C(norm): $\bar{x}$, $n=6$. *: $p \leqslant 0.05$ (Ss vs. Sn and Nn vs. Ns).

nicotine, with which they are not familiar, may dominate under additional situation-specific and emotionally negatively colored influences. Thus, in both cases psychic influences probably play a substantial role. If certain constitutional and psychic characteristics (such as extraversion, anxiety, and a high level of neuroticism) predispose a person to habitual smoking, a difference in the absorption pattern or behavior between smokers and nonsmokers cannot be excluded (16, 256). Hence, stringent protocol does not always render the most relevant results when a number of experimental factors are interacting at the same time.

Ethanol. The acute influence of ethanol on the gastrointestinal physiology primarily consists of a prolongation of the transit time. Ethanol delays gastric emptying (257). This effect can be increased indirectly by an enhancement of gastric acid secretion, which is caused by ethanol and mediated by gastrin, and leads to a lowering of the pH in the duodenum (241, 257). The tone of the muscles in the duodenum, the bile duct, and the pancreatic duct is increased (241). The motility of the ileum and the colon is unaffected (241). The blood flow in the intestinal wall is enhanced (258–260). Ethanol lowers the transmural potential difference of the gastric mucosa, indicating enhanced permeability (261). The extent of the delay of gastric emptying exhibits great individual variation, and depends on dose and concentration of ethanol and time of ingestion relative to drug intake (257, 262).

Table 7. Influence of Ethanol on the Bioavailability of Drugs[a]

Drug	Bioavailability		Reference
	Rate	Extent	
Acetylsalicylic acid	∅	∅	(263, 264)
Chloral hydrate	+	+	(265, 266)
Chlordiazepoxide	(+)	+	(267)
Chlorpromazine	∅	( )	(268)
Clobazam	+	+	(269)
Diazepam	+	∅	(270)
	∅	∅	(257)
	+	(∅)	(271)
	∅	+	(272)
	(−)[b]	(−)	(273, 274)
	(−)[b]	∅	(275)
Glutethimide	(−)	(−)	(276)
Indomethacin	∅	∅	(263)
Meprobamate	−	−	(277)
Nitrofurantoin	∅	∅	(55, 174)
Nomifensine	∅	∅	(278)
Oxazepam	−	∅	(279)
Phenylbutazone	∅	∅	(263)
Sulfaperine	∅	+	(55, 56, 174)

[a]The following symbols are used in the table: − = decreased; + = improved; ∅ = not affected; ( ) = questionable;
Prolongation of lag-time.

The trial conditions of the studies listed in Table 7 differ considerably. This leads to contradictory results, as is evident with diazepam. The prolongation of the transit time by ethanol is pronounced when, at the same time, food is ingested (257). When the bioavailability of a poorly soluble drug improves under the influence of ethanol, it is likely that the prolongation of the transit time favors better dissolution and enhanced drug absorption.

1.1.4 *Posture and Physical Activity*

When the supine posture is maintained for a long period of time, cardiac output and blood flow rate in the liver and the kidney increase (280–282), the volume of plasma and of the extracellular fluids decreases (283, 284), and the gastric emptying rate is reduced, especially if a person is lying on the left side (285, 286). Blood flow rate and tone of the skeletal muscles are decreased (287). Varying changes of gastrointestinal motility and of the plasma protein concentrations have also been reported (288, 289). Examples of the influence of the supine position on the bioavailability of drugs are listed in Table 8.

Physical activity especially raises the sympathetic tone (3). At the same time the body temperature increases slightly (294), and the blood flow in the splanchnic region including the liver is reduced (295). The motility of the gastrointestinal tract depends on the extent of physical exercise and the state of training. In persons who are only moderately trained, a workload of 80–100 watts for 20 minutes increases the rate of gastric emptying, and above 100 watts the pyloric passage is reduced. In persons who are well-trained, the rate of stomach emptying is unaffected even under a workload of 130 watts (296). Colon motility may be increased (3). The secretion of gastric acid is reduced to half of the basal value under increasing workloads (296).

Under a heavy workload, the excretion of urine is reduced to half of its normal value and the urinary pH falls slightly, causing the renal excretion of substances that are predominantly eliminated by the kidneys, especially when their elimination is dependent on the urinary pH, to be delayed without

Table 8. Influence of the Supine Position on the Bioavailability of Drugs[a]

Drug	Bioavailability		Reference
	Rate	Extent	
Acetaminophen	–[b]	Ø	(290)
Acetylsalicyclic acid	–	(Ø)	(291)
Cephradin	–	(Ø)	(292)
Fenoprofen	–	(Ø)	(98)
Phenazone	±	(–)	(293)
Sodium salicylate	–	–	(52, 170)
Sulfacarbamide	(Ø)	–[c]	(52, 170)
Sulfisomidine	(Ø)	–	(52, 170)
Tolbutamide	(Ø)	–[c]	(52, 170)

[a]The following symbols are used in the table: + = improved; – = decreased; Ø = not affected; ( ) = questionable.
[b]Reduced lag-time.
[c]In the fasting state or with a light breakfast.

Table 9. Influence of Physical Activity/Exercise on the Bioavailability of Drugs[a]

Drug	Bioavailability		Reference
	Rate	Extent	
Acetylsalicylic acid	Ø	Ø	(128)
Antipyrine	+	Ø	(295)
Atenolol	Ø	(+)	(298)
Benzylpenicillin	+	Ø	(299)
Diazepam	+	Ø	(300)
Doxycycline	+	Ø[c]	(297)
Sulfamethiazole	+	Ø[c]	(297)
Sulfaperine	(−)[b]	Ø	(55, 56, 174)
Tetracycline	+	Ø[c]	(297)
Vitamin A	(Ø)	−	(301)

[a]The following symbols are used in the table: − = decreased; + = improved; Ø = not affected; ( ) = questionable.
[b]Prolongation of lag-time.
[c]By comparison with cumulative renal elimination.

a reduction of the cumulative renal elimination (297). A similar decrease in renal clearance during an exercise phase that probably reduced renal blood flow was observed for atenolol (298).

Very strong and protracted physical exercise may lead to hemoconcentration and a reduction in hepatic first-pass metabolism. For most of the examples listed in Table 9, an increase of the absorption rate was observed during exercise. In these cases, the workload might have accelerated gastric emptying.

Protocols for bioavailability studies should define adequate physical activity for the subjects (to avoid, for example, that some subjects sleep between blood samplings and others exhaustingly play table tennis).

1.1.5 *Psychic Stress*

Specific investigations of the influence of psychic stress on the bioavailability of drugs are not available. Studies in psychophysiology, physiology, and occupational medicine demonstrated that mental or psychic stress—which may be caused by pain and noise or triggered by a specific situation—has the following influences on physiological factors: the sympathetic tone is increased, which leads to an overall decrease in gastrointestinal motility (302–304). The secretion of gastric juice is inhibited, whereas the production of gastric acid may be enhanced (32, 305). The blood flow in the splanchnic region is reduced (60). The variability of physiological reaction profiles as responses to a complex psychic stress situation is large because of confounded reaction manners (306–308).

This is the reason for the variable influence of psychic stress on gastric emptying. In more aggressively colored emotional states combined with internal tension a rapid pyloric passage prevails; in more depressive emotional states combined with anxiety or fear gastric emptying is often delayed (6).

Psychic stress can be induced by various experimental procedures. In a study with indomethacin (55, 309), psychic stress was induced by an acoustic vigilance test (signal recognition under white noise) given for 2 hours. Figure 3 illustrates that the absorption of indomethacin is delayed under the stress situation, and that the absorption deficit is rapidly compensated after the stress ceases. The same effect could be shown for sulfaperine (55, 310, 311). Under complex psychic stress of limited duration, the gastrointestinal absorption is delayed, and the extent of absorption is practically unaffected. Different results may be obtained under prolonged psychic stress.

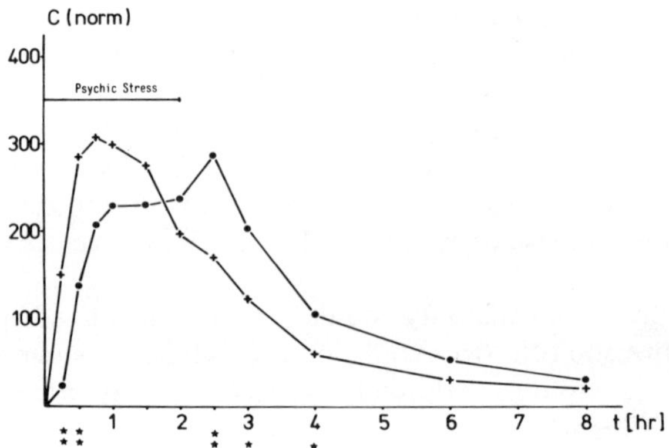

Figure 3. Influence of psychic stress on GI-absorption of 100 mg indomethacin. Mean plasma concentration–time curves [C(norm)] after oral administration of 2 × 50 mg Amuno®-capsules under and without psychic stress. C(norm) = see Figure 1. Psychic stress: acoustical vigilance test of 2 hours duration (identifying discrete signals under white noise of 90 dB). $\bar{x}$: $n = 16$ volunteers (8 with high level of neuroticism and 8 with low level of neuroticism). Two-way-cross-over: *: $p \leq 0.1$; ⁑: $p \leq 0.05$. +——+ Control, ●——● under psychic stress

1.2 Environment Related

1.2.1 *Climatic Variations*

Temperature, atmospheric pressure, humidity, and local weather conditions can influence the physiological functions of the organism and thus modify the bioavailability of drugs (9, 312).

1.2.2 *Chronobiologic Factors*

The influence of chronobiologic factors (circadian and seasonal variations) has lead to the development of such new research fields as clinical chronopharmacology, chronopharmacokinetics, and chronobioavailability (313–318). It may be necessary, for example, to investigate pharmacokinetics and bioavailability of a hypnotic agent under clinically relevant conditions, which means drug application at night.

1.2.3 *Atmosphere of the Clinical Environment*

The atmosphere of the clinical environment (surroundings, recreation facilities, and contact with the staff) is also important. When the subjects are familiar with the study situation and know the staff well, tension is not likely to develop. It is also necessary to avoid conflict-producing situations (e.g., to provide for a no-smoking area or a sufficient number of armchairs) (56, 319).

2. CHARACTERISTICS OF VOLUNTEERS

The characteristics of volunteers, which are important criteria for the selection of subjects, can be divided into three groups: somatic, psychic, and habits and living conditions. Each individual aspect within these groups can influence one or more factors of the biopharmaceutical LADME*-system and thus modify results of bioavailability/bioequivalency studies.

2.1 Somatic Characteristics

2.1.1 *Anthropometric Data*

These comprise the usual anthropometric data of volunteers, that is specication of race, sex (pregnancy), age, weight, height, ponderal index, and so

*LADME: Liberation, Absorption, Distribution, Metabolism, Elimination.

forth. The influence of these characteristics on pharmacokinetics and bioavailability has been extensively reviewed (race, 320; sex, 321–323; age, 324–331; weight, 332–334).

2.1.2 *Physical State*

The clinical examination ensures that the volunteers are actually healthy. Volunteers sometimes tend to conceal or diminish former or present limitations of their physical condition. This implies the obligation to search very carefully by anamnesis, medical examination, and laboratory analyses for past diseases, disposition toward allergies, and present limitations of the physical state.

2.1.3 *Physiological Functions*

Special attention must also be paid to several physiological functions. Even moderate functional disorders of the gastrointestinal tract, the thyroid, the liver, or the kidneys may result in clinically relevant distortion of pharmacokinetic results. It may also be favorable to know in advance genetic differences in the activity of drug metabolizing enzyme systems of the volunteers, or to exclude volunteers with known enzymatic deficiencies (335–337). For example, when acetylation of a drug will be an important metabolic step in man, the study should involve a group of volunteers with a defined or ethnically balanced number of slow and fast acetylators. With sulfadimidine, it is easily possible to assess the individual acetylator phenotype of volunteers (338). Pharmacogenetics and ethnopharmacokinetics are important

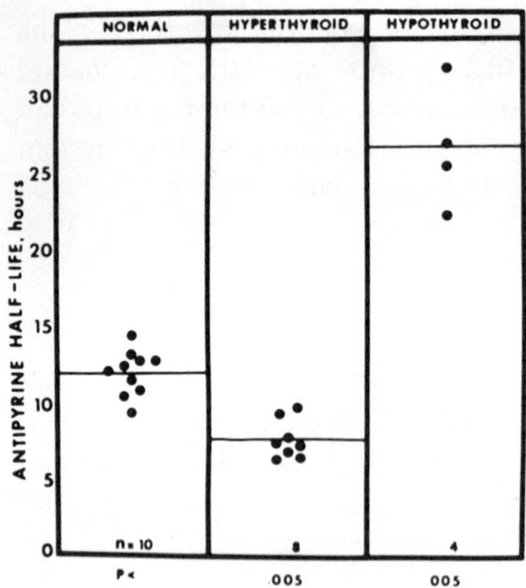

Figure 4. Values for plasma antipyrine half-life in normal subjects and in patients with hyperthyroidism and hypothyroidism. Each closed circle represents the value for a single individual (341).

and growing areas of research (330, 339, 340). Volunteers with undetected achlorhydria can easily be prevented from taking part in a study (34). Disturbances of the thyroid function (hypothyroidism and hyperthyroidism) can lead to changes in the characteristic parameters of drug metabolism and elimination [Figure 4 (341)].

2.2 Psychic Characteristics

The importance of determining the somatic characteristics of volunteers for a well-defined and balanced protocol is widely accepted. This is not true for the psychic characteristics, which are not given sufficient consideration. It is evident that personality traits—such as the level of neuroticism, which is assessed by special questionnaires (342) and correlates well with the degree of emotional lability and instability in the autonomic nervous system (343)—clearly modify the results of pharmacodynamic studies. The results of pharmacokinetic studies can be thus influenced as well. Nakano et al. (344, 345) demonstrated that the rate and extent of diazepam absorption was significantly greater in volunteers exhibiting a high level of neuroticism, and that this was probably due to enhanced gastric motility and faster gastric emptying (Figure 5).

In the studies mentioned in 1.1.5 (Figure 3), which were designed to investigate the influence of complex psychic stress situations on the bioavailability of sulfaperine and indomethacin (55, 56), an identical number of emotionally stable and unstable volunteers, equally unexperienced with respect to such trials, were involved. In these cases, the delay of absorption observed under the influence of the complex psychic stress situation was greater in the emotionally unstable volunteers. Not only must the actual period of stress be regarded as psychic stress, but also the trial situation

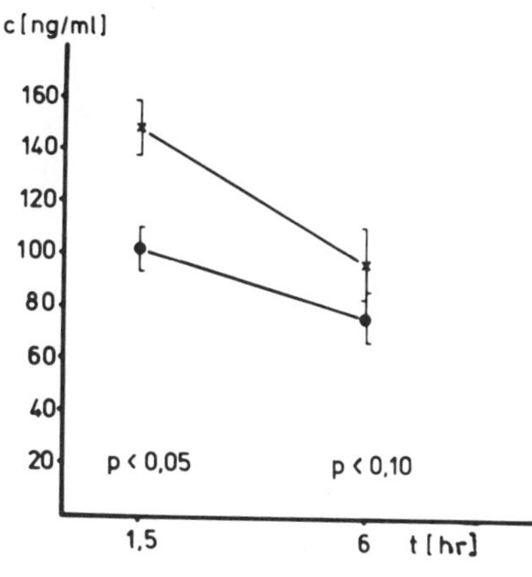

Figure 5. Influence of neuroticism level on diazepam absorption; 12 volunteers of low neuroticism level (●——●); 12 volunteers of high neuroticism level (×——×); single dose of 5 mg diazepam after a standard breakfast; plasma concentrations of diazepam, $\bar{x} \pm$ S.E.M. (344, 345).

itself. The general circumstances and conditions associated with participation in bioavailability studies—especially if new and unfamiliar to the subjects—may cause mental stress. The subjects who were in the crossover design first exposed to the stress condition exhibited a greater influence on GI-absorption than those who experienced initially the control situation. This indicates that the psychic stress caused by the stress model is virtually augmented by the trial situation itself. In acute indications, when after oral application of a drug, fast and sufficient enteral absorption is therapeutically necessary, a delay of absorption caused by psychic stress may become clinically relevant. This is especially so in cases where the disease itself exhibits a strong psychic component. It was repeatedly demonstrated that the absorption of acetylsalicylic acid is delayed or even reduced in migraine patients during acute episodes (346). In these situations, gastric emptying can be normalized by metoclopramide (347). Ergotamine absorption is delayed as well during a migraine attack (348). It is also well-known that x-ray opaque material is, under the influence of pain (especially migraine), retained for unusually long periods in the stomach (349, 350).

For practical reasons, the individual attitude of volunteers toward a trial may be very important. The lack of motivation, cooperation, and compliance—especially in the case of very complex protocols—can reduce the quality of the results.

2.3 Habits and Conditions of Living

These factors are now becoming increasingly important. This group does not comprise the external conditions during a study, but the individual habits and conditions of living and environment that have persistantly (chronically) affected the internal milieu of a volunteer before a study.

2.3.1 Dietary Factors

Kappas et al. (351) demonstrated that a variation from normal food to a high protein/low carbohydrate diet was accompanied by a significant reduction of the elimination half-life of theophylline, whereas a change back to a low protein/high carbohydrate diet led, within 2 weeks, to a restoration of the original half-life (Figure 6).

The same is true for antipyrine (17, 351–353), but not for phenytoin (354). This is in agreement with the observations of Fraser et al. (355), who found a longer elimination half-life for antipyrine in vegetarians than in non-vegetarians. The mechanism responsible for the change in microsomal enzyme activities caused by differences introduced in the protein–carbohydrate relationship of food is not clear. We do know, however, why diets

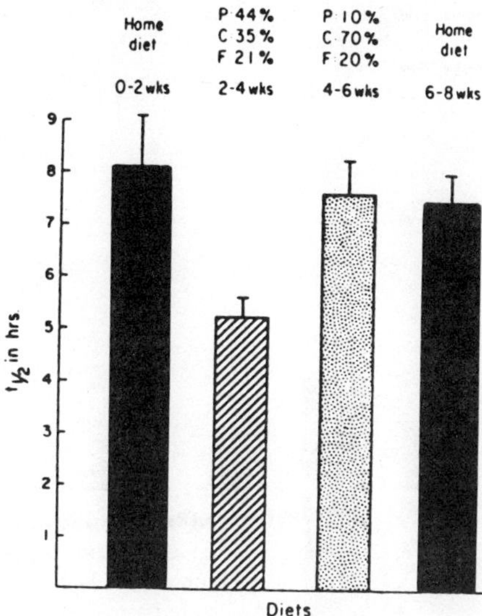

Figure 6. Theophylline half-lives in six normal subjects maintained on their usual home diets and two test diet periods. Each bar represents mean ± SE for the six subjects. The abbreviations are: P = protein; C = carbohydrate; and F = fat. After 2 weeks on their usual home diets (diet 1), subjects were maintained on the low C—high P diets (diet 2) for 2 weeks, followed by 2 weeks on the high C—low P diets (diet 3), followed by 2 weeks on their usual home diets (diet 4). The values for diets 1, 3, and 4 are not significantly different from each other. The value for diet 2 is significantly different from that of diet 1 ($p < 0.05$) and diet 3 ($p < 0.01$) (351).

rich in charcoal-broiled beef or in cabbage induce drug metabolizing enzymes. Figure 7 shows that a diet rich in charcoal-broiled beef results, after four days, in a significant reduction of the area under the plasma concentration–time curve of phenacetin (352). The situation is quite similar for antipyrine and theophylline (352, 356). Polycyclic hydrocarbons present in the smoke of charcoal fire are responsible for the induction of the drug metabolizing enzymes. Pantuck et al. (357) described the enzyme inducing effect of diets containing cabbage and brussels sprouts—it enhanced the metabolism of antipyrine and phenacetin. Figure 8 shows the relative changes in the half-life of antipyrine and the area under plasma concentration–time curve of phenacetin. Compounds with indole structure, which are common in cabbage and brussels sprouts, are responsible for the enzyme induction.

Healthy volunteers fasting for weight reduction should not take part in bioavailability studies. Reidenberg (352) reviewed the changes that occur in the elimination half-lives of some drugs during fasting.

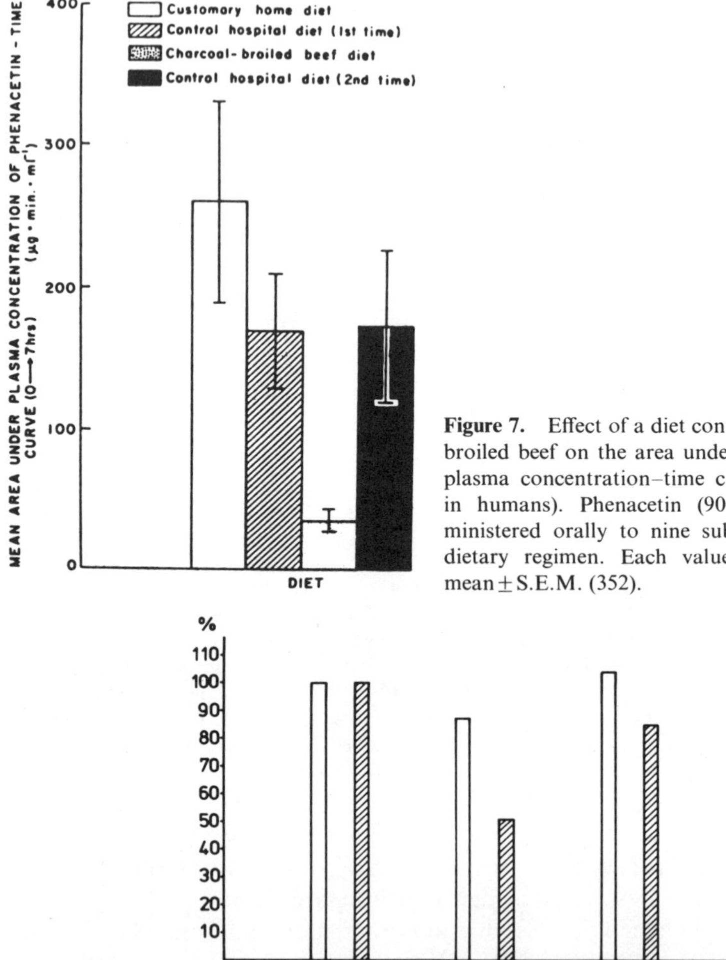

Figure 7. Effect of a diet containing charcoal-broiled beef on the area under the phenacetin plasma concentration–time curve (0–7 hours in humans). Phenacetin (900 mg) was administered orally to nine subjects after each dietary regimen. Each value represents the mean ± S.E.M. (352).

Figure 8. Effect of a diet containing cabbage and brussels sprouts on antipyrine and phenacetin metabolism in man (17, 357). Antipyrine: 1.8 mg/kg orally on day 7, 17, and 27. Phenacetin: 900 mg orally on day 10, 20, and 30. Results as relative changes of: antipyrine half-life—open columns; phenacetin $AUC_{(0\text{-}7\ \text{hours})}$—hatched columns. (Ten Subjects.)

2.3.2 *Social Drugs*

Another factor to be considered is the habitual and regular consumption of "social drugs." Since Pantuck et al. (358) demonstrated in 1972 lower plasma concentrations of phenacetin in cigarette smokers, many similar findings have been reported. The influence of smoking on pharmacokinetics has been extensively reviewed by Jusko (16, 359). Figure 9 demonstrates, for example, that the elimination half-life of theophylline is significantly smaller in smokers than in nonsmokers. Enhancement of the clearance rate is directly proportional to the daily cigarette consumption (16). When smoking is stopped, it takes 3 months or longer until the elimination characteristics for theophylline in ex-smokers become similar to those in nonsmokers (360). Polycyclic hydrocarbons present in the tobacco smoke are responsible for the induction of primarily hepatic microsomal enzymes.

Another important social drug is ethanol. The drinking habits of volunteers should be carefully explored and documented and the liver function should be checked. The influence of chronic ingestion of alcohol on pharmacokinetics has been extensively reviewed by Sellers and Holloway (15) and Linnoila et al. (260). As an example, Figure 10 shows that tolbutamide is eliminated significantly faster from the blood of alcoholics as compared to nondrinking adults (361). During abstinence this difference disappears (362). The influence of chronic alcohol consumption depends very much on type, concentration, daily volume, and duration of regular intake.

Methylxanthine-containing beverages (primarily coffee and tea) play a major role as mild stimulants and influence, for example, theophylline

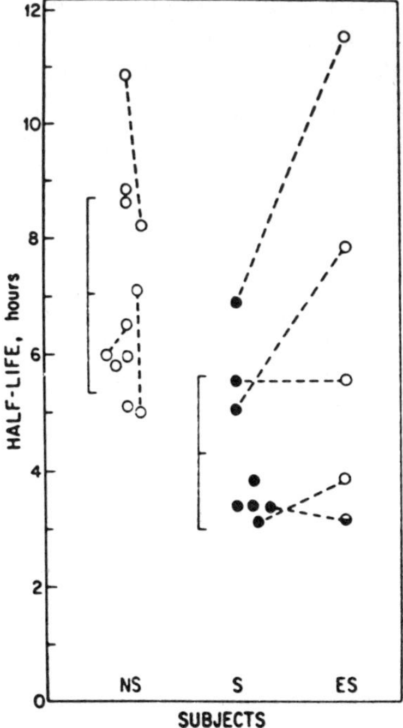

Figure 9. Elimination half-life of theophylline in nonsmokers (NS) and cigarette smokers (S). Some of the smoking subjects were studied after stopping smoking for 3 months (ES), but one of the latter did not fully quit smoking (◒). Broken lines connect data from repeated studies in individual subjects. The vertical lines depict the mean ± 1 standard deviation of the data sets (360).

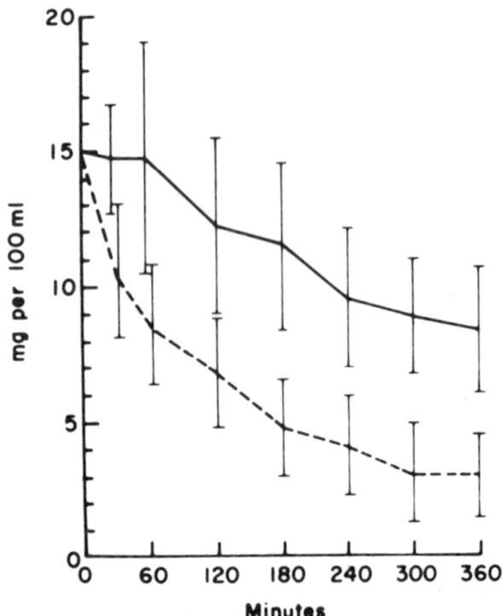

Figure 10. Ten alcoholic subjects (——) drinking more than 200 g ethanol daily were studied 3 days after cessation of alcohol. Six nondrinking adults (---), all male and all with no history of any drug intake, were given 1 g tolbutamide intravenously at zero time and subsequent blood levels of tolbutamide were measured. All values (mean and SD) after 3 hours are significantly different at the $p \leqslant 0.05$ level, which indicates that such alcoholic subjects remove tolbutamide from the blood faster than normal subjects (361).

kinetics (363). The daily consumption of methylxanthines—besides smoking and drinking habits—should also be recorded as a characteristic feature of each volunteer. This is important, because there probably is a tendency to more intensive consumption of more than one "social drug." Heavy smokers, for example, tend to drink more coffee. Heavy smoking presumably causes a higher clearance rate for caffeine, which in turn is compensated by a higher

Table 10. Summary of Associations Among Metabolic Clearance Rate (MCR), Age, and Habits[a]

	MCR	Age	Smoking	Caffeine	Alcohol
MCR	—				
Age	↓	—			
Smoking	↑	↓	—		
Caffeine	↑	↓	↑	—	
Alcohol	0	↓	↑	↑	—

[a]Simple associations by χ^2 analysis. The arrows give the direction of the association and all are statistically significant at $p<0.025$; 0 indicates no significant association (365).

consumption of coffee (364). The simultaneous influence of several factors on the metabolism of antipyrine was investigated by Vestal et al. (365). Table 10 summarizes the associations that were observed between metabolic clearance rate, age, and habits by multiple analyses of variance. The metabolic clearance of antipyrine is reduced with rising age and increased with smoking and drinking coffee. Under moderate consumption of alcohol, no change could be observed. This table also shows that smoking is associated with a higher consumption of coffee.

2.3.3 *Drugs*

The recent ingestion of other drugs by the volunteers has to be carefully checked. It is especially important to search for substances that the volunteers often do not spontaneously recognize as drugs. This means such commonly used drugs as laxatives, antacids, analgesics, vitamins, hypnotics, sedatives, and oral contraceptives. The combined influence of oral contraceptives and smoking on the elimination half-life of antipyrine is shown in Figure 11. Although the use of contraceptive pills generally causes a prolongation of the half-life, smoking reduces it. Both effects are obviously independent (366).

2.3.4 *Micturition and Defecation*

For practical reasons, it might be important to select for bioavailability studies subjects whose normal frequency of defecation and ability for optimal control of micturition meet the requirements of the protocol.

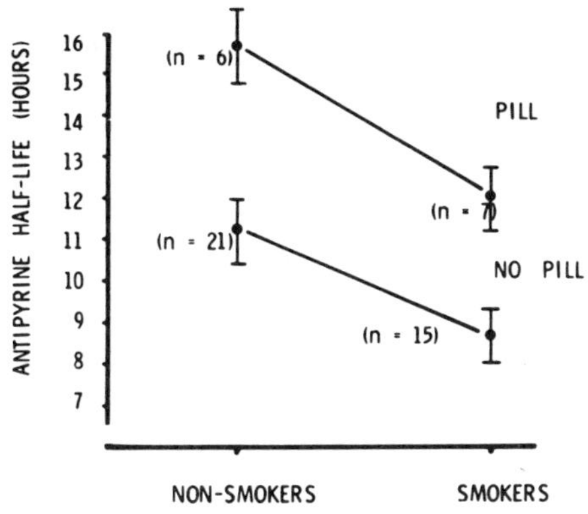

Figure 11. Antipyrine half-life in nonvegetarian women in relation to smoking habits and use of the contraceptive pill (mean ± SEM) (366).

2.3.5 *Employment*

The employment or profession of the subject might indicate possible hepatic enzyme induction by environmental or occupational exposure (367, 368).

3. SPECIAL CHARACTERISTICS OF PATIENTS

On some occasions, it might be reasonable and necessary to investigate whether the bioavailability/bioequivalence of a drug is altered by pathophysiological conditions or by interaction with other drugs. As it is not possible within the scope of this chapter to discuss these groups of factors in detail, attention is focused on several reviews:

3.1 Influence of Pathophysiologic Conditions (Disease) on Pharmacokinetics

Topic	Reference
Disease and pharmacokinetics	(369, 370)
Cardiac failure and pharmacokinetics	(371)
Pulmonary disease and pharmacokinetics	(372)
Disease and gastric emptying	(262)
Disease and drug distribution volume	(373)
Disease and drug protein binding	(374–377)
Renal disease and pharmacokinetics	(378–380)
Hepatic disease and pharmacokinetics	(381–383)

3.2 Drug Interactions and Pharmacokinetics

Topic	Reference
Clinical effects of interaction between drugs	(384)
Evaluations of drug interactions	(385)
Drug interactions	(11)
Antacid therapy and drug kinetics	(386)

4. THE COMBINED INFLUENCE OF EXPERIMENTAL FACTORS ON THE BIOAVAILABILITY OF DRUGS

It is not sufficient to know about the isolated influences of the different experimental factors; it is also necessary to learn more about their combined effect. If one adds to this all possible physicochemical and galenic factors of drugs and drug products, it is not surprising that solid information in this field is still scanty. Some results have been obtained (387–389), and have led to the new field of population pharmacokinetics (390).

Jusko and coworkers (391) recently described their method of investigating the significance of individual and interacting factors affecting theophylline clearances: age, tobacco, marijuana, cirrhosis, congestive heart failure, obesity, oral contraceptives, benzodiazepines, barbiturates, and ethanol. This approach tries to better characterize the determinants of the biotransformation rate of a drug.

A means of estimating the population characteristics of pharmacokinetic parameters from routine clinical data was described by Sheiner et al. (392), and a population-based approach to bioavailability studies in patients was outlined by Riegelman et al. (393).

In conclusion, it is important in bioavailability/bioequivalency studies to avoid results that are distorted or irrelevant to the clinical situation by carefully attending to a great number of experimental factors, to the external trial conditions, and to the characteristics of the subjects. The importance of each individual factor varies with regard to objective and type of the study. It is impossible and even unnecessary to control all factors in one study. However, when writing a protocol the investigator must check each experimental factor by considering the objectives of the trial, the biopharmaceutic principles, and the relevant preclinical data to determine which factor might be critical in a given situation.

Tappeiner (19) said, "All these conditions imply great uncertainty!" Drug delivery systems that make drug absorption independent of at least a few of these factors can lead to more efficient and safer therapy. Nevertheless, efficient therapy—especially pharmacotherapy comprising the choice of appropriate drugs and adequate dosage and monitoring—will remain one of the essentials of medical skill.

REFERENCES

1. D. H. Smith. In T. B. Binns (ed.), *Absorption and Distribution of Drugs*, Livingstone, Edinburgh, 1964.

2. J. G. Wagner, *Biopharmaceutics and Relevant Pharmacokinetics*, Drug Intelligence Publications, Hamilton, 1971.

3. J. G. Wagner, *Fundamentals of Clinical Pharmacokinetics*, Drug Intelligence Publications, Hamilton, 1975.

4. L. F. Prescott. Concepts in Biochemical Pharmacology, Part 3, In J. R. Gillette and J. R. Mitchell (eds.), *Handbook of experimental Pharmacology*, 3rd ed., Vol. 28, Springer, Berlin, 1975.

5. S. Riegelman. *Pharmacology* **8**:118 (1972).

6. M. Mayersohn. In J. Blanchard, R. J. Sawchuk, and B. B. Brodie (eds.), *Drug Bioavailability*, S. Karger, Basel, 1979.

7. M. Rowland. In J. Swarbrick (ed.), *Current Concepts in the Pharmaceutical Sciences: Dosage Form Design and Bioavailability*, Lea and Febiger, Philadelphia, 1973.

8. E. W. Martin. *Hazards of Medication*, J. B. Lippincott Company, Philadelphia, 1971.

9. W. A. Ritschel. *Angewandte Biopharmazie*, Wissenschaftliche Verlagsgesellschaft, Stuttgart, 1973.

10. W. A. Ritschel. In H. P. Kuemmerle, T. K. Shibuya, and E. Kimura (eds.), *Advances in Clinical Pharmacology*, Vol. 13, Urban & Schwarzenberg, Munich, 1977.

11. P. D. Hansten. *Drug Interactions*, 4th ed., Lea and Febiger, Philadelphia, 1979.

12. T. R. Bates and M. Gibaldi. In J. Swarbrick (ed.), *Current Concepts in the Pharmaceutical Sciences: Biopharmaceutics*, Lea and Febiger, Philadelphia, 1970.

13. L. Diamond, J. T. Dolusio, and W. G. Crouthamel. *Eur. J. Pharmacol.* **11**:109 (1970).

14. P. G. Welling. *J. Pharmacokin. Biopharm.* **5**:291 (1977).

15. E. M. Sellers and M. R. Holloway. *Clin. Pharmacokin.* **3**:440 (1978).

16. W. J. Jusko. *J. Pharmacokin. Biopharm.* **6**:7 (1978).

17. A. H. Conney, E. I. Pantuck, C. B. Pantuck, M. Buening, D. M. Jerina, J. G. Fortner, A. P. Alvares, K. E. Anderson, and A. Kappas. In R. W. Estabrook and E. Lindenlaub (ed.), *The Induction of Drug Metabolism*, F. K. Schattauer, Stuttgart, 1979.

18. G. W. Liddle. *Klin. Wschr.* **56**: 3 (1978) (Suppl. I).

19. H. Tappeiner. *Lehrbuch der Arzneimittellehre und Arzneiverordnungslehre*, 3rd ed., F. C. W. Vogel, Leipzig, 1899.

20. H. Glatzel. *Die Gewürze. Ihre Wirkungen auf den Gesunden und Kranken Menschen.* Nicholaische Verlagsbuchhandlung, Herford, 1968.

21. J. L. Brandt, L. Castleman, H. D. Ruskin, J. Greenwald, J. J. Kelly Jr., and A. Jones. *J. Clin. Invest.* **34**:1017 (1955).

22. T. F. Burks. **Ann. Rev. Pharmacol. Tox. 16**:15 (1976).

23. W. Crouthamel, J. T. Dolusio, R. E. Johnson, and L. Diamond. *J. Pharm. Sci.* **59**:878 (1970).

24. W. Crouthamel, L. Diamond, L. W. Dittert, and J. T. Dolusio. *J. Pharm. Sci.* **64**:664 (1975).

25. L. Diamond, J. T. Dolusio, and G. Crouthamel. *Eur. J. Pharmacol.* **11**:109 (1970).

26. J. S. Fordtran and J. H. Walsh. *J. Clin. Invest.* **52**:645 (1973).

27. W. Forth and W. Rummel. *Pharmacology of intestinal absorption: Gastrointestinal absorption of drugs. International Encyclopedia of Pharmacology and Therapeutics*, Vols. I and II, Section 39b, Pergamon Press, Oxford, 1975.

28. J. N. Hunt. *Gastroenterol.* **45**:149 (1963).

29. J. N. Hunt and M. T. Knox. *Am. J. Dig. Dis. (n.s.)* **13**:372 (1968).

30. J. N. Hunt and M. T. Knox. in C. F. Code (ed.), *Handbook of Physiology*, Vol. 4, Section 6, American Society, Washington, DC, 1968.

31. M. J. Kendall. *Br. Med. J.* **II**:179 (1973).

32. S. Kuna. *Arch. Int. Pharmacodyn.* **151**:79 (1964).

33. L. F. Prescott. *Br. J. Clin. Pharmacol.* **1**:189 (1974).

34. L. F. Prescott. *Med. Clin. North Am.* **58**:907 (1974).

35. S. J. Rune. *Digestion* **8**:261 (1973).

36. T. J. Sernka and E. D. Jacobson. *Gastrointestinal Physiology, The Essentials*, Williams & Wilkins, Baltimore, 1979.

37. H. G. Boxenbaum, I. Bekersky, M. L. Jack, and S. A. Kaplan. *Drug Metabol. Rev.* **9**:259 (1979).

38. D. Winne. *Pharmacol. Ther.* **6**:333 (1979).

39. N. S. Track. *Can. Med. Assoc. J.* **122**:287 (1980).

40. P. G. Burhol, H. L. Waldum, R. Jorde, and I. Lygren. *Scand. J. Gastroenterol.* **14**:939 (1979).

41. D. A. Roe, *N.Y. State J. Med.* **63**:1835 (1963).

42. D. A. Roe. In J. N. Hathcock and J. Coon (Eds.), *Nutrition and Drug Interrelations*, Academic Press, N.Y., 1978.

43. P. G. Pierpaoli. *Drug Intell. Clin. Pharm.* **6**:89 (1972).

44. A. Krondl. *Can. Med. Assoc. J.* **103**:360 (!970).

45. R. J. Petrick and K. Kleinmann. *Am. J. Hosp. Pharm.* **32**:1008 (1978).

46. M. Mitchard. *J. Sci. Fd. Agric.* **26**:1047 (1975).

47. Editorial. *Br. Med. J.* **I**:1304 (1977).

48. A. N. Kudrin and O. N. Davydowa. *Klin. Med. (Moskau)* **53**:13 (1) (1975).

49. P. G. Welling. *Postgrad. Med.* **62**:73 (1977).

50. P. G. Welling. *Pharm. Intl.* **1**:14 (1980).

51. R. D. Toothaker and P. G. Welling. *Ann. Rev. Pharmacol. Toxicol.* **20**:173 (1980).

52. E. Weber and U. Gundert-Remy. In E. Gladtke and G. Heimann (eds.), *Pharmacokinetics*, G. Fischer, Stuttgart, (1980).

53. A. Melander. *Clin. Pharmacokin.* **3**:337 (1978).

54. B. Beermann. International Conference on Drug Absorption, Edinburgh, 1979, p. 50, abstract comm.

55. G. Leopold, H. M. Burow, A. Breitstadt, and H. Nowak. In E. Gladtke and G. Heimann (eds.), *Pharmacokinetics*, G. Fischer, Stuttgart, (1980).

56. G. Leopold. *Modifizierung der Bioverfügbarkeit von Pharmaka durch äußere Faktoren*, Habilitation Publication, University of Frankfurt, 1979.

57. A. Hopkins. *J. Physiol. (London)* **182**:144 (1966).

58. J. N. Hunt and I. MacDonald. *J. Physiol. (London)* **126**:459 (1954).

59. K. Kramer. In O. H. Gauer, K. Kramer, and R. Jung (eds.), *Physiologie des Menschen*, 2nd ed., Vol. 8, Urban & Schwarzenberg, Munich, 1977.

60. S. Silbernagl and A. Despopoulos. *dtv-Atlas der Physiologie*, dtv.-G. Thieme, Munich, 1979.

61. H. W. Davenport. *Physiology of the Digestive Tract*, Chicago Year Book Publishers, Chicago, 1961.

62. C. S. Marcus and F. W. Lengemann. *J. Nutr.* **77**:155 (1962).

63. W. A. Ritschel and E. Erni. *Int. J. Clin. Pharmacol.* **15**:172 (1977).

64. G. Levy and W. J. Jusko. *J. Pharm. Sci.* **55**:285 (1966).

65. A. J. McLean, P. J. McNamara, P. du Souich, M. Gibaldi, and D. Lalka. *Clin. Pharmacol. Ther.* **24**:5 (1978).

66. A. J. McLean, A. Bobik, and F. J. Dudley. Abstract Communication No. 0201, World Conference on Clinical Pharmacology and Therapeutics, London, 1980.

67. A. S. D. Spiers and H. F. Malone. *Lancet* **1**:440 (1967).

68. J. H. Wood. *Lancet* **2**:212 (1967).

69. P. Paull, R. Day, G. Graham, and D. Champion. *Med. J. Aust.* **1**:617 (1976).

70. C. Bogentoft, I. Carlsson, G. Ekenved, and A. Magnusson, *Eur. J. Clin. Pharmacol.* **14**:351 (1978).

71. P. M. Brooks, M. S. Roberts, and B. Patel, *Br. J. Clin. Pharmac.* **5**:337 (1978).

72. E. Schmid and G. Fricke. *Pharmacol. Clin.* **1**, 110 (1969).

73. P. G. Welling, H. Huang, P. A. Koch, W. A. Craig, and P. O. Madsen. *J. Pharm. Sci.* **66**:549 (1977).

74. J. O. Klein and M. Finland. *Am. J. Med. Sci.* **245**:544 (1963).

75. L. Magni and J. Sjövall. *Farm. Tid.* **32**:645 (1972).

76. C. A. Fernandez, J. P. Menezes, and J. Ximenes. *J. Ing. Med. Res.* **1**:530 (1973).

77. H. C. Neu. *J. Infect. Dis. (Suppl.)* **129**:123 (1974).

78. F. N. Eshelman and D. A. Spyker. *Antimicrob. Agents Chemother.* **14**:539 (1978).

79. A. Melander, P. Stenberg, H. Liedholm, B. Schersten, and E. Wahlin-Boll. *Eur. J. Clin. Pharmacol.* **16**:327 (1979).

80. C. Post and A. Walan. *Scand. J. Gastroenterol.* **12** (Suppl. 45): 72 (1977).

81. C. T. Dollery. *Lancet* **I**:296 (1960).

82. B. R. Meyers, K. Kaplan, and L. Weinstein. *Clin. Pharmacol. Ther.* **10**:810 (1969).

83. W. M. M. Kirby, C. E. Roberts, and R. E. Burdick. *Antimicrob. Agents Chemother.* **1**:286 (1961).

84. J. Schreiner and W. A. Altemeier. *Surg. Gynecol. Obstet.* **114**:9 (1962).

85. J. E. Rosenblatt, J. E. Barrett, J. L. Brodie, and W. M. M. Kirby. *Antimicrob. Agents Chemother.*, 134 (1966).

86. P. G. Welling, P. A. Koch, C. C. Lau, and W. A. Craig. *Antimicrob. Agents Chemother.* **11**:462 (1977).

87. A. Pilbrant and A.-K. Gruber. International Conference on Drug Absorption, Edinburgh, 1979, p. 99, abstract comm:

88. J. W. Smith, R. W. Dyke, and R. S. Griffith. *J. Am. Med. Assoc.* **151**:805 (1953).

89. R. Mäntylä, A. Ailo, H. Allonen, and J. Kanto. *Ann. Clin. Res.* **10**:258 (1978).

90. R. S. Griffith and H. R. Black. *Am. J. Med. Sci.* **247**:69 (1964).

91. H. A. Hirsch and M. Finland. *Am. J. Med. Sci.* **237**:693 (1959).

92. W. E. Clapper, M. Mostyn, and G. H. Meade. *Antibiot. Med. Clin. Ther.* **7**:91 (1960).

93. P. G. Welling, R. L. Elliott, M. E. Pitterle, H. P. Corrick-West, and L. L. Lyons. *J. Pharm. Sci.* **68**:150 (1970).

94. P. G. Welling, H. Huang, P. F. Hewitt, and L. L. Lyons. *J. Pharm. Sci.* **67**:764 (1978).

95. Y. J. Lin, D. J. Weidler, D. C. Garg, and J. G. Wagner. *Res. Commun. Chem. Pathol. Pharmacol.* **13**:713 (1976).

96. P. G. Welling, L. L. Lyons, R. Elliott, and G. L. Amidon. *J. Clin. Pharmacol.* **17**:199 (1977).

97. P. K. Wilkinson, A. J. Sedman, E. Sakmar, Y. J. Lin, and J. G. Wagner. *J. Pharmacokin. Biopharm.* **5**:41 (1977).

98. S. M. Chernish, A. Rubin, B. E. Rodda, A. S. Ridolfo, and C. M. Gruber, Jr. *J. Med. Exp. Clin.* **3**:249 (1972).

99. I. L. Cohen, L. E. Irwin, G. J. Marshall, H. Darvey, and J. R. Bateman. *Cancer Chemother. Rep.* **58**:723 (1974).

100. H. W. Emori, H. Paulus, and R. Bluestone. *Ann. Rheum. Dis.* **35**:333 (1976).

101. A. Melander, K. Danielson, A. Hanson, L. Jansson, C. Rerup, B. Schersten, T. Thulin, and E. Wahlin. *Acta Med. Scand.* **200**:93 (1976).

102. N. G. Gillespie, I. Mena, G. C. Cotzias, and M. A. Bell. *J. Am. Diet. Assoc.* **62**:525 (1973).

103. K. W. Wenzel and H. E. Kirschsieper. *Metabolism* **26**:1 (1977).

104. C. E. McCall, N. H. Steigbigel, and M. Finland. *Am. J. Med. Sci.* **254**:144 (1967).

105. P. Neuvonen, M. Mattila, G. Gothini, and R. Hackman. *Scand. J. Clin. Lab. Invest.* **27** (Suppl. 116): 76 (1971).

106. J. O. Klein and M. Finland. *Am. J. Med. Sci.* **246**:10 (1963).

107. C. Watanakunakorn. *Antimicrob. Agents Chemother.* **11**:1007 (1977).

108. C. G. McCarthy and M. Finland. *New Engl. J. Med.* **263**:315 (1960).

109. N. G. Heatly. *Antibiot. Med. Clin. Ther.* **2**:33 (1956).

110. G. H. McCracken, Jr., C. M. Ginsburg, J. C. Clahsen, and M. L. Thomas. *Pediatrics* **62**:738 (1978).

111. G. A. Cronk, D. E. Naumann, H. Albright, and W. B. Wheatley. *Antibiotics Annual, 1959–1960*, Medical Encyclopedia, Inc., N.Y., 1960 p. 133.

112. G. A. Cronk, W. B. Wheatley, G. F. Fellers, and H. Albright. *Am. J. Med. Sci.* **240**:219 (1960).

113. L. Verbist. *Antimicrob. Agents Chemother.* **6**:588 (1974).

114. M. Gibaldi and B. Grundhofer. *Clin. Pharmacol. Ther.* **18**:457 (1974).

115. G. Ekenved, A. Magnusson, G. Bodemar, and A. Walan. *Scand. J. Gastroenterol.* **12**:963 (1977).

116. D. I. Siegler, M. Bryant, D. M. Burley, K. M. Citron, and S. M. Standen. *Lancet* **2**:197 (1974).

117. J. Ekstrand and M. Ehrnebo. *Eur. J. Clin. Pharmacol.* **16**:211 (1979).

118. P. Kahela, M. Anttila, R. Tikkanen, and H. Sundquist. *Acta Pharmacol. Toxicol.* **44**:7 (1979).

119. O. L. Peterson, M. Finland, and A. N. Ballou. *Am. J. Med. Sci.* **204**:581 (1942).

120. L. E. Khologov and E. T. Linin. *Khim. Farm. Zh.* **12**:22 (1978).

121. G. Bianchetti, H. Caqueret, G. Gomeni, J. Larribaud, J. Coquelin, and J. J. Thebault. World Congress on Clinical Pharmacology and Therapeutics, Abstract No. 0280, London, 1980.

122. J. L. Schelling, S. Müller-Hess, and F. Thonney. *Lancet* **2**:968 (1973).

123. F. J. Oelshlegel, Jr. and G. J. Brewer. *Clin. Res.* **23**:222A (1975).

124. A. Pecoud, P. Donzel, and J. L. Schelling. *Clin. Pharmacol. Ther.* **17**:469 (1974).

125. J. J. Jaffe, J. L. Colaizzi, and H. Barry. *J. Pharm. Sci.* **60**:1646 (1971).

126. I. J. McGilveray and G. L. Mattok. *J. Pharm. Pharmacol.* **24**:615 (1972).

127. G. L. Mattok and I. J. McGilveray. *Rev. Can. Biol.* **32**:77 (1973).

128. G. N. Volans. *Brit. J. Clin. Pharmacol.* **1**:137 (1974).

129. P. Kahela and M. Anttila. World Conference on Clinical Pharmacology and Therapeutics, Abstract No. 0616, London, 1980.

130. L. T. Sennello, R. C. Sonders, and N. Friedman. *Clin. Pharmacol. Ther.* **23**:414 (1978).

131. T. G. Vitti, M. J. Gurwith, and A. R. Ronald. *J. Infect. Dis. (Suppl.)* **129**:149 (1974).

132. K. H. Bauer, D. Förster, D. Hoff, and H. Weuta. *Pharm. Ind.* **38**:1153 (1976).

133. M. Homeida, K. R. Hunter, and G. J. C. Roberts. *Br. J. Clin. Pharmacol.* **3**:969P (1976).

134. P. C. Johnson, G. A. Braun, and W. A. Cressman. *Arch. Intern. Med.* **131**:199 (1973).

135. A. Glynne, R. A. Goulbourn, and R. Ryden. *J. Antimicrob. Chemother.* **4**:343 (1978).

136. P. E. Gower and C. H. Dash. *Br. J. Pharmacol.* **37**:738 (1969).

137. C. Harvengt, P. de Schepper, F. Lamy, and J. Hansen. *J. Clin. Pharmacol.* **13**:36 (1973).

138. T. R. Tetzlaff, G. H. McCracken Jr., and M. L. Thomas. *J. Pediatr.* **92**:292 (1978).

139. T. W. Mischler, A. A. Sugerman, D. A. Willard, L. J. Brannick, and E. S. Neiss. *J. Clin. Pharmacol.* **14**:604 (1974).

140. R. W. Spence, D. R. Creak, and L. R. Celestin. *Digestion* **14**:127 (1976).

141. R. E. Pounder, J. G. Williams, C. G. Russell, G. J. Milton-Thompson, and I. I. Misiewicz. *Gut* **17**:161 (1976).

142. G. Bodemar, B. Norlander, L. Fransson, and A. Walan. *Scand. J. Gastroenterol.* **12** (Suppl. 45): 12 (1977).

143. R. M. de Hann, W. K. Vanden Bosch, and C. M. Metzler. *J. Clin. Pharmacol. J. New Drugs* **12**:205 (1972).

144. D. J. Greenblatt, M. D. Allen, D. S. MacLaughlin, J. S. Harmatz, and R. I. Shader. *Clin. Pharmacol. Ther.* **24**:600 (1978).

145. J. T. Doluisio, J. C. La Piana, G. R. Wilkinson, and L. W. Dittert. *Antimicrob. Agents Chemother.* **9**:49 (1969).

146. G. Leopold, J. Pabst, W. Ungethüm, W. Schad, and R. Meub. In N. Rietbrock and K. Greeff (eds.), *Digitoxin als Alternative in der Therapie der Herzinsuffizienz*, Schattauer, Stuttgart, 1979.

147. J. Pabst, G. Leopold, W. Schad, and R. Meub. *Naunyn Schmiedeberg's Arch. Pharmak.* **307** (Suppl.):R70 (1979).

148. R. J. White, D. A. Chamberlain, M. Howard, and T. W. Smith. *Br. Med. J.* **1**:380 (1971).

149. N. Sanchez, L. B. Sheiner, H. Halkin, and K. L. Melmon. *Br. Med. J.* **4**:132 (1973).

150. D. J. Greenblatt, D. W. Duhme, J. Koch-Weser, and T. W. Smith. *Clin. Pharmacol. Ther.* **16**:444 (1974).

151. B. F. Johnson, J. O'Grady, G. A. Sabey, and C. Bye. *Clin. Pharmacol. Ther.* **23**:315 (1978).

152. S. Cronenberg, A. Hanson, and B. Ode. *Läkartidningen* **76**:3427 (1979).

153. L. D. Bechtol, C. T. Bessent, and M. B. Perkal. *Curr. Ther. Res.* **25**:618 (1979).

154. M. R. Kelly, R. E. Cutler, A. W. Forrey, and B. M. Kimpel. *Clin. Pharmacol. Ther.* **15**:178 (1974).

155. A. Melander, L.-O. Almér, G. Sartor, B. Schersten, and E. Wahlin-Boll, World Conference on Clinical Pharmacology and Therapeutics, Abstract No. 0411, London, 1980.

156. W. W. Wallusch, H. Nowak, G. Leopold, and K. J. Netter. *Int. J. Clin. Pharmacol.* **16**:40 (1978).

157. V. Tamassia, G. Corvi, L. M. Fuccella, E. Moro, G. Tosolini, and E. Tremoli. *Eur. J. Clin. Pharmacol.* **15**:329 (1979).

158. V. Tamassia, G. Corvi, E. Moro, G. P. Tosolini, and L. M. Fuccella. *Int. J. Clin. Pharmacol.* **15**:389 (1977).

159. R. F. McGehee, C. B. Smith, C. Wilcox, and M. Finland. *Am. J. Med. Sci.* **256**:379 (1968).

160. A. Melander, G. Kahlmeter, C. Kamme, and B. Ursing. *Eur. J. Clin. Pharmacol.* **12**:69 (1977).

161. J. O. Klein and M. Finland. *New Engl. J. Med.* **269**:1019 (1963).

161a. S. D. Sharma, A. D. Mehra, and B. J. Vakils. *Curr. Ther. Res.* **27**:576 (1980).

162. R. B. Smith, L. W. Dittert, W. O. Griffen, Jr., and J. T. Doluisio. *J. Pharmacokin. Biopharm.* **1**:5 (1973).

163. R. Gugler, W. Höbel, F. Bodem, and H. J. Dengler. *Clin. Pharmacol. Ther.* **17**:127 (1975).

164. T. Ishizaki, T. Nomura, and T. Abe. *J. Pharmacokin. Biopharm.* **7**:369 (1979).

165. D. Ben-Ishay and K. Engelmann. *Clin. Pharmacol. Ther.* **14**:250 (1973).

166. M. Uribe, S. W. Schalm, W. H. J. Summerskill, and V. L. W. Go, *Gastroenterol.* **71**:362 (1976).

167. W. D. McKnight and M. L. Murchy. *South Med. J.* **69**:851 (1976).

168. E. Woo and D. J. Greenblatt. *Clin. Pharmacol. Ther.* **27**:188 (1980).

169. L. Verbist and A. Gysellen. *Am. Rev. Resp. Dis.* **98**:923 (1968).

170. U. Gundert-Remy and E. Weber. *Arch. Pharmacol.* **294**:R28 (1976).

171. H. MacDonald, V. A. Place, H. Falk, and A. Darken. *Chemotherapia* **12**:282 (1976).

172. M. T. Bush, G. Berry, and A. Hume. *Clin. Pharmacol. Ther.* **7**:373 (1966).

173. B. Möller-Reinhardt. Experimentelle Untersuchungen über die Biologische Verfügbarkeit eines Pharmakons am Beispiel des Sulfaperins (Pallidin®) bei bestimmten Kostformen, MD Thesis, University of Frankfurt, 1977.

173a. A. H. C. Chun, D. J. Hoffmann, N. Friedmann, and P. J. Carrigan. *J. Clin. Pharmacol.* **20**:30 (1980).

174. G. Leopold, J. Pabst, H. Nowak. In N. Rietbrock and B. Schnieders (eds.), *Bioverfügbarkeit von Arzneimitteln*, G. Fischer, Stuttgart, 1979.

175. M. N. Musa and L. L. Lyons. *Curr. Ther. Res.* **20**:630 (1976).

176. A. Melander, A. Berlin-Wahlen, N. O. Bedin, K. Danielson, B. Gustafsson, S. Lindgren, and D. Westerland. *Acta Med. Scand.* **202**:119 (1977).

177. M. C. Jordan, J. de Maine, and W. Kirby. *Antimicrob. Agents Chemother.* **2**:438 (1970).

178. K. Roholt, B. Nielsen, and E. Kristensen. *Antimicrob. Agents Chemother.* **6**:563 (1974).

179. B. Beermann, M. Groschinsky-Grind, and B. Lindström. *Acta Med. Scand.* **204**:291 (1978).

180. G. Sartor, A. Melander, B. Schersten, and E. Wahlin-Boll. *Eur. J. Clin. Pharmacol.* **17**:285 (1980).

181. P. J. Neuvonen. *Drugs* **11**:45 (1976).

182. C. G. C. MacArthur, A. J. Johnson, M. V. Chadwick, and H. J. Wingfield. *J. Antimicrob. Chemother.* **4**:509 (1978).

183. H. A. Hirsch, C. V. Pryles, and M. Finland. *Am. J. Med. Sci.* **239**:198 (1960).

184. R. S. Griffith, M. Joiner, and H. Kottlowski. *Antibiot. Med. Clin. Ther.* **7**:320 (1960).

185. M. J. Badian, W. Heptner, W. Rupp, and W. Sittig. International Conference on Drug Absorption, Abstracts Communications, p. 98, Edinburgh, 1979.

186. H. Larsson et al., cited in reference 223.

187. L. A. Howard and M. Coleman. *J. Asthma Res.* **8**:197 (1971).

188. A. Melander, K. Danielson, B. Schersten, and E. Wahlin. *Acta Soc. Med. Suec.* **85**:47 (1976) (abstract).

189. A. Melander, K. Danielson, J. Vessman, and E. Wahlin. *Acta Pharmacol. Tox.* **40**:584 (1977).

190. C. P. Dawes, M. J. Kendall, and P. G. Welling. *Br. J. Clin. Pharmacol.* **7**:299 (1979).

191. F. B. Peck, Jr. and R. S. Griffith. *Antibiotics Annual, 1957–1958*, Medical Encyclopedia, Inc., N.Y., 1958 p. 1004.

192. J. L. Kiger, D. Lavéne, M. F. Guillaume, M. Guerret, and J. Langchampt. *Int. J. Clin. Pharm.* **13**:228 (1976).

193. K. Roholt. *J. Antimicrob. Chemother. Suppl. B* **3**:71 (1977).

194. R. Verbesselt, A. Mullie, T. B. Tjandramagen, P. J. de Schepper, and P. Dessain. *Acta Ther.* **2**:27 (1976).

195. D. A. H. Lee, G. M. Taylor, J. G. Walker, and V. H. T. James. *Br. J. Clin. Pharmacol.* **7**:523 (1979).

195a. A. V. Tembo, E. Sakmar, M. R. Hallmark, D. J. Weidler, and J. G. Wagner. *J. Clin. Pharmacol.* **16**:620 (1976).

196. A. Melander, E. Wahlin, K. Danielson, and A. Hanson. *Acta Med. Scand.* **201**:41 (1977).

197. C. Kamme, G. Kahlmeter, and A. Melander. *Scand. J. Infect. Dis.* **10**:135 (1978).

198. A. Melander, E. Wahlin, K. Danielson, and C. Rerup. *Acta Med. Scand.* **200**:497 (1976).

199. P. G. Welling, L. L. Lyons, W. A. Craig, and G. A. Trochta. *Clin. Pharmacol. Ther.* **17**:475 (1975).

200. R. L. Parsons, G. A. Hossack, G. M. Paddock, and J. R. Trounce. *Br. J. Clin. Pharmacol.* **4**:406P (1977).

201. R. L. Parsons, G. A. Hossack, and G. M. Paddock. *Br. J. Clin. Pharmacol.* **4**:267 (1977).

202. R. H. Levy, W. H. Pitlick, A. S. Troupin, J. R. Green, and J. M. Neal. *Clin. Pharmacol. Ther.* **17**:657 (1975).

203. A. Melander and E. Wahlin. *Eur. J. Clin. Pharmacol.* **14**:441 (1978).

204. L. T. Tenconi, G. Buniva, E. Beretta, and V. Pagani. *Int. J. Clin. Pharmacol.* **15**:485 (1977).

205. A. S. Malmborg. *J. Antimicrob. Chemother.* **5**:591 (1979).

206. T. Beveridge, R. L. Galeazzi, E. Nüesch, and W. Pacha. World Conference on Clinical Pharmacology and Therapeutics, Abstract No. 0618, London, 1980.

207. R. G. Crounse. *J. Invest. Dermatol.* **37**:529 (1961).

208. R. G. Crounse. *Arch. Dermatol.* **87**:176 (1963).

209. P. Kabasakalian, M. Katz, B. Rosenkrantz, and E. Townley. *J. Pharm. Sci.* **59**:595 (1970).

210. W. J. Jusko and G. P. Lewis. *J. Pharm. Sci.* **62**:69 (1973).

211. A. Melander, K. Danielson, A. Hanson, B. Rudell, B. Schersten, T. Thulin, and E. Wahlin. *Clin. Pharmacol. Ther.* **22**:104 (1977).

212. B. Beermann and M. Groschinsky-Grind. *Eur. J. Clin. Pharmacol.* **13**:129 (1978).

213. B. Beermann and M. Groschinsky-Grind. *Eur. J. Clin. Pharmacol.* **13**:385 (1978).

214. R. Mäntylä, H. Allonen, J. Kanto, T. Kleimola, and R. Sellman. *Br. J. Clin. Pharmacol.* **9**:435 (1980).

215. J. Jeppson and J. Sjögren. *Acta Psychiatr. Scand.* **51**:285 (1975).

216. H. Ehrsson, S. O. Nielsson, M. Ehrnebo, I. Wallin, and G. Wennersten. *Clin. Pharmacol. Ther.* **25**:167 (1979).

217. A. Melander, K. Danielson, B. Schersten, and E. Wahlin. *Clin. Pharmacol. Ther.* **22**:108 (1977).

218. P. Lundborg, C.-G. Regardh. International Conference on Drug Absorption, Abstracts Communications, p. 105, Edinburgh, 1979.

219. T. R. Bates, J. A. Sequeira, and A. V. Tembo. *Clin. Pharmacol. Ther.* **16**:63 (1974).

220. H. A. Rosenberg. Biopharmaceutical studies on nitrofurantoin, PhD Thesis, State University of New York at Buffalo, 1975.

221. H. A. Rosenberg and T. R. Bates. *Clin. Pharmacol. Ther.* **20**:227 (1976).

222. P. Männistö, *Int. J. Clin. Pharmacol.* **16**:223 (1978).

223. A. Melander, G. Brante, Ö. Johansson, T. Lindberg, and E. Wahlin-Boll. *Eur. J. Clin. Pharmacol.* **15**:269 (1979).

224. P. G. Welling, L. L. Lyons, F. L. S. Tse, and W. A. Craig. *Clin. Pharmacol. Ther.* **19**:559 (1975).

225. M. N. Musa and L. L. Lyons. *Curr. Ther. Res.* **19**:669 (1976).

226. T. Beveridge, E. E. Ohnhaus, E. Nüesch, and W. Pacha. International Conference on Drug Absorption, Abstracts Communications, p. 111, Edinburgh, 1979.

227. G. Levy and W. Jusko. *J. Pharm. Sci.* **55**:285 (1966).

228. W. J. Jusko and G. Levy. *J. Pharm. Sci.* **56**:58 (1967).

229. A. Melander, K. Danielson, B. Schersten, T. Thulin, and E. Wahlin. *Clin. Pharmacol. Ther.* **22**:100 (1977).

230. J. Böhm. Der Einfluß des Füllungszustandes von Magen und Darm auf die enterale Resorption von Methylsulfadiazin, MD Thesis, University of Giessen, 1976.

231. J. J. Jaffe, J. L. Colaizzi, and H. Barry. *J. Pharm. Sci.* **60**:1650 (1971).

232. P. A. Koch, C. A. Schultz, R. J. Wills, S. L. Hahlquist, and P. G. Welling. *J. Pharm. Sci.* **67**:1533 (1978).

233. V. Görisch. *Österr. Apoth. Ztg.* **21**:20 (1967).

234. H. W. Börger, A. Schafmayer, R. Arnold, H. D. Becker, and W. Creutzfeldt. *Dtsch. Med. Wschr.* **101**:455 (1976).

235. M. M. Cohen, H. T. Debas, I. B. Holubitzky, and R. C. Harrison. *Gastroenterology* **61**:440 (1971).

236. H. T. Debas, M. M. Cohen, I. B. Holubitzky, and R. C. Harrison. *Scand. J. Gastroenterol.* **6**:453 (1971).

237. J. M. Berkowitz, J. E. Shields, I. H. Andersen, and M. Praisman. *Gastroenterology* **66**:666 (1974).

238. F. E. Stieve, *Heilkunst* **78**:54 (1965).

239. E. Beubler and F. Lembeck. *Naunyn-Schmiedeberg's Arch. Pharmacol.* **292**:73 (1976).

240. G. Czok, W. Midani, and R. I. Finke. In G. Czok and K. Lang (eds.), *Physiologische, Pharmakologische und Klinische Wirkungen des Kaffees*, Steinkopf, Darmstadt, 1972.

241. W. Rösch. In R. Ottenjann (ed.), *Fortschritte und Tendenzen in der Gastroenterologie*, Witzstrock, Baden-Baden, 1975.

242. D. Robertson, J. C. Frölich, R. K. Carr, J. T. Watson, J. W. Hollifield, D. G. Shand, and J. A. Oates. *New Engl. J. Med.* **299**:181 (1978).

243. B. H. Thomas, B. B. Coldwell, W. Zeitz, and G. Solomonraj. *Clin. Pharmacol. Ther.* **13**:906 (1972).

244. D. Berde, A. Cerletti, H. J. Dengler, and M. A. Zoglis. In A. L. Cochrane (ed.), *Background to Migraine*, W. Heinemann Medical Books, London, 1970.

245. R. Schmidt and A. Fanchamps. *Eur. J. Clin. Pharmacol.* **7**:213 (1974).

246. J. G. Schnedorf and A. C. Ivy. *J. Am. Med. Assoc.* **112**:898 (1939).

247. H. Schievelbein. In H. Schievelbein (ed.), *Nikotin*, G. Thieme, Stuttgart, 1968.

248. S. Rattan and R. K. Goyal. *Gastroenterology* **69**:154 (1975).

249. N. W. Read and P. Grech. *Br. Med. J.* **3**:313 (1973).

250. D. S. Grimes and J. Goddard. *Br. Med. J.* **2**:460 (1978).

251. E. Wobser, O. Stadelmann, A. Löffler, and S. E. Miederer. *Dtsch. Med. Wschr.* **99**:900 (1974).

252. H. T. Debas, M. M. Cohen, I. B. Holubitzky, and R. C. Harrison. *Gut* **12**:93 (1971).

253. D. P. Whitecross, A. D. Clarke, and D. W. Piper. *Scand. J. Gastroenterol.* **9**:399 (1974).

254. G. Mazzacca, G. Budillon, F. De Marco, and G. N. Perillo. *Eur. Soc. Clin. Invest.* **4**:380 (1974).

255. J. R. Hoon. *Gastrointest. Endosc.* **15**:172 (1969).

256. C. C. Selzer. *Ann. N.Y. Acad. Sci.* **142**:322 (1967).

257. J. J. Barboriak and R. C. Meade. *Am. J. Clin. Nutr.* **23**:1151 (1970).

258. M. P. Magnusson and H. H. Frey. *Naunyn-Schmiedeberg's Arch. Pharmacol.* **257**:39 (1967).

259. S. W. Stein, C. S. Lieber, and C. M. Leavy. *Am. J. Clin. Nutr.* **13**:64 (1963).

260. M. Linnoila, M. J. Mattila, and B. S. Kitchell. *Drugs* **18**:299 (1979).

261. W. F. Caspary, *Dtsch. Med. Wschr.* **100**:1263 (1975).

262. W. S. Nimmo. *Clin. Pharmacokin.* **1**:189 (1976).

263. M. Linnoila, T. Seppala, and M. J. Mattila. *Br. J. Clin. Pharmacol.* **1**:477 (1974).

264. K.-H. Frömming and L. Schwabe. *Drug. Res.* **30**:836 (1980).

265. H. L. Kaplan, R. B. Forney, F. W. Hughes, and N. C. Jain. *J. Forensic Sci.* **12**:295 (1967).

266. E. M. Sellers, M. Lang, J. Koch-Weser, A. E. Le Blanc, and H. Kalant. *Clin. Pharmacol. Ther.* **13**:37 (1972).

267. M. Linnoila, S. Otterstrom, and M. Anttila. *Ann. Clin. Res.* **6**:4 (1974).

268. F. M. Forrest, I. S. Forrest, and B. S. Finkle. *Aggressiologie* **13**:67 (1971).

269. K. Taeuber, M. Badian, H. F. Brettel, Th. Royen, W. Rupp, W. Sittig, and M. Nihlein. *Br. J. Clin. Pharmacol.* **7**:91S (1979).

270. M. Linnoila and M. J. Mattila. *Eur. J. Clin. Pharmacol.* **5**:186 (1973).

271. R. Rangno, D. S. Sitar, R. I. Ogilvie, and J. Kreeft. *Clin. Res.* **24**:652A (1976).

272. S. L. Hayes, G. Pablo, T. Radomsky, and R. F. Palmer. *New Engl. J. Med.* **296**:186 (1977).

273. S. M. MacLeod, H. G. Giles, G. Patzalek, J. J. Thiessen, and E. M. Sellers. *Eur. J. Clin. Pharmacol.* **11**:345 (1977).

274. S. M. MacLeod, H. G. Giles, G. Patzalek, J. J. Thiessen, and E. M. Sellers. *Alcoholism* **1**:295 (1977).

275. D. J. Greenblatt, R. I. Shader, D. R. Weinberger, and M. D. Allen. *Clin. Pharmacol. Ther.* **23**:(1), 114 (1977).

276. G. P. Mould, S. H. Curry, and T. B. Binns. *J. Pharm. Pharmacol.* **24**:894 (1972).

277. J. M. Cobby and J. R. Ashford. *J. Stud. Alcohol* **7**:162 (1975) (suppl.).

278. K. Taeuber, W. Rupp, H.-F. Brettel, G. Gammel, and R. Bender. *Blutalkohol* **13**:171 (1976).

279. H. J. Mallach, A. Moosmayer, K. Gottwald, and M. Staak. *Drug. Res.* **25**:1840 (1975).

280. S. Bevegard, A. Holmgren, and B. Johnson. *Acta Physiol. Scand.* **49**:279 (1960).

281. J. W. Culbertson, R. W. Wilkins, F. J. Ingelfinger, and S. E. Bradley. *J. Clin. Invest.* **30**:305 (1951).

282. E. E. Selkurt. Circulation (Section 2). In W. F. Hamilton and P. Dow (eds.), *Handbook of Physiology*, Vol. 2, Williams and Wilkins, Baltimore, 1963.

283. P. B. Miller, R. L. Johnson, and L. E. Lamb. *Aerosp. Med.* **35**:1194 (1964).

284. F. B. Vogt and P. C. Johnson. *Aerosp. Med.* **38**:21 (1967).

285. C. A. Chang, R. D. McKenna, and I. T. Beck. *Gut* **9**:420 (1968).

286. V. Y. H. Yu. *Arch. Dis. Child.* **50**:500 (1975).

287. J. P. Clausen and N. A. Lassen. *Cardiovasc. Res.* **5**:245 (1971).

288. G. Levy. *J. Pharm. Sci.* **56**:928 (1967).

289. E. König and A. Lemp. *Klin. Wschr.* **44**:862 (1966).

290. W. S. Nimmo and L. F. Prescott. *Br. J. Clin. Pharmacol.* **5**:348 (1978).

291. B. K. Martin, *Adv. Pharm. Sci.* **3**:107 (1971).

292. A. J. Rommel, R. A. Vukovich, J. R. Knill, and A. A. Sugarman. *Clin. Pharmacol. Ther.* **23**:127 (1978).

293. J. Elfström and S. Lindgren. *Eur. J. Clin. Pharmacol.* **23**:379 (1978).

294. P. A. Bradbury, R. H. Fox, R. Goldsmith, and I. F. G. Hampton. *J. Physiol.* **171**:384 (1964).

295. R. D. Swartz, F. R. Sidell, and S. A. Cucinell. *J. Pharmacol. Exp. Ther.* **188**:1 (1974).

296. N. Ramsbottom and J. N. Hunt. *Digestion* **10**:1 (1974).

297. P. Ylitalo, H. Hinkka, and J. P. Neuvonen. *Eur. J. Clin. Pharmacol.* **12**:367 (1977).

298. W. D. Mason, G. Kochak, N. Winer, and J. Cohen. *J. Pharm. Sci.* **69**:344 (1980).

299. H. Schmidt and K. Roholt. *Acta Path. Microbiol. Scand.* **68**:396 (1966).

300. J. A. S. Gamble. *Proc. Roy. Soc. Med.* **68**:22 (1975).

301. E. C. Texter, C. C. Chou, H. C. Laureta, and G. R. Ventroppen. *Physiology of the Gastrointestinal Tract*, C. V. Mosby Co., St. Louis, 1968.

302. W. B. Cannon. *Bodily Changes in Pain, Hunger, Fear and Rage*, 2nd ed., Appleton, New York, 1929.

303. E. L. Smith and D. A. Laird. *J. Acoust. Soc. Am.* **2**:94 (1930/31).

304. T. Almay. In M. H. Sleisenger and J. S. Fordtran (eds.), *Gastrointestinal Disease: Pathophysiology, Diagnosis and Treatment*, Saunders, Philadelphia, 1973.

305. D. A. Laird. *Med. J. Rec.* **135**:461 (1932).

306. J. Fahrenberg. *Psychologische Persönlichkeitsforschung*, Hofgrefe, Göttingen, 1967.

307. F. Alexander. *Psychosomatische Medizin*, de Gruyter, Berlin, 1951.

308. J. I. Lacey, D. E. Bateman, and R. Van Lehn. *Psychosom. Med.* **15**:8 (1953).

309. A. Breitstadt. *Einfluß von Psychischer Belastung auf die Enterale Resorption von Indometacin*, MD Thesis, University of Frankfurt, 1979.

310. H.-M. Burow and G. Leopold. *Naunyn-Schmiedeberg's Arch. Pharmacol.* **287**:R96 (1975) (suppl.).

311. H.-M. Burow. *Einfluß von Psychischer Belastung auf die Enterale Resorption von Methylsulfadiazin*, MD Thesis, University of Heidelberg, 1976.

312. B. E. Ballard. *J. Pharm. Sci.* **63**:1345 (1974).

313. A. Reinberg and F. Halberg. *Ann. Rev. Pharmacol.* **11**:455 (1971).

314. M. C. Moore. *Clin. Pharmacol. Ther.* **14**:925 (1974).

315. A. Reinberg. In J. Aschoff, F. Ceresa, and F. Halberg (eds.), *Chronobiological Aspects of Endocrinology*, Schattauer, Stuttgart, 1974.

316. A. Reinberg. *Arch. Toxicol.* **36**:327 (1976).

317. A. Reinberg. *Drug. Res.* **28**:1861 (1978).

318. F. Halberg, H. F. Kabat, and P. Klein. *Am. J. Hosp. Pharm.* **37**:101 (1980).

319. G. Levy and L. E. Hollister. *J. Pharm. Sci.* **53**:1446 (1964).

320. W. Kalow. *Clin. Pharmacokin.* **7**:373 (1982).

321. J. F. Giudicelli and J. P. Tillement. *Clin. Pharmacokin.* **2**:157 (1977).

322. R. Kato. *Drug. Metabol. Rev.* **3**:1 (1974).

323. B. Krauer and F. Krauer. *Clin. Pharmacokin.* **2**:167 (1977).

324. P. L. Morselli. *Clin. Pharmacokin.* **1**:81 (1976).

325. A. Rane and J. T. Wilson. *Clin. Pharmacokin.* **1**:2 (1976).

326. G. Heimann. In E. Gladtke and G. Heimann (eds.), *Pharmacokinetics*, G. Fischer, Stuttgart, 1980.

327. E. J. Triggs, R. L. Nation, A. Long, and J. J. Ashley. *Eur. J. Clin. Pharmacol.* **8**:55 (1975).

328. E. J. Triggs and R. L. Nation. *J. Pharmacokin. Biopharm.* **3**:387 (1975).

329. J. Crooks, K. O'Malley, and I. H. Stevenson. *Clin. Pharmacokin.* **1**:280 (1976).

330. D. P. Richey. In R. Goldman and M. Rockstein (eds.), *The Physiology and Pathology of Human Aging*, Academic Press, New York, 1975.

331. D. P. Richey and A. D. Bender. *Ann. Rev. Pharmacol. Toxicol.* **17**:49 (1977).

332. M. Weiß, W. Sziegoleit, and W. Förster. *Int. J. Clin. Pharmacol.* **15**:572 (1977).

333. M. M. Reidenberg. *Clin. Pharmacol. Ther.* **22**:729 (1977).

334. P. Gal, W. J. Jusko. A. M. Yurchak, and B. A. Franklin. *Clin. Pharmacol. Ther.* **23**:438 (1978).

335. H. J. Dengler and M. Eichelbaum. *Drug. Res.* **27**:1836 (1977).

336. M. Eichelbaum, N. Spannbrucker, B. Steincke, and H. J. Dengler. *Eur. J. Clin. Pharmacol.* **16**:183 (1979).

337. T. Inaba, S. V. Otton, and W. Kalow. *Clin. Pharmacol. Ther.* **27**:547 (1980).

338. T. Talseth and K. H. Landmark. *Eur. J. Clin. Pharmacol.* **11**:33 (1977).

339. A. P. Alvares, A. Kappas, I. L. Eiseman, K. E. Anderson, C. B. Pantuck, E. I. Pantuck, K.-C. Hsiao, W. A. Garland, and A. H. Conney. *Clin. Pharmacol. Ther.* **26**:407 (1979).

340. P. K. M. Lunde, K. Frislid, and V. Hansten. *Clin. Pharmacokin.* **2**:182 (1977).

341. E. S. Vesell, J. R. Shapiro, G. T. Passanati, H. Jorgensen, and C. A. Shively. *Clin. Pharmacol. Ther.* **17**:48 (1975).

342. H. J. Eysenck and S. B. G. Eysenck. *Manual for the Eysenck Personality Inventory*, University Press, London, 1964.

343. G. D. Wilson. In H. J. Eysenck and G. D. Wilson (eds.), *Human Psychology*, MRP Press, Lancaster, 1976.

344. S. Nakano, N. Ogawa, and Y. Kawazu. *Clin. Pharmacol. Ther.* **25**:239 (1979).

345. S. Nakano and N. Ogawa. International Conference on Drug Absorption, Abstract Communication p. 103, Edinburgh, 1979.

346. G. N. Volans. *Clin. Pharmacokin.* **3**:313 (1978).

347. G. N. Volans. *Br. J. Clin. Pharmacol.* **2**:57 (1975).

348. D. Orton. In *Proceedings of the Migraine Trust*, International Symposium, London, 1976.

349. A. F. Hurst and M. J. Stewart. *Gastric and Duodenal Ulcer*, Oxford University Press, London, 1929.

350. L. S. Carstairs. *Proc. Roy. Soc. Med.* **51**:790 (1958).

351. A. Kappas, K. E. Anderson, A. H. Conney, and A. P. Alvares. *Clin. Pharmacol. Ther.* **20**:643 (1976).

352. A. H. Conney, E. I. Pantuck, R. Kuntzman, A. Kappas, K. E. Anderson, and A. P. Alvares. *Clin. Pharmacol. Ther.* **22**:707 (1977).

353. K. E. Anderson, A. H. Conney, and A. Kappas. *Clin. Pharmacol. Ther.* **26**:493 (1979).

354. C. Balabaud, G. Vinon, and J. Paccalin. *Br. J. Clin. Pharmacol.* **8**:369 (1979).

355. H. S. Fraser, J. C. Mucklow, C. J. Bulpitt, C. Kahn, G. Mould, and C. T. Dollery. *Clin. Pharmacol. Ther.* **22**:799 (1977).

356. A. Kappas, A. P. Alvares, K. E. Anderson, E. I. Pantuck, C. P. Pantuck, R. Chang, and A. H. Conney. *Clin. Pharmacol. Ther.* **23**:445 (1978).

357. E. I. Pantuck, C. P. Pantuck, W. A. Garland, B. H. Min, W. L. Wattenberg, K. E. Anderson, A. Kappas, and A. H. Conney. *Clin. Pharmacol. Ther.* **25**:88 (1979).

358. E. I. Pantuck, R. Kuntzman, and A. H. Conney. *Science* **175**:1248 (1972).

359. W. J. Jusko. *Drug Metabol. Rev.* **9**:221 (1979).

360. S. N. Hunt, W. J. Jusko, and A. M. Yurchak. *Clin. Pharmacol. Ther.* **19**:546 (1976).

361. R. M. H. Kater, F. Tobon, and F. L. Iber. *J. Am. Med. Assoc.* **207**:363 (1969).

362. M. E. Kostelnik and F. L. Iber. *Am. J. Clin. Nutr.* **26**:161 (1973).

363. T. J. Monks, J. Caldwell, and R. L. Smith. *Clin. Pharmacol. Ther.* **26**:513 (1979).

364. W. D. Parsons and A. H. Neims. *Clin. Pharmacol. Ther.* **24**:40 (1978).

365. R. E. Vestal, A. H. Norris, J. D. Tobin, B. H. Cohen, N. W. Shock, and R. Andres. *Clin. Pharmacol. Ther.* **18**:425 (1975).

366. H. S. Fraser, J. C. Mucklow, C. J. Bulpitt, C. Kahn, G. Mould, and C. T. Dollery. *Br. J. Clin. Pharmacol.* **7**:237 (1979).

367. B. Kolmodin, D. L. Azarnoff, and F. Sjöquist. *Clin. Pharmacol. Ther.* **10**:638 (1969).

368. J. C. Mucklow, H. S. Fraser, C. J. Bulpitt, C. Kahn, G. Mould, and C. T. Dollery. *Br. J. Clin. Pharmacol.* **10**:67 (1980).

369. L. Z. Benet (ed.), *The Effect of Disease States on Drug Pharmacokinetics*, American Pharmaceutical Association, Washington, D.C., 1976.

370. E. S. Vesell. *Drug Metabol. Rev.* **8**:265 (1978).

371. N. L. Benowitz and W. Meister. *Clin. Pharmacokin.* **1**:389 (1976).

372. P. du Souich, A. J. McLean, D. Lalka, S. Erill, and M. Gibaldi. *Clin. Pharmacokin.* **3**:257 (1978).

373. U. Klotz. *Clin. Pharmacokin.* **1**:204 (1976).

374. M. M. Reidenberg. *Clin. Pharmacokin.* **1**:121 (1976).

375. J. P. Tillement, F. Lhoste, and J. F. Guidicelli. *Clin. Pharmacokin.* **3**:144 (1978).

376. K. M. Piafsky. *Clin. Pharmacokin.* **5**:246 (1980).

377. R. Gugler and D. L. Azarnoff. *Clin. Pharmacokin.* **1**:25 (1976).

378. J. Fabre and L. Balant. *Clin. Pharmacokin.* **1**:99 (1976).

379. L. Dettli. *Clin. Pharmacokin.* **1**:126 (1976).

380. M. M. Reidenberg and D. E. Drayer. *Drug Metabol. Rev.* **8**:293 (1978).

381. A. S. Nies, D. G. Shand, and G. R. Wilkinson. *Clin. Pharmacokin.* **1**:136 (1976).

382. A. W. Harman, D. B. Folwin, B. G. Priestly, and C. B. J. Alexander. *Br. J. Clin. Pharmacol.* **7**:45 (1979).

383. E. A. Neal, P. F. Meffin, P. B. Gregory, and T. F. Blaschke. *Gastroenterology* **77**:96 (1979).

384. L. E. Cluff and J. C. Petrie (eds.), *Clinical Effects of Interaction between Drugs*, Excerpta Medica, Amsterdam, 1975.

385. APhA, *Evaluations of Drug Interactions*, 2nd ed., 1976, American Pharmaceutical Association, Washington, D.C.; *Supplement*, 1978.

386. A. Hurwitz. *Clin. Pharmacokin.* **2**:269 (1977).

367. A. P. Alvares, E. I. Pantuck, E. E. Anderson, A. Kappas, and A. H. Conney. *Drug Metabol. Rev.* **9**:185 (1979).

388. C. T. Dollery, H. S. Fraser, J. C. Mucklow, and C. J. Bulpitt. *Drug Metabol. Rev.* **9**:207 (1979).

389. R. E. Vestal and A. J. J. Wood. *Clin. Pharmacokin.* **5**:309 (1980).

390. W. J. Jusko. In E. Gladtke and G. Heimann (eds.), *Pharmacokinetics*, G. Fischer, Stuttgart, 1980.

391. W. J. Jusko, M. J. Gardner, A. Mangione, J. J. Schentag, J. R. Koup, and J. W. Vance. *J. Pharm. Sci.* **68**:1358 (1979).

392. L. B. Sheiner, B. Rosenberg, and V. V. Marathe. *J. Pharmacokin. Biopharm.* **5**:445 (1977).

393. S. Riegelman, L. B. Sheiner, and S. L. Beal. In E. Gladtke and G. Heimann (eds.), *Pharmacokinetics*, G. Fischer, Stuttgart, 1980.

CHAPTER 2

Animal Studies and the Bioavailability Testing of Drug Products

R. M. J. INGS

Hoechst UK, Ltd.
Bucks, England

CONTENTS

The primary objective for developing any dosage formulation is to deliver the required concentration of an active drug substance to the site of action to elicit a desired therapeutic response. Furthermore, it should be designed to maintain these drug levels for a sufficient period to achieve maximum efficacy. Since many drugs are administered orally, it is necessary to design formulations that will release the drug not only at the desired rate but also at the correct site for optimum absorption. Many factors influence this decision, and these have been established for a large number of drugs (1–4). This has led to the concept of bioavailability, which can be defined generally as the rate and extent that an intact drug appears from its dosage form into the systemic circulation. Variations in bioavailability, unless controlled, should be avoided since they can lead to therapeutic ineffectiveness if availability is reduced (5–8), and toxicity, even resulting in fatalities, if it is increased (9).

Bioavailability testing, therefore, plays an important and integral part in any drug development program. In this chapter, the problems and relevance of incorporating animal bioavailability studies into a drug development program are discussed. It does not include absorption, distribution, metabolism, and excretion studies (ADME), normally undertaken as part of a drug metabolism program, since these invariably involve the use of radiolabeled compound with little or no attempt to quantitatively differentiate between the levels of intact drug and metabolites. Although such studies provide useful and valuable information, it would be erroneous to equate absorption of a radiolabel with that of the bioavailability of an intact drug substance when no specific measurements of the latter had been made (10).

1. WHY USE ANIMALS?

The bioavailability of a drug can be affected by many variables resulting from either the inherent physical chemical properties of the drug (pK_a, solubility, and stability) or the way it is formulated (disintegration and dissolution). Hence, it is necessary to establish the bioavailability and the factors that may affect bioavailability at an early stage of a drug's development. However, since it is generally agreed that man remains the best species for testing drugs for human use, it must also follow that man is the best species for bioavailability testing. In that case, why should we revert to using animals? There are many reasons:

1. Limited toxicological data.
2. A narrow or poorly defined therapeutic window.
3. The necessity for an early assessment of *absolute* bioavailability.

4. The study of the interaction of one drug on the bioavailability of another.
5. The determination of the effect of disease on bioavailability.
6. The investigation of the absorption process, such as the site of absorption and presystemic metabolism.

Although animal models for bioavailability testing may play a useful role at any stage of a drug's development, they are more likely to be used earlier rather than later when there is relatively limited toxicological data available, and when efficacy in man still has to be proven. This is exemplified by Figure 1, which shows a very simple network plan for the early stages of a drug's development.

Sometimes absorption studies using animals form part of a pharmacological screen, such as the search for orally active antibiotics (11–13). More often, however, they are employed when there is insufficient toxicological information to dose a new compound to man, even though an early selection of a formulation using in-vivo data is necessary for future clinical studies. Also, it is frequently advantageous to have an idea of the absolute bioavailability of a compound, and this is normally obtained by comparing oral and intravenous data. If man is used for these determinations, a suitable intravenous formulation is developed and undergoes considerable toxicity testing. This is costly, and investigators are reluctant to embark on such work, especially when there is no intention of producing an intravenous formulation for clinical use. The use of animals requires much less toxicity data, thereby providing a means of estimating in-vivo absolute bioavailability at considerably less cost.

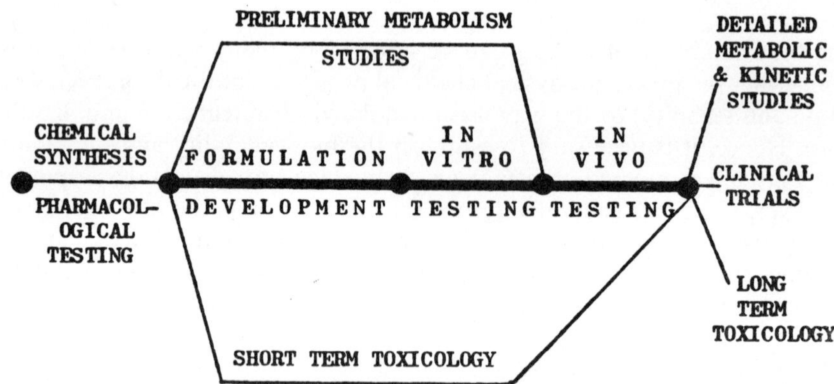

Figure 1. A simplified network plan of the early stages of a drug's development. The heavy line shows the pathway for the initial development of a dosage formulation.

The intensity of a reversible pharmacological response for many drugs is directly related to the concentration of the drug at the receptor site within the body (14), which in turn can be in equilibrium with blood or plasma. If such an equilibrium has been achieved, the time-course of the pharmacological activity correlates with the time-course of the blood or plasma levels of the drug. This phenomenon has been described for many drugs, including the β blockers (15, 16), furosemide (17, 18), and hypnotic agents (19). If a drug is administered orally, a minimum blood or plasma level must be reached before a desired pharmacological (therapeutic) response can be elicited. This is termed the minimum effective or threshold concentration of the drug. As the blood or plasma levels increase, a concentration is eventually reached at which either the same pharmacological response becomes too intense, or other secondary undesirable pharmacological responses manifest themselves, causing side effects or toxicity (Figure 2). This is the toxic threshold, and the difference between the therapeutic and toxic threshold (therapeutic window) gives the margin of safety for a particular drug.

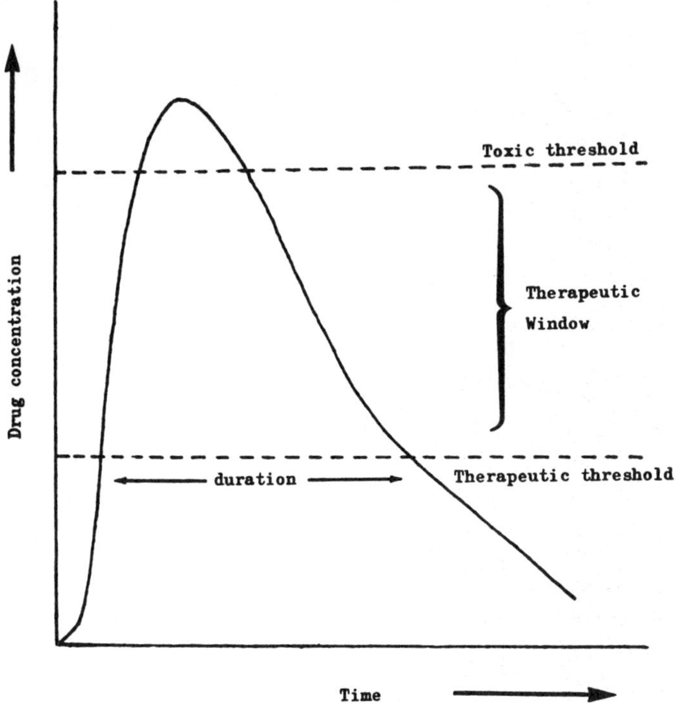

Figure 2. A diagrammatic representation of the relationship between blood or plasma level and therapeutic response of a drug.

For drugs with a large therapeutic window, such as the penicillins (20) and the benzodiazepines (21), there is little problem in undertaking bioavailability studies in man. However, for drugs with a narrow therapeutic window, such as the cytotoxic agents, ethical problems may arise with bioavailability testing in man. Animals may, therefore, provide the only acceptable alternative.

Another ethical problem becomes apparent when scientists wish to establish the bioavailability of a compound in the neonate. Sodium cromoglycate is effective in a variety of allergic conditions, including milk allergy (22). Since this indication principally applies to infants, preclinical safety evaluation studies were needed to support oral administration of the compound to the young. After considering the ethics, Smith and Fisher (23) chose to undertake these studies in rats. Also, since sodium cromoglycate is not metabolized (24), a dual isotope technique was used for this investigation. An age-related decrease in bioavailability between 5 and 75-day-old animals was clearly demonstrated (Figure 3), which was attributed to both an increase in clearance and a decrease in the absorption of the drug in the older animals.

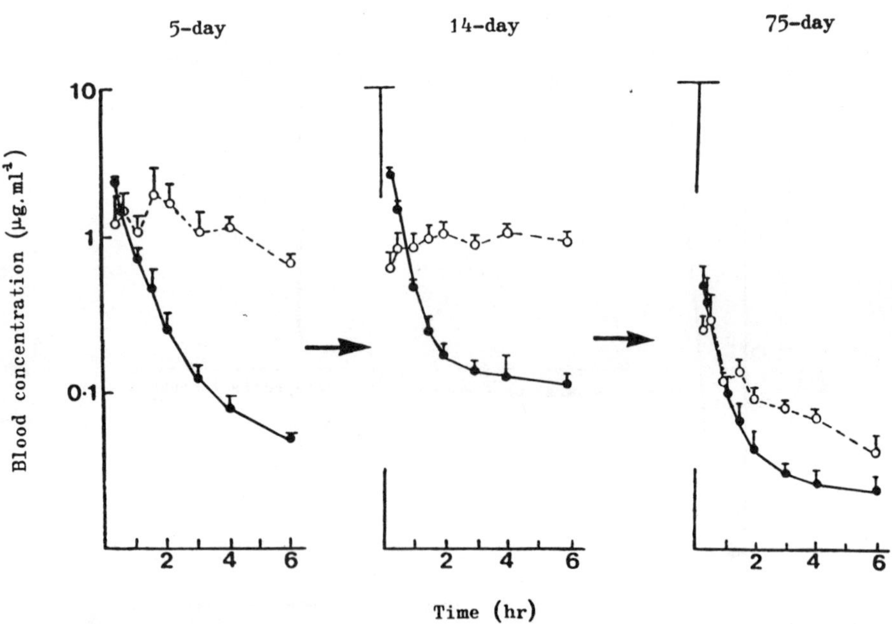

Figure 3. The absorption and elimination of sodium cromoglycate in the young rat at different times after birth.

2. IN-VIVO ANIMAL MODELS

When reviewing animal models for bioavailability testing, most authors start with in-vitro models and then move to the in-vivo situation. For this review, however, the order is reversed, since emphasis has already been put on the in-vitro aspects in excellent reviews by Barr (25), Bates and Gibaldi (26), and Kaplan and Jack (27). Apart from some smaller reviews on in-vivo animal models for bioavailability testing (28, 29), these have received relatively little attention. Also, since in-vivo models use the intact animal, many of the problems associated with these models apply to in-vitro models as well, whereas the converse may not be true.

There are occasions when in-vivo toxicological studies can supply a crude estimate of bioavailability, such as a comparison of the LD_{50} after oral and intravenous dosing. Dittert et al. (30) used this technique to show that the bioavailability of 4-acetamidophenyl 2,2,2,-trichloroethyl carbonate increased with decreasing particle size of the powder. Goldfish have also been used to test the absorption and toxicity of chemical compounds such as the phenothiazines (31), *n*-alkyl esters of *p*-aminobenzoic acid (32), and derivatives of lidocaine (33). The pharmacological end point for these experiments can be either the time of loss of righting reflex or the time of death.

If it has been decided that a more precise in-vivo animal model is needed for bioavailability testing, the difficult choice of animal species must be decided. Any use of animals as a model for man involves the risk of major differences in the handling of drugs, which are, unfortunately, often conveniently hidden in the phrase "extrapolation to man." Thus, before choosing the species of experimental animal, thought should be given to what factors will affect the bioavailability from one species to another. These factors can be broadly divided into two categories, the physiological and the metabolic or pharmacokinetic.

2.1 Physiological Factors

2.1.1 *Size*

One important factor in determining the choice of animal species for bioavailability testing is its size, since, in most circumstances, it would not be possible to study the bioavailability of an intact, solid pharmaceutical formulation (tablets and capsules) in small rodents such as mice, rats, or hamsters. This, therefore, limits the choice of species to the larger rabbits, dogs, and monkeys.

Another problem associated with the smaller species of animal is that of repetitive blood sampling, although several methods have been described for the rat. Upton (34) used a relatively simple surgical procedure for implanting a one-piece jugular cannula cut from commercial silicone polymer tubing, thus allowing multiple blood sampling from the unanesthetized, unrestrained animal for about 5 weeks. Brown and Breckenridge (35), however, advocate a more sophisticated technique, cannulating the jugular vein and mounting the cannula on the skull. These authors claim that their preparations, again using the freely behaving rat, allow blood sampling for up to a year.

A tail bleeding technique is favored in the author's laboratories (36), since it is extremely simple and involves relatively little trauma to the animal. By the use of microhematocrit tubes, it is possible to obtain and measure the drug concentration in both blood and plasma. Also, it is possible to perform crossover experiments comparing, for example, an aqueous oral formulation with that of an intravenous formulation to determine absolute bioavailability. It should be stressed, however, that sensitive assay procedures are usually needed for the drug, since the volume of plasma obtained (50 μl) is relatively small.

Urine measurements of drug excretion can be employed for all animal species to determine bioavailability, overcoming many of the blood sampling difficulties. A reasonable proportion of the drug, however, must be excreted unchanged via the kidney to make the results meaningful. In addition, extensive first pass metabolism would preclude this approach if the total metabolite excretion is being used.

2.1.2 *Gastrointestinal pH*

The principle of the pH-partition hypothesis (37–39), which assumes that primarily the lipid soluble nonionized molecules of a drug cross the intestinal wall, has found widespread acceptance among scientists studying drug absorption. Consequently, it would be expected that the pH of the gastrointestinal tract, and hence the degree of ionization of the drug molecule, would have a profound effect on the absorption of different drugs, although ionized molecules have shown significant absorption, albeit at a slower rate (40). The gastrointestinal pH should, therefore, be an important determinant in the selection of animal species.

Despite the obvious importance of gastrointestinal pH, there is limited information in the literature comparing the gastrointestinal pH of different species of animal with that in man. Smith (41) compared the pH in the contents of different parts of the alimentary tract of 15 different species, including dog, monkey, rabbit, rat, and mouse, as part of his comprehensive review on the microflora in the alimentary tract. Crouthamel et al. (42)

Table 1. Intestinal pH of Different Animal Species

Intestinal section	pH Values				
	Rat	Rabbit	Dog	Monkey	Man
Duodenum (no bile flow)	6.6±0.2	7.8±0.1	—	—	—
Duodenum (normal bile flow)	6.5±0.3	—	—	5.6	4.7–6.5
Upper jejunum	6.4±0.1	7.5±0.1	6.2±0.1	5.8–6.0	6.2–6.7
Lower jejunum	7.2±0.1	—	—	6.0	6.2–7.3

also examined the intestinal pH of three species of animal (rat, dog, and rabbit), using an in-situ method of Doluisio et al. (43) in which the intestine was exposed by a midline incision, and the section to be examined was cannulated using a small polythene cannula. Care was taken to reduce trauma to a minimum and to maintain an intact blood supply. A plastic syringe barrel was attached to the end of each cannula and isotonic saline placed into the intestinal loop. The pH of the solution was determined once equilibrium had been reached (50, 60, and 100 minutes for dog, rat, and rabbit, respectively). The results summarized in Table 1 (by comparison with the values from man and monkey) suggested that although rat and dog correlated reasonably well with man, rabbit did not. Hence, the authors recommend rat and dog for bioavailability testing, but could not recommend rabbit, despite the advantages of relatively low cost and sufficient size for testing solid formulations.

2.1.3 *Gastrointestinal Motility*

The long gastric emptying time for rabbits (44) makes it difficult to ensure that the stomach is empty by conventional fasting techniques, causing another problem in absorption studies.

All animal species suffer from the disadvantage of a shorter gastrointestinal transit time compared to man, ranging from 6 to 8 hours in rat (45) and from 14 to 18 hours in dog (46). This could have profound consequences on the bioavailability of drugs that are only absorbed from a narrow section of the intestinal tract, since the amount absorbed will depend on the residence time of the drug at that site. The study of sustained or delayed release preparations can present similar problems. It is conceivable that a sustained release formulation designed to give complete dissolution of the drug in man [gastrointestinal transit time 21–72 hours (47)] could be voided in the feces of some animal species long before dissolution is complete. Animal data would therefore indicate incomplete absorption, which, if extrapolated to man, would be an erroneous conclusion. Special care is needed in the design and interpretation of such experiments; consequently, it is recommended that, when measuring the bioavailability of sustained release preparations, man should be used whenever possible.

Garcia (48) examined controlled release preparations of indomethacin and overcame these problems by using unanesthetized, restrained rhesus monkeys fitted with a plastic cannula surgically implanted in the stomach. In these animal models, the passage of the intestinal contents to the large bowel was prevented, and the contents were collected from the ileum for readministration at the upper jejunum. This technique also established that the enterohepatic recycling of indomethacin in the monkey (49.8%) was virtually identical to that reported for man (50%).

2.1.4 *The Unstirred Layer*

Another possible variable between different animal species and man, which could affect the interpretation of bioavailability data, is the thickness of the unstirred layer. This was studied by Winne (49), who demonstrated that the absorption of butanol, antipyrine, salicylic acid, and urea from rat jejunal loops was increased by up to 64% if the intralumenal contents were mixed efficiently to reduce the effective thickness of the unstirred layer.

The effective thickness of the intestinal unstirred layer was measured in several species and the values obtained include: rat small intestine in-vitro, 180–220 μm for unstirred solution and 140–160 μm for stirred solution (50–52); rabbit small intestine in-vitro, 330 μm for unstirred solution and 110μm for stirred solution (53, 54); rat jejunum in-vivo, 420 μm (55); and human jejunum in-vivo, 620–630 μm (56–58).

2.1.5 *Intestinal Blood Flow*

Many drugs are not readily absorbed from the gastrointestinal tract and the rate determining step is the transfer through the intestinal wall. For drugs that are readily absorbed, however, equilibrium between each side of the intestinal wall can be rapid, and the rate at which the drug is removed from the absorption site by the blood becomes the rate determining factor (59). Blood flow thus becomes the important determinant of their absorption, as recently reviewed by Winne (60). The absorption of antipyrine (61), salicylamide (62), digitoxin, and digoxin (63) were all correlated with blood

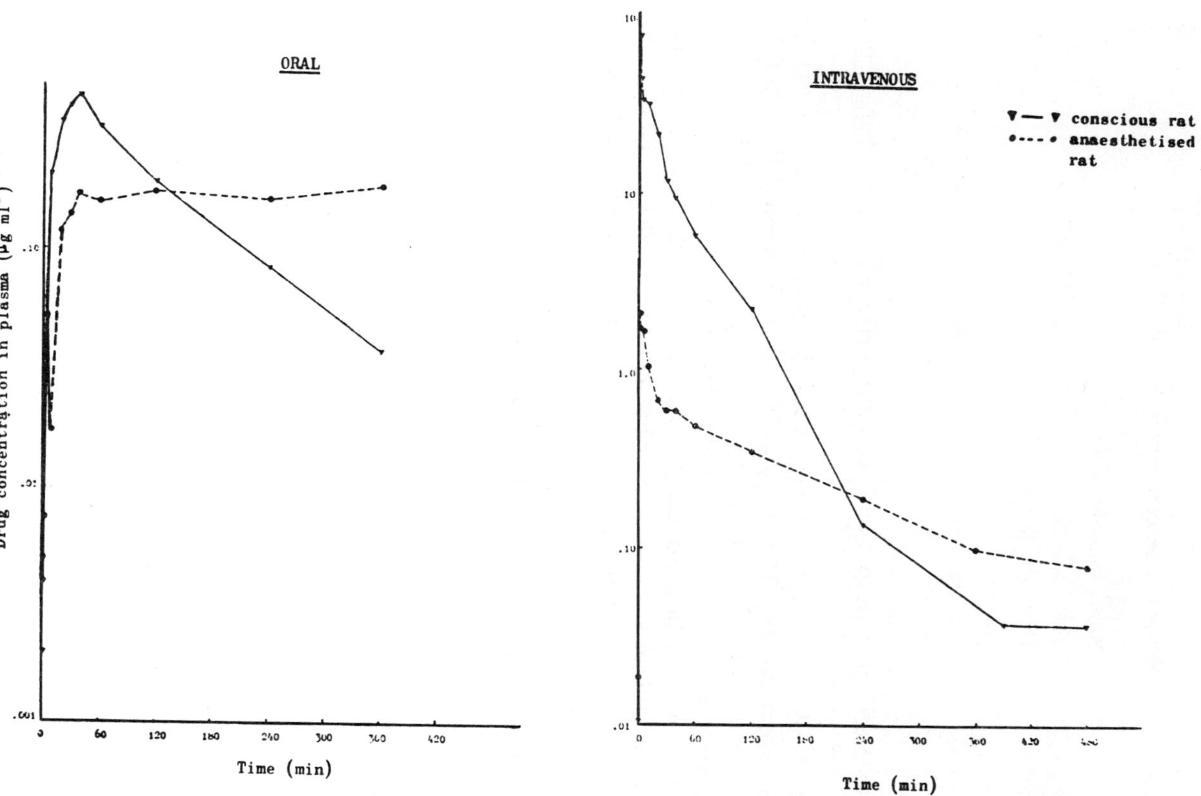

Figure 4. The effect of urethane anesthesia on the absorption and elimination kinetics of a candidate drug.

Table 2. Hepatic Blood Flow of Different Animal Species

Species	Method of Determination	Blood flow ($ml\ min^{-1}$)	Reference
Man	Bromosulfophthalein	1405 (1040–2080)	65
Dog	Blood collection	415 (266–612)	66
Rabbit	Thermal dilation	100 ± 5.7	67
Rat	Thermoelectric	268 (251–308)	68
Monkey	Microspheres	218 ± 78	69

flow, whereas ouabain (63) and mannitol (64) were independent of blood flow.

Hepatic blood flow can vary considerably between animal species (Table 2) from approximately 1400 ml min^{-1} in man to about 270 ml min^{-1} in rat. In addition, if anesthetized animals are used, the anesthetic can alter blood flow, which may affect both the absorption and elimination kinetics, and hence bioavailability, of drugs. This was exemplified by a study undertaken in the author's laboratories, showing that the kinetics of a nonmetabolized compound, following oral and intravenous administration, were altered by anesthesia (Figure 4).

2.1.6. *Gastrointestinal Microflora*

Microorganisms in the gastrointestinal tract can metabolize a large range of compounds. If this occurs before the compounds are absorbed, their bioavailability is reduced. Examples of the reactions undertaken by these microorganisms include hydrolysis (70), dehydroxylation (71), *O*-demethylation (72), and reduction of nitro- (73, 74) and azo-groups (75). Microbial metabolism of drugs has been reviewed in detail by several authors (76–79).

There are significant quantitative and qualitative differences in the population of the microflora in different species of animals (Table 3), with the consequent risk of variations in the routes and rates of metabolism of foreign compounds (77). The cause of these differences is due to the contrast in diet, and it could be expected that carnivores and herbivores would be quite distinctive in this respect (41). For example, when rats were fed a normal diet, *Clostridium welchii* counts were very low or absent, whereas those fed raw pork had considerable numbers. Rats given no cereals had low counts of Lactobacilli, and those receiving a high protein diet were practically devoid of yeasts in their gastrointestinal tract (41).

Coprophagy is one of the most important factors when considering the effect of gastrointestinal microflora on the metabolism and bioavailability

Table 3. The Distribution of Microflora Within Various Sections of Gastrointestinal Tract of Different Animal Species[a]

Species and Bacteria	Stomach	Proximal Intestine	Distal Intestine	Cecum	Feces
Man					
E. Coli	—	—	—	—	—
Cl. welchii	N[b]	N	N	—	N–5
Streptococci	N–5	N–5	3–4	—	2–6
Lactobacilli	N–4	N–2	3–6	—	2–7
Yeasts	N	N	N	—	N–4
Bacteriodes	N–4	N–5	5–7	—	9–11
Rat					
E. coli	N–2.0	N–3.4	3.6–4.5	5.2	5.6
Cl. welchii	N	N	N	2.0	1.7
Streptococci	4.2–5.0	3.0–4.7	4.7–5.0	6.0	6.2
Lactobacilli	7.5–8.4	7.0–7.4	7.8–8.0	8.4	8.6
Yeasts	6.0–6.2	6.0–6.7	6.7–6.8	7.3	7.0
Bacteriodes	N	N	N	8.2	8.4
Rabbit					
E. coli	N	N	N	N	N
Cl. welchii	N	N	N	N	N
Streptococci	N	N	N	4.0	4.7
Lactobacilli	N	N	N	N	N
Yeasts	N	N	N	N	N
Bacteriodes	4.2	3.8–4.1	5.0–6.7	8.5	8.7
Dog					
E. coli	4.4–4.5	2.7–3.4	4.4–5.2	7.2	7.2
Cl. welchii	5.2	4.5–4.8	5.2–6.2	7.7	7.8
Streptococci	5.5	5.6–5.9	5.8–7.0	8.2	9.3
Lactobacilli	4.2–4.5	3.3–4.7	4.7–5.8	8.7	9.0
Yeasts	N	N	N	N	N
Bacteriodes	N	N	N	8.5	9.3
Monkey					
E. coli	2.6–3.0	2.4–3.4	3.4–4.7	5.7	6.4
Cl. welchii	1.7	N–2.0	N–2.4	2.6	N
Streptococci	5.0–6.5	5.0–5.7	6.4–6.7	8.0	7.8
Lactobacilli	8.0–8.7	7.8–8.6	8.6–9.0	9.7	9.5
Yeasts	5.2–5.3	5.1–5.8	5.6–5.7	6.4	5.2
Bacteriodes	N	N	N	9.0	9.0

[a] Log_{10} viable count per g contents.
[b] N—indicates none isolated.

of drugs, since many commonly used laboratory animals (e.g., rat and rabbit) exhibit this practice. In these animals, the stomach and upper portion of the intestinal tract contain significant numbers of bacteria, whereas in man and in animals prevented from indulging in coprophagy, these areas are essentially sterile (41).

Thus, when metabolism of a drug by gastrointestinal microflora is suspected, and animal bioavailability studies are to be performed, due consideration must be given to the type of metabolism and the responsible microorganisms in the test species, if the results are to be extrapolated to the situation in man.

2.2 Metabolic and Pharmacokinetic Factors

2.2.1 *Metabolism*

The preceding discussion concentrated on the physiological differences between animal species that may affect bioavailability, and the implication of different gastrointestinal microflora on the presystemic metabolism of drugs was considered in Section 2.1.6. This section emphasizes differences in the handling of drug substances by various animal species, the best documented aspect of which is species differences in drug metabolism.

Numerous reviews have appeared on this subject (80–85), reflecting its importance to both the efficacy of a drug (86, 87) and its safety (87). The main function of Drug Metabolism Departments throughout the pharmaceutical industry is to examine the metabolism of candidate drug products in different animal species prior to selecting animal species for long-term toxicity studies. Once the most suitable species is chosen, the expensive toxicity testing can proceed, based on the knowledge that the animal species used are exposed to the same metabolites as patients who will receive the drug clinically. Just as species differences in drug metabolism can influence toxicity testing, so too they can affect bioavailability testing. To make an extrapolation of the results from animal bioavailability studies meaningful for man, the test species should metabolize the drug product in a similar manner.

The basic pattern of drug metabolism can be considered as biphasic, with the products from phase 1 metabolism proceeding to the phase 2 reactions (88). Phase 1 reactions consist mainly of oxidation, reduction, and hydrolysis, whereas phase 2 processes are largely synthetic (Table 4). The objective in metabolizing foreign compounds is to make them more polar, thereby increasing their water solubility and facilitating their elimination from the body by the normal excretory processes. Although these reactions are often termed "detoxification," there are many instances where they enhance the toxicity (84).

Table 4. Classification of Metabolic Reactions for Foreign Compounds

Phase I	Phase II
Aromatic hydroxylation	Glucorinic acid conjugation
Oxidation at aliphatic carbon	Sulphate conjugation
Oxidation of alcoholic hydroxyl to carboxyl	Glycoside conjugation
N-oxidation	Mecapturic acid formation
S-oxidation	Acetylation
N-dealkylation	Methylation
S-dealkylation	Amino acid conjugation
O-demethylation	
Deamination	
Decarboxylation	
Hydrolysis	

There are, however, some predictable differences in metabolic reactions between species, since some species are apparently unable to undertake certain reactions. Cats have difficulty forming glucuronides owing to a deficiency of hepatic glucuronyl transferases, making this species very susceptible to phenolic compounds. 2,6-Dimethyoxyphenol is relatively nontoxic to rats, and studies using ^{14}C-labeled compound (89) showed that it was largely excreted in the urine as 2,6-dimethyoxyphenylglucuronide and 2,6-dimethoxyphenylsulphate. In cats, however, 2,6-dimethyoxyphenol is highly toxic and causes a dark discoloration of the urine. Metabolic studies using this species (90, 91) demonstrated that 2,6-dimethyoxyquinol, either free or conjugated with sulphate, was the major metabolite. The formation of quinones from quinol would, therefore, explain both the high toxicity and colored urine when 2,6-dimethoxyphenol was administered to cats.

Dogs do not excrete significant quantities of acetylated metabolites from aromatic amines. This may be due to either an inhibitor of arylamine acetyl transferance in liver and kidney (92) or a high aromatic deacetylase activity in this species. Dogs can, however, acetylate aliphatic amino groups and, when dosed with sulfanilamide, excrete N^1-acetylsulfanilamide but not N^4-acetylsulfanilamide (93) (Figure 5). Another anomalous species is the guinea pig, which does not readily form mercapturic acids as a result of a deficiency in the enzyme acetylating aryl cysteine (83).

Unfortunately, most species differences in drug metabolism are less well-defined than those described above and can only be identified by comparing the metabolism of a candidate drug in one species with that of another and eventually with that of man. Although it is not necessary to screen every

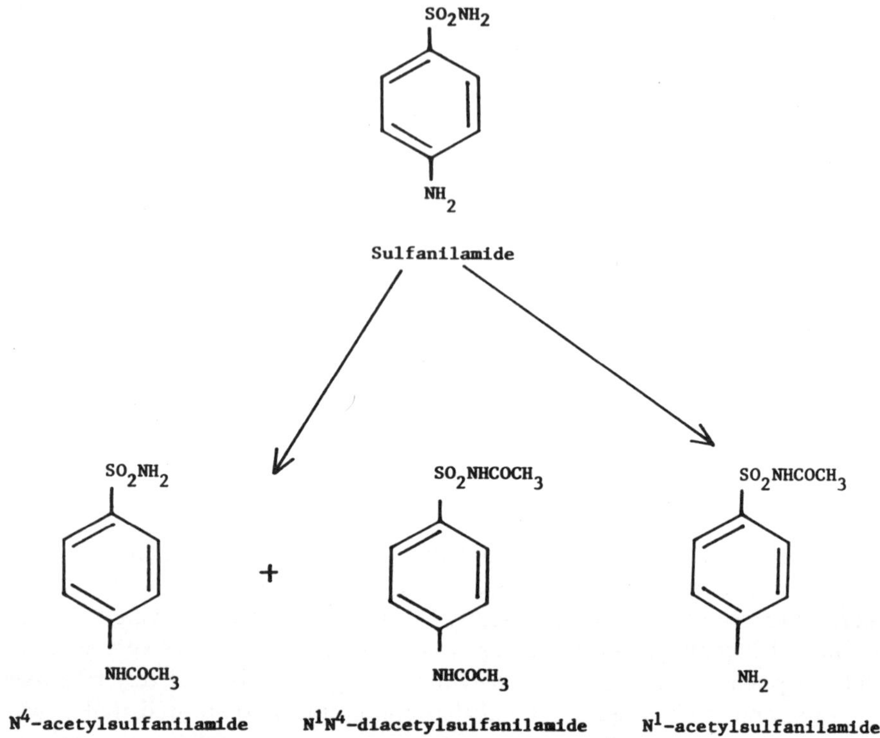

Figure 5. The metabolic pathways of sulfanilamide.

possible animal species to find one whose metabolism corresponds to man, or even to go to the lengths taken when studying the metabolism of sulfadimethoxine (94) (Table 5), it is essential to compare the main toxicological species (rat and dog) with man and, if necessary, to extend this comparison to species such as rabbit and monkey.

Such studies have been undertaken for many compounds, and in many instances significant differences were found between the main toxicological species and man, as the following examples show.

Amphetamine. Dring et al. (95–97) demonstrated that man, monkey, and dog excrete virtually 30% of the drug unchanged and, as a result of deamination and oxidation, another 30% as free and conjugated benzoic acid (Figure 6). Hydroxylation is only a minor route of metabolism in these species, whereas in rat it accounts for 60% of the dose. In rabbit, deamination to phenylacetone is the main reaction, followed by conjugation with sulphate after enolization on reduction to benzyl methyl carbinol. Some oxidation to benzoic acid also takes place (Figure 7).

Table 5. The Formation of Sulfadimethoxine N^1-glucuronide in Various Species

24-Hour excretion as N^1-glucuronide			
Nonprimates (%)		Primates (%)	
Dog	19	Man	65
Cat	0	Rhesus Monkey	66
Ferret	0	Green Monkey	30
Rabbit	0	Baboon	63
Rat	8	Squirrel Monkey	44
Mouse	12	Capuchin	48
Guinea pig	4	Bushbaby	62
Fruit bat	10	Slow Loris	49
Hen	16	Tree Shrew	52

Lidocaine. Lidocaine is used to control ventricular arrhythmias and is extensively metabolized by all species examined (98, 99). In man and dog, the major route of metabolism involves removal of the diethylaminoacetyl side chain to form 4-hydroxy-2,6-xylidine. However, in dog glycine xylidide is an important excretion product. Furthermore, although hydroxylation of lidocaine to 3-hydroxylidocaine and 3-hydroxydeethyl-lidocaine is a minor metabolic pathway in dog, it represents the major route in rat. The relative proportions of each metabolite in each species are shown in Table 6.

Nomifensine. Nomifensine is a new antidepressant agent used in a number of countries. A radioactive tracer technique established that the majority of the administered radioactivity from ^{14}C-nomifensine ($>50\%$) was eliminated in the urine of all species examined, including man (100). The main excretion products were unchanged drug and conjugates. However, three

Table 6. The Metabolism of Lidocaine in Various Species

Excretion Product	Man	Rat	Dog
Lidocaine	<3	<3	<3
4-Hydroxy-2,6-xylidine	73	12	35
Glycine xylidide	2–3	2–3	12
3-Hydroxylidocaine	—	30	6
3-Hydroxydeethyl-lidocaine	—	37	3

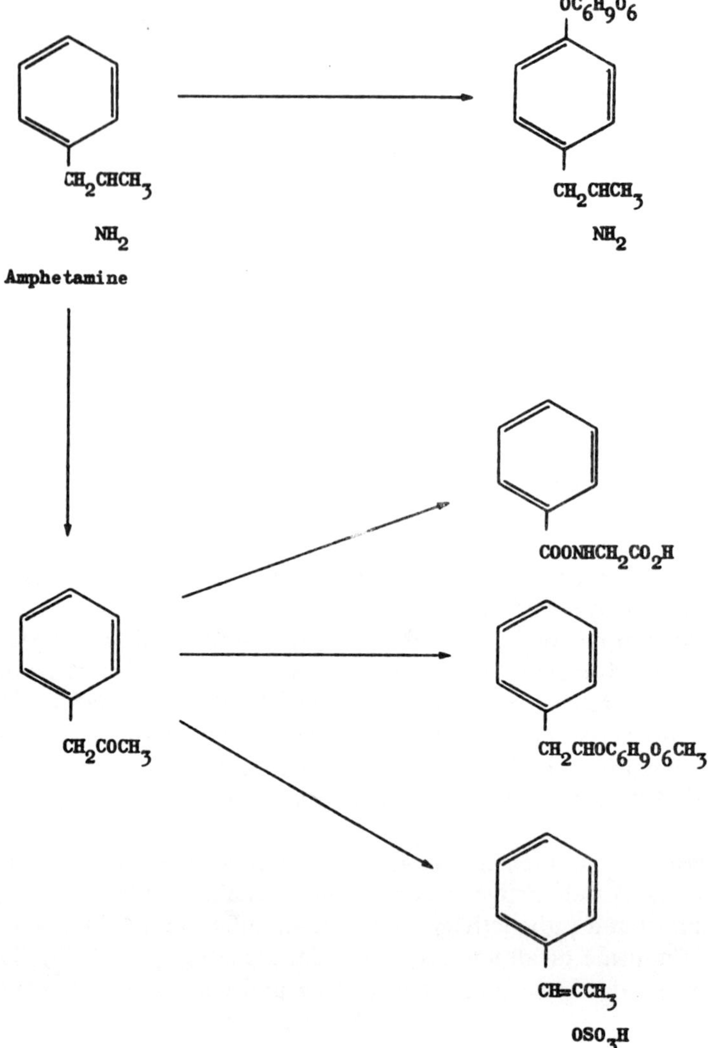

Figure 6. The metabolic pathways of amphetamine.

additional metabolites were found in man (Figure 8) and accounted for 20% of the dose. These products were also found in monkey to the level of 15% of the dose, but were absent from rabbit, dog, pig, and guinea pig.

Isoxepac. Isoxepac is one of a series of substituted dibenzoxepines showing considerable promise as an anti-inflammatory and analgesic agent from both

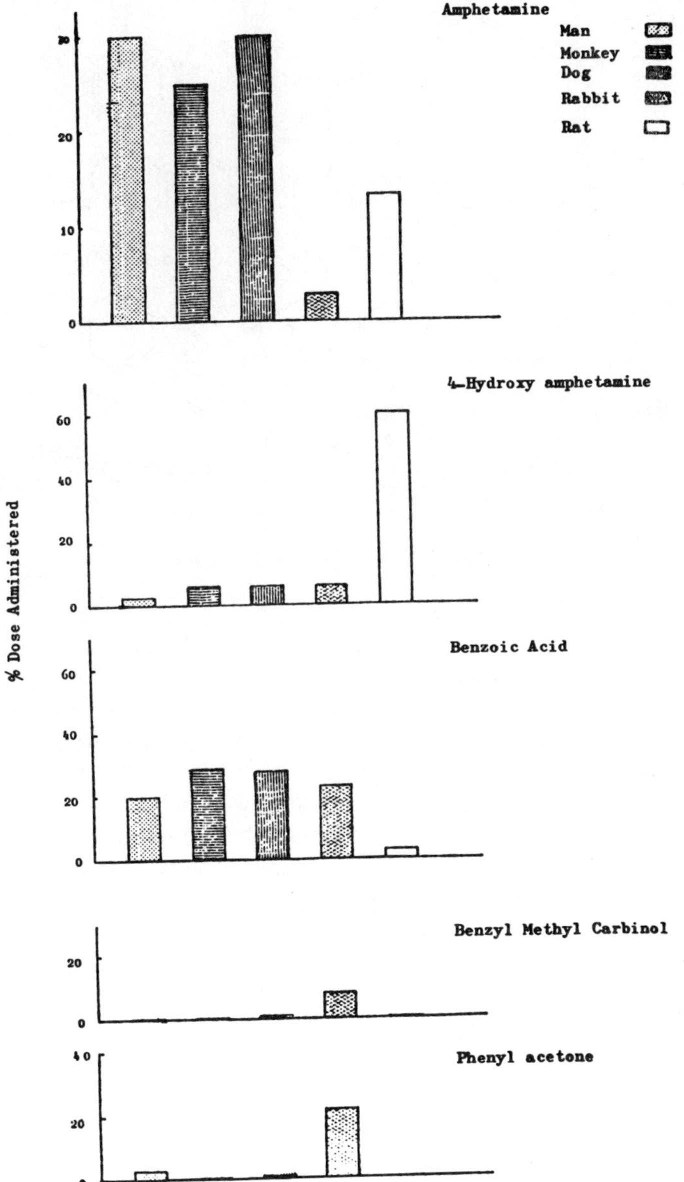

Figure 7. The amounts of amphetamine and its metabolites excreted by different animal species in 24-hour urine.

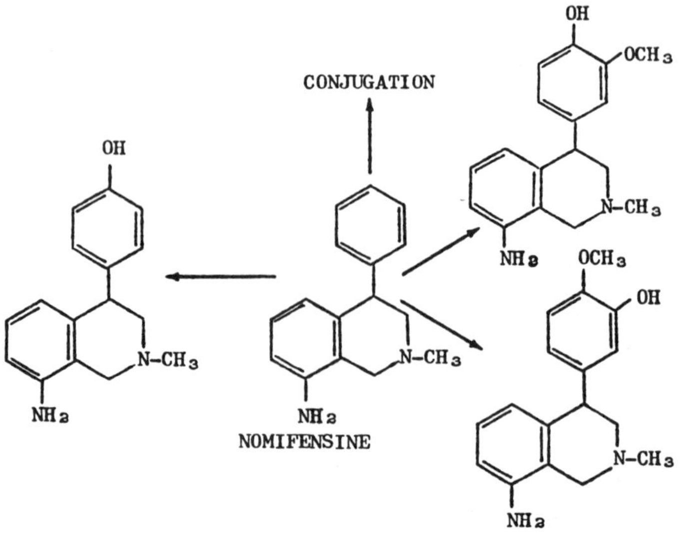

Figure 8. The metabolic pathways of nomifensine.

animal and human tests (101, 102). Extensive metabolism and disposition studies have been carried out to determine the most suitable species for long-term toxicity trials (103). ^{14}C-Isoxepac was used to investigate its metabolism in rat, rabbit, dog, monkey, and man, demonstrating significant species differences both in the route by which ^{14}C-products were eliminated from the body (Figure 9) and by which the drug was metabolized (Figure 10). Hence, it was considered unwise to extrapolate the results from rat and rabbit to man, and that the best species for such a purpose was monkey.

With the possible exception of lidocaine, the species that most closely resembled man in the metabolism of all these products was monkey. Smith and Caldwell (85) included a table with ratings for the suitability of rat, other nonprimates, and monkey as metabolic models for man in their review of drug metabolism in the nonhuman primate. By updating this list with nomifensine and isoxepac, and expressing the results as percentages (Table 7), it becomes apparent that monkey is far more likely to mimic man metabolically than the other species examined. For monkey, there was a good correlation with man for 76% of the drugs studied and a fair correlation (many similarities but with some significant differences) for 20% of the cases. The proportion of good correlations was reduced to 20% for rabbit, dog, and guinea pig, with 24% being invalid. Rats had the worst record, despite being a standard toxicological species, by only giving good correlations for 9% of the cases and invalid correlations for 39%.

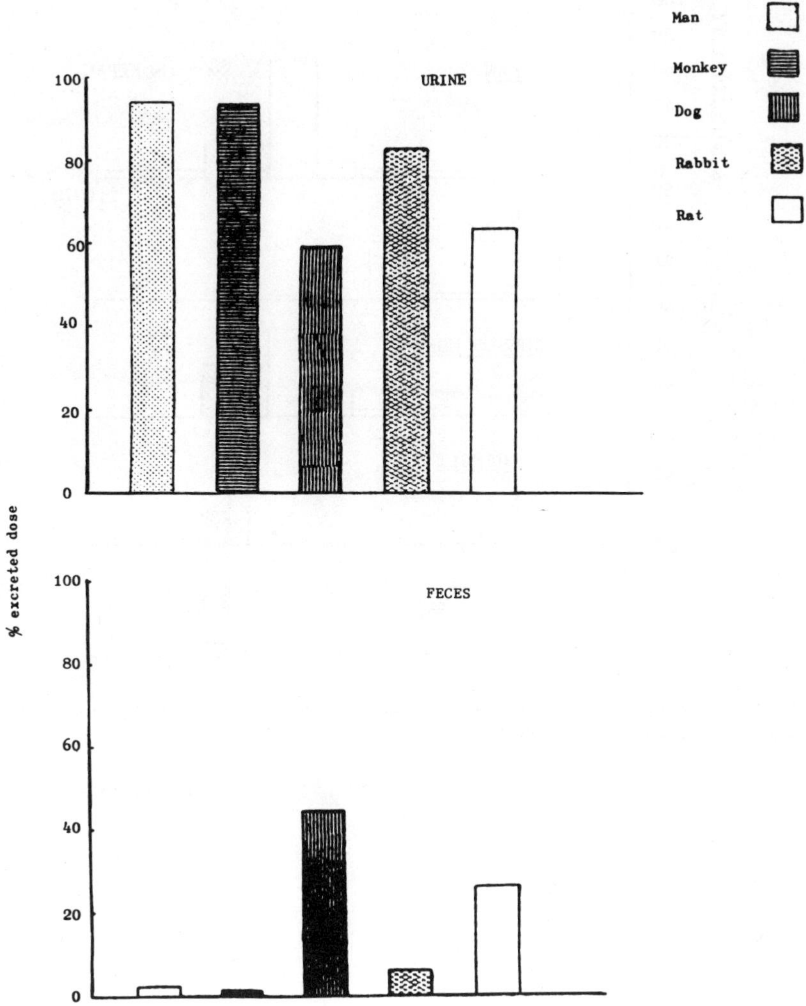

Figure 9. The routes of elimination of isoxepac in different animal species.

Smith and Caldwell (85) point out, however, that although monkey is the best metabolic animal model for man, the rates of metabolism between these species can differ considerably. With the exception of drugs that have a relatively short half-life in man ($\leqslant 5$ hours), the half-life in monkey tends to be shorter than that in man. It is suggested that for drugs with a half-life longer than 30 hours in man, none of the animal species provides a suitable kinetic model.

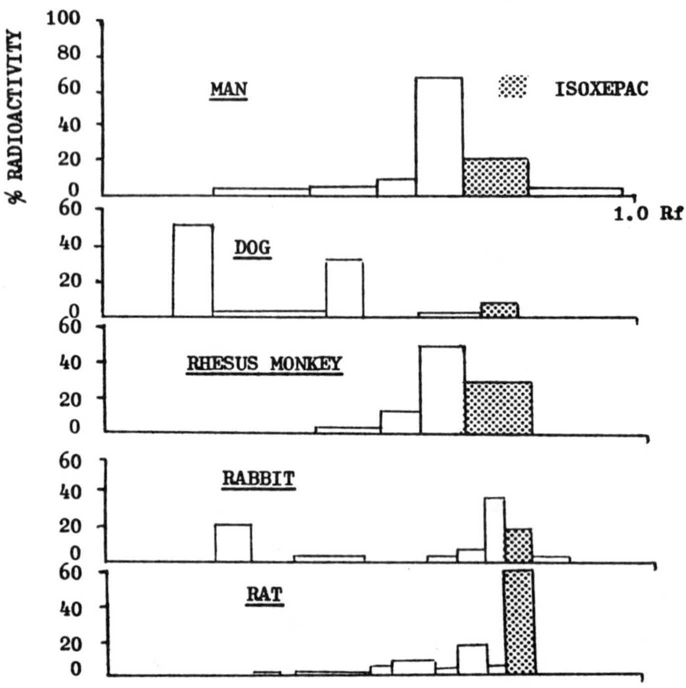

Figure 10. A histogram of a thin-layer chromatogram showing the variation in metabolism of isoxepac by different animal species.

Table 7. The Suitability of Various Animal Species as a Metabolic Model for Man[a]

Rating	Monkey (%)	Rat (%)	Dog, Rabbit, and Guinea Pig (%)
Good	76	17	20
Fair	20	9	28
Poor	4	35	28
Invalid	0	39	24

[a]The table incorporates data from Smith and Caldwell (85).

2.2.2 *Biliary Excretion and Enterohepatic Circulation*

Although the excretion of foreign compounds into bile was first reported in the early nineteenth century, it was not until about 1950 that the significance of bile as an excretory pathway was generally recognized. This corresponded to the increased use of compounds with relatively high molecular weights (>300) for drugs, food additives, and agricultural chemicals. Now that the importance of the biliary route (as opposed to just the urinary) is more fully realized, several reviews have appeared on the subject (104–107). Yet, the mechanism by which foreign compounds are excreted into bile is still poorly understood. It is, however, thought to occur in several stages, including transfer across a freely permeable sinusoid wall, uptake by the parenchymal cells often followed by metabolism, and concentrative passage from the liver cell into the bile (106).

The uptake of anionic compounds by the parenchymal cells may be facilitated by selective binding onto two proteins, designated the X and Y proteins (108). The Y protein, which constitutes the major proportion of the two intracellular acceptors, is present exclusively in liver. Moreover, its concentration increases after phenobarbitone pretreatment with a concomitant increase in the uptake of organic anions by the liver (109).

Brauer (110) classified compounds that appear in bile into three groups: A, with a bile to plasma concentration ratio of about 1; B, with a bile to plasma concentration ratio >1; and C, with a bile to plasma concentration ratio <1. When considering the biliary excretion of drugs, group B is the most interesting, since compounds in this group are secreted into bile against a concentration gradient. Several theories have been postulated to clarify this process. Schanker (111) proposed an energy dependent active transport system to explain the saturable and competitive nature of the biliary excretion of some compounds. Clarke et al. (112) felt that it was an effect of selective reabsorption, a theory accounting for molecular size, since it is based on the assumption that small compounds are readily reabsorbed from the bile and higher molecular weight compounds are reabsorbed at a slower rate. The incorporation of compounds into a salt/phospholipid/cholesterol micelle has also been proposed by Hirom (113).

There are certain requirements for a compound to be excreted into bile. Polarity plays an important role, and a strongly polar group (such as a carboxyl, sulfate, quaternary ammonium, or glycoside group) appears to be essential for biliary excretion. Structural factors are also implicated, as these may change lipid solubility, the shape of the molecule, or the spatial relationship between the polar and nonpolar groups on the molecule (113). However, although these are important determinants in the extent of biliary excretion of a compound, the most important factor by far appears to be molecular weight.

Accumulated evidence has shown, with the exception of some quaternary ammonium compounds, that for compounds of endogenous and exogenous origin, molecular weight must exceed 300 if extensive biliary excretion is to occur. Endogenous compounds such as the glucuronide conjugates of the steroid hormones, bilirubin, and thyroxine (molecular weights approximately 500–1000) are extensively secreted in bile, whereas the low molecular weight endogenous metabolites are not. Similarly for foreign compounds, those with a molecular weight <300 are poorly excreted into bile; those with a molecular weight >500 are well excreted by this route. There does appear to be an upper threshold, since very high molecular weight compounds, such as proteins, are poorly excreted in bile (110).

A critical aspect of biliary excretion, as far as the design of bioavailability studies using animals is concerned, is the species variations for biliary excretion of compounds with a molecular weight between 300 and 500 (Table 8). Rat and dog, the two most commonly used laboratory animals, have a molecular weight threshold of approximately 325, whereas that for man is about 500. Rat is also different from man in that it does not possess a gall bladder. The implications of these molecular weight threshold differences can be quite serious for absorption studies, since drugs that are extensively biliary excreted are also capable of undergoing enterohepatic circulation (Figure 11). Thus, when the administered drug is absorbed, taken up by the liver, and excreted into the bile, it can be transported back to the intestine where it is available for reabsorption. Even metabolism of a drug may not break this sequence, since, if the drug undergoes direct conjugation prior to biliary excretion, the intestinal microflora are quite adept at hydrolyzing conjugates, thereby releasing the parent compound for reabsorption.

The main consequence of enterohepatic circulation is to reduce the rate of elimination of the drug, as shown by digitoxin, which has a half-life of 14 hours in sham operated dogs but a half-life of 6 hours in dogs where enterohepatic circulation was prevented by a biliary fistula (114). The delayed

Table 8. The Approximate Molecular Weight Thresholds for Biliary Excretion of Compounds in Different Animal Species

Species	Molecular Weight
Rat	325
Dog	325
Guinea pig	400
Rabbit	475
Monkey	500
Man	500

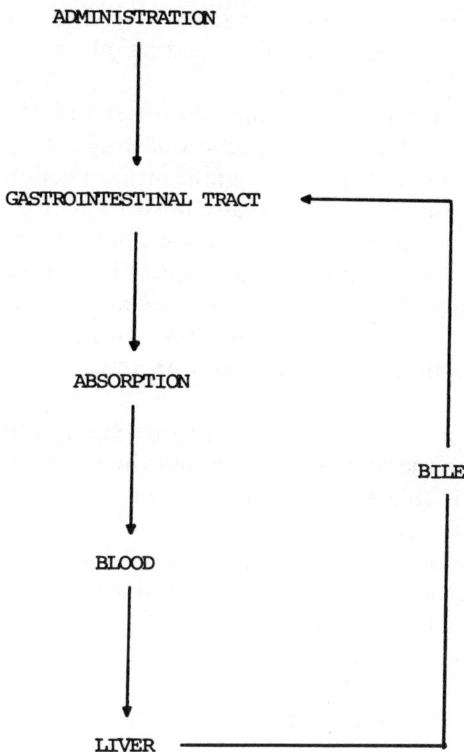

Figure 11. A schematic representation of the events occurring with enterohepatic circulation.

excretion of stilbestrol (115) and butylated hydroxytoluene (116) was also attributed to enterohepatic circulation.

Enterohepatic circulation can also make the pharmacokinetic interpretation of data extremely complex, especially if bile is stored in the gall bladder and suddenly released into the intestine after a suitable stimulus such as food. This can result in significant amounts of drug entering the intestinal tract for reabsorption, and is often reflected by a series of secondary peaks in the blood or plasma level curves. These problems were discussed by many workers and several pharmacokinetic models proposed (117–119). More important, Pang and Gillette (119) predicted on theoretical grounds that enterohepatic circulation could affect both area under the curve and bioavailability measurements.

Since biliary excretion of compounds with a molecular weight between 300 and 500 varies between species, and as it can affect the interpretation of bioavailability studies, it is necessary to select a species with a similar biliary threshold to meaningfully extrapolate the animal results to man. However, only rabbit and monkey fit this criteria, which would be unnecessarily restrictive if biliary excretion was not particularly extensive in different species. Thus, methods are needed to measure biliary excretion in the proposed test species for bioavailability testing.

Several methods, both direct and indirect, are available for determining the relative importance of the biliary route in the excretion of drugs. That biliary excretion is important is first indicated by the significant proportion of the dose appearing in the feces after parenteral administration (e.g., intravenous). This could, however, be misleading, since some drugs can be secreted either into the saliva or directly into the gastrointestinal tract. Metronidazole, which is used for the treatment of amoebic dysentary, shows the latter effect, with most of the drug appearing in feces arising from secretion directly into the gastrointestinal tract, and biliary excretion being only a relatively minor route (120).

Direct measurements of biliary excretion are obviously preferred, and these normally involve anesthetizing the animal, cannulating the common bile duct, and collecting the bile for subsequent analysis. However, if the bile is collected while the animal is still under anesthesia, the anesthetic may reduce the bile flow. Also, the temperature of the animal has to be carefully maintained, since temperature can influence biliary output (121). Thus, it is preferable to use unanesthetized animals, and a brief summary of methods for three of the most commonly used species is given.

Rat. Many workers, when examining biliary excretion of drugs from rat, cannulate the common bile duct and, when the animal has recovered from the anesthetic, restrain them in a Bollman style cage (122) for the bile collection. This can distress the animal which, in turn, can have an adverse effect on the results of the study. Johnson and Rising (123) describe a method used routinely at the author's laboratories, which enables biliary excretion studies to be performed in the conscious unrestrained rat. This has many advantages, including overcoming the problems associated with the anesthetic, temperature, and stress and allowing the animals to feed normally and to be maintained in standard metabolism cages for urine and fecal collections. It also permits bile collection for up to 6 days, which is considerably longer than any of the other methods discussed. Finally, it can easily be modified for enterohepatic circulation studies.

Bile is collected in a glass reservoir housed in the peritoneal cavity of the animal. The technique involves cannulation of the common bile duct proximal to the liver while the rat is under halothane anesthesia. A hollow spike is introduced, from the inside to the outside, through the dorsal body wall close to the liver and backbone, but avoiding major blood vessels. A wide side arm of the glass reservoir is placed in the open end of the spike, pushed through the body wall (shielded by the spike), and held in place by a rubber collar. The reservoir is then positioned carefully in the peritoneal cavity, and the free end of the biliary cannula is placed at the bottom of the reservoir via a narrow side arm prior to sealing in position with silicone tubing to prevent leakage of bile (Figure 12). The incisions are closed, the anesthetic is discontinued, and the rats are allowed to recover for a period not less than 16 hours. Biliary excretion studies are only carried out if (*1*) the bile flow is 6–10 ml per 100 g in 24 hours, (*2*) the rats can defecate easily, (*3*) the animals appear healthy, and (*4*) there is adequate food intake.

The technique can be easily modified to study enterohepatic circulation by inserting two cannulae into the bile duct: a hepatic cannula, as described previously, and a duodenal cannula for the infusion of bile from a donor rat into the duodenum. This latter procedure, however, necessitates restraining the animals.

The success rate of this procedure is >95%, and the reproducibility is good for all compounds tested. Examples of biliary excretion and enterohepatic circulation studies are given in Figure 13 and Table 9, respectively.

Dog. The procedure for implantation of a chronic biliary fistula into dog is somewhat more complicated than that for rat, although a method has been developed and used routinely over a number of years with a high degree of

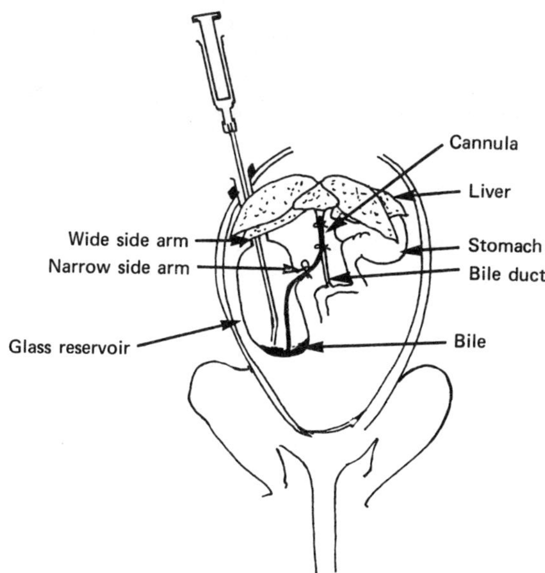

Figure 12. The collection of bile into a glass reservoir housed in the peritoneal cavity of a freely behaving rat, as described by Johnson and Rising (123).

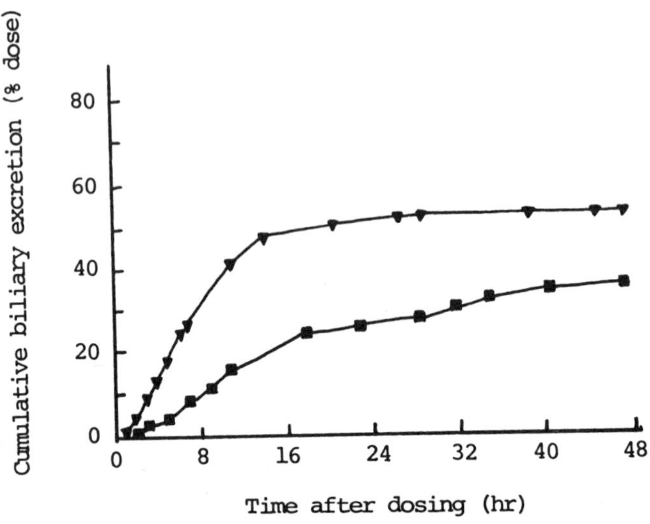

Figure 13. The biliary excretion of radioactive products when ^{14}C-fendosal was administered orally to rats.

Table 9. Enterohepatic Circulation of Radioactivity from ^{14}C-Fendosal and ^{14}C-Isoxepac in Rats[a]

	Radioactivity Recovered from Recipient Animal (%)	
Drug Administered to Donor Animal	Fendosal	Isoxepac
Urine	ND[b]	14–19
Bile	27–34	24–30
Gastrointestinal tract	25–40	14–20
Feces	12–15	23

[a]Data taken from Johnson and Rising (123).
[b]ND—not determined.

success (103). The method, developed by Steward, is based on an operation described by Herrera et al. (124) for examining pancreatic function.

Halothane anesthesia is again used, the cystic duct is ligated, and the gall bladder is removed. The segment of duodenum in which the bile duct enters is transected, and an end to end anastomosis is performed on the remaining two ends of duodenum. The two ends of the isolated duodenal segment where the bile duct enters are also sutured to form an enclosed pouch.

A side arm of a stainless steel cannula is then inserted into the isolated pouch, with one end of the cannula introduced into the duodenum and the other exteriorized (Figure 14). Metronidazole, neomycin, and chloramphenical are used prophylactically to minimize the risk of bacterial infection.

The cannula is constructed to accept a bolt (Figure 14). A short bolt is used when the animal is not under test and allows free passage of the bile into the duodenum. A specially adapted bolt is used for most experimental studies, which allows not only the collection of bile by diverting the flow from the duodenum, but also the infusion of replacement bile or bile from a donor animal through it into the duodenum (Figure 14).

Monkey. Meszaros et al. (125) describe a method of permanent bile duct cannulation for Rhesus monkey in which a silicone rubber cannula is introduced into the common bile duct just short of the cystic duct. A second cannula is also introduced through the stomach wall and pylorus to the entrance of the common bile duct in the duodenum. Further movement of the cannulae is prevented by silicone rubber collars. The two cannulae are exteriorized between the sternum and umbelicus via a plexiglass U-tube end-piece. When the animals are not being used, ends of each cannulae are joined by the U-tube to allow normal bile flow. For the study of biliary excretion and/or enterohepatic circulation, the monkeys are restrained so that drugs or bile can be infused into the duodenum through the inlet cannula and bile collected from the outlet cannula. Postoperative examination has established, however, that collateral tissue channels can form through which bile can reach the duodenum. Once this shunt occurs, bile can no longer be collected, although this usually takes about 3 months to happen. However,

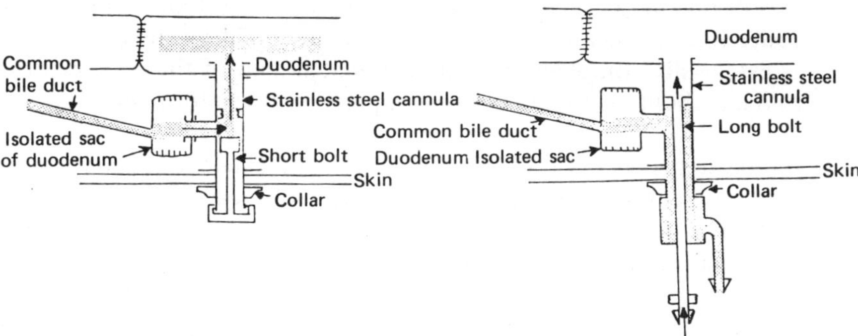

Figure 14. A schematic representation of the positions of the bolts fitted into a biliary cannula of a dog. Position A represents the short bolt allowing normal bile flow to the duodenum, and position B, the specially adapted cannula allowing infusion and collection of bile for enterohepatic circulation studies.

as the monkeys are in good condition after removal of the cannula to restore normal bile flow, they are still available for other purposes (125).

An alternative approach used for studying the disposition of diethylstilbestrol utilizes the insertion of a Latex T-tube to just below the juncture of the left and right hepatic bile ducts, the distal length of the T-tube being exteriorized. Prior to this, however, the cystic duct is isolated from the common bile duct, although the gall bladder is left in place. A second T-tube is inserted into the proximal third of the duodenum, and again the distal portion is exteriorized. After surgery, the hepatic and duodenal loops are connected to permit normal biliary flow from the liver, bypassing the gall bladder, to the duodenum. With this preparation, however, it is necessary to include a peristaltic pump to maintain the bile flow or phospholipids and cholesterol will precipitate and block the tubes (177).

2.2.3 *Pharmacokinetic Considerations*

Inevitably, when determining the bioavailability of drug products in animals or man, it is necessary to make some assumptions about the pharmacokinetic parameters used to measure bioavailability.

Most in-vivo studies use blood or plasma level data to determine bioavailability, although urine measurements can also be used in one of two ways:

1. If sufficient drug is excreted unchanged in the urine, total urine collections can be made until elimination is virtually complete, and the cumulated amount of drug recovered can be compared between formulations.
2. If substantial presystemic metabolism can be excluded, total urine collections can again be made until elimination of drug and metabolites is essentially complete, and the cumulated sum of the urinary drug and metabolite amounts can be compared between formulations.

For blood and plasma level data, however, the extent of absorption is usually determined from area under the curve (AUC) measurements extrapolated to infinite time. Absolute bioavailability is calculated from oral and intravenous data using the Dost principle (126) (equation 1).

$$\text{Absolute bioavailability } (F\%) = \frac{\text{AUC PO}}{\text{AUC IV}} \cdot \frac{\text{Dose IV}}{\text{Dose PO}} \cdot 100 \qquad (1)$$

Similarly, when comparing one oral formulation with another, the relative bioavailability is obtained from the ratio of AUC of each formulation, normalized for dose.

A fundamental assumption of both these procedures is that the pharmacokinetics of the drug are linear. Most laboratory animals weigh considerably less than the standard 70 kg man (rabbit approximately 3 kg, monkey approximately 6 kg, and beagle dog approximately 15 kg) and consequently, if the animals are dosed with a formulation designed for man, the dose level is proportionally higher than that envisaged for clinical use. The risk of nonlinear kinetics must, therefore, increase.

Nonlinearity can be caused by saturation or Michaelis-Menten kinetics involving either an enzymatic or an active excretory process (127, 128). This, in turn, has implications on the area–dose relationships as considered by Chan (129). However, nonlinear kinetics of extensively plasma protein bound drugs has also been seen when the degree of plasma protein binding is concentration dependent (130–132).

Thus, before conducting bioavailability testing using animals, the linearity of kinetics for the species of interest must be established. Wagner (133) enumerated a comprehensive list of tests to establish this, and all require that several dose levels of the drug be given, preferably by the intravenous route. Obviously, the dose levels should encompass that proposed for the bioavailability study. Two tests that can readily distinguish between linear and nonlinear kinetics are superimposition of the blood or plasma level curves and the linear relationship between AUC and dose. The former involves normalizing the blood or plasma level data to one dose level and determining if the blood (plasma) level curves are superimposable. This can be performed either graphically or statistically, using a split-plot analysis (134). The relationship between AUC and dose can also be examined graphically or statistically, the latter best performed by linear regression analysis on logarithmically transformed data and testing if the slope of the regression line differs from 1 (135). If the slope is significantly different from 1, the kinetics are nonlinear, and when the dose is changed, the AUC will change disproportionally.

Nonlinearity of kinetics in animals can occur reasonably frequently, and two examples are given from the author's laboratories when the linearity of kinetics was tested in dogs. Isoxepac, the anti-inflammatory agent, showed linear kinetics with the plasma profiles being superimposable and the AUC being directly proportional to dose (Figure 15). For another example (a psychotropic agent), however, nonlinear kinetics was demonstrated at a dosage level normally used for the bioavailability testing of clinical formulations. In this case, the plasma profiles were not superimposable, and there was a disproportionate increase of AUC with increasing dose (Figure 16).

Additional information can also be obtained from these preliminary studies, especially if the intravenous route of administration is used and if the blood levels can be calculated. This permits the determination of the

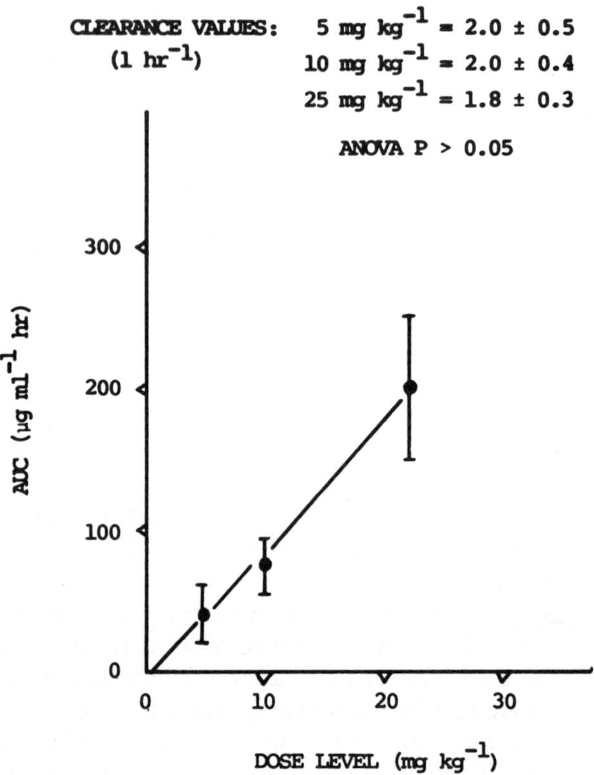

Figure 15. The linear elimination kinetics of isoxepac in dogs, as demonstrated by a proportional increase in area under the curve with intravenous dose level.

total blood clearance (*Cl*), which is a function of hepatic blood flow (*Q*) and the extraction ratio of the liver (*ER*). It therefore becomes possible to calculate the extraction ratio of the drug and to ascertain if it is liable to undergo first pass metabolism (equation 2).

$$ER = \frac{Cl}{Q} \qquad (2)$$

2.3 Summary

Before embarking on any in-vivo bioavailability testing using animals, investigators should ask themselves three questions:

1. What information is needed—can we use man?
2. What species is most appropriate?
3. Are the kinetics in that species linear at the dose level to be used?

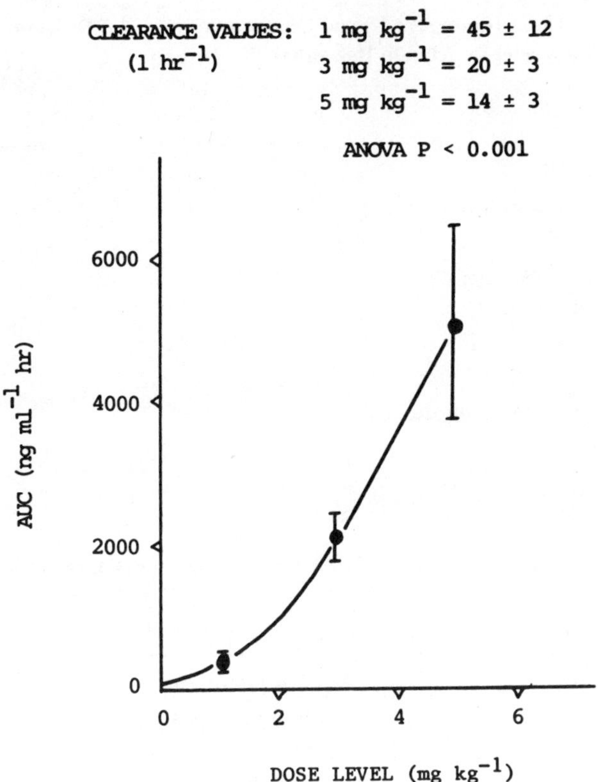

Figure 16. The nonlinear elimination kinetics of a candidate psychotropic agent in dogs, as demonstrated by a disproportional increase in area under the curve with intravenous dose level.

Once the objectives of the study are defined and it is decided to use animals, the most difficult decision is the choice of animal species. None are ideal and each has its advantages and disadvantages (Table 10). In fact, with the number of variables possible the reader might be forgiven for asking whether the study is worth pursuing. Despite this, many investigators have used animals for bioavailability testing and have obtained invaluable information which has helped in their understanding of their drug product (Table 11). It should also be stressed that factors such as metabolism, biliary excretion, and linearity of kinetics of drugs should all form an integral part of the drug development program for the design and interpretation of toxicological studies and, as such, very little additional work would be needed to assist in the choice of animal species for bioavailability testing.

Of the species listed in Table 10, rabbit appears to be the least suitable animal model for bioavailability testing, despite its relatively large size (large enough to test solid formulations) and low cost. This is because it has

Table 10. The Advantages (+) and Disadvantages (−) of Different Animal Species as a Model for Man in Bioavailability Testing

	Rat	Rabbit	Dog	Monkey
Cost	+	+	−	−
Ease of urine collection	+	+	+	−
Ease of blood sampling	−	+	+	+
Ease of handling	+	+	+	−
Intact solid formulation	−	+	+	+
Intestinal pH	+	−	+	+
Gastrointestinal transit time	−	−	−	−
Gastrointestinal microflora	−	−	+	+
Drug metabolism	−	(− +)	(− +)	+
Biliary excretion	−	+	−	+

Table 11. Examples of Uses of In-Vivo Animal Models for Bioavailability Testing

Species	Drug	Comments	Reference
Dog	Digoxin	Antacid interation	136
Dog	Dicumarol	Effect of particle size	137
Dog	Dicumarol	Effect of particle size and crystalline form	138
Dog	Sulfadimethoxine	Bioavailability from oral suspension	139
Dog	Levodopa	Influence of route of administration	140
Rat	Griseofulvin Sulfisoxazole acetyl Dicumarol	Effects of lipids on bioavailability	141
Rat	Sulfafurazol	Effect of pharmaceutical additives	142
Rabbit	Griseofulvin	Relationship between dissolution rate and bioavailability	143
Rat	Penicillin and cephalosporins	Absorption of β-lactum antibiotics	13

a long gastric emptying time and both its gastrointestinal pH and microflora bear little resemblance to that in man. Rat has the major disadvantage of being too small to test most solid formulations, as well as being difficult to obtain relatively large blood samples from repetitively, especially in those countries where bleeding from the retrobulbar venous plexus is discouraged.

In addition, the gastrointestinal microflora is different from that of man. This species does have the advantage, however, of having a gastrointestinal pH similar to that in man and, if urinary data are used for bioavailability testing, it is easy to obtain total urine collections using all-glass metabolism cages.

In most respects, monkey offers the closest physiological and metabolic model for man and would be first choice if not for its extremely high cost and difficulties with handling. Handling difficulties not only apply to the animals themselves, as they usually have to be restrained during the experiment, but also to the biological samples (urine, blood, and plasma) after collection, since these are capable of transmitting several human pathogens. Obviously, if primate facilities are routinely available, the use of this species becomes more attractive.

Dogs offer a reasonable compromise, since (*1*) they are large enough to test solid formulations, (*2*) their gastrointestinal pH is similar to man, (*3*) they are easy to bleed repetitively, (*4*) they are easy to handle, and (*5*) there are no special precautions needed when handling the biological samples after collection. There are occasions, however, when metabolic and enterohepatic circulation considerations preclude their use as a test species for bioavailability testing. If this should occur, the choice usually becomes limited to monkey, if applicable, or man.

3. IN-VITRO AND IN-SITU MODELS

No review of animal models for bioavailability testing is complete without some consideration of in-vitro and in-situ techniques for investigating drug absorption, although these have received considerable attention from other authors (25–27).

3.1 Everted Intestinal Sac

This in-vitro technique, originally developed by Wilson and Wiseman (144), provides one of the simplest methods for rapidly examining absorption of drugs. The original method involves removing a segment of the small intestine from a small rodent, usually rat, and everting it on a glass rod so that the mucosa are on the outside and the serosa on the inside. After sealing one end, the sac is filled with a suitable volume of physiological buffer, the free end sealed, and the enclosed sac incubated at 37°C in a fairly large volume of oxygenated buffer containing the test drug. After a predetermined time, the contents of the sac are assayed for the drug. This technique has the major advantage of producing a large change of drug concentration in the serosal fluid, even if absorption is comparatively low, which in turn facilitates the drug analysis. Its great disadvantage, however, is that it only allows for one drug measurement per intestinal segment. Consequently, the method was modified, as described by Crane and Wilson (145), and later improved by Kaplan and Cotler (146). Both these modifications allow the serosal fluid to be sampled repetitively during the experiment. The apparatus used for these repeated sampling experiments is based on that shown in Figure 17. Virtually all of the small intestine is everted for these modified methods and, when stretched, 5–15 cm lengths of the area of intestine to be examined are cut. The distal end of the everted segment is ligated and the proximal end tied to a cannula (*c*). The sac is then immersed in a known volume of continuously oxygenated mucosal fluid (*b*) prior to the introduction of a small volume (1 ml per 5 cm length) of buffer into the serosal chamber. Test drug is then added to the mucosal fluid and samples taken from the serosal side via the sampling tube (*a*) for the determination of drug concentration. For sampling, the total volume of the serosal fluid is removed and replaced by an equal volume of drug-free buffer.

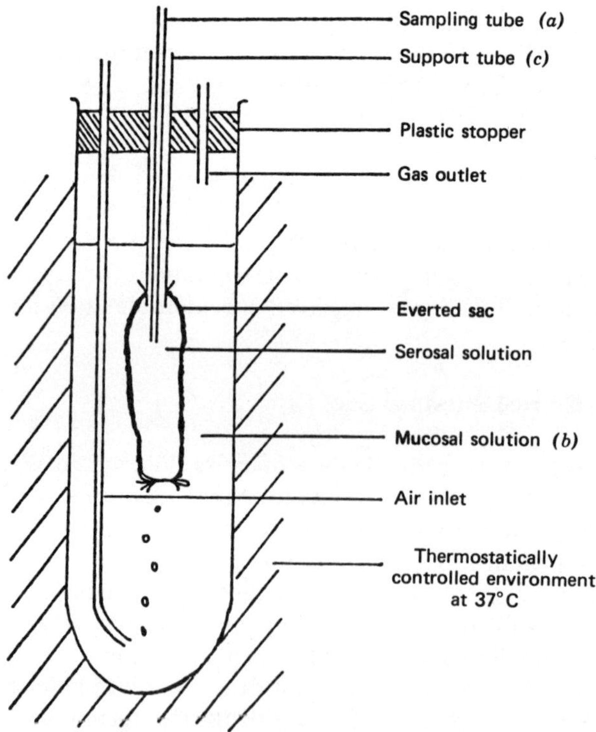

Figure 17. A typical apparatus for the repetitive sampling of serosal fluid in everted intestinal sac experiments.

Table 12. Examples of the Use of the Everted Intestinal Sac for Absorption Studies

Investigator	Objective	Reference
Barr and Riegelman	Intestinal metabolism of salicylamide	62
Matthews and Bell	Identification of absorption rates	147
Perrier and Gibaldi	Absorption of antibiotics	148
Chowhan and Amaro	Absorption of new drugs	149
Dixon and Mizen	Absorption of amino penicillins	150
Miyazaki et al.	Absorption of ampicillin derivatives	151
Penzotti and Poole	Absorption of β-lactam antibiotics	152
Wiseman	Active transport of amino acids	153
Schanker and Tocco	Active transport of pyrimidines	154
Reuning and Levy	Effects of complexing agents	155
Benet et al.	Effect of buffer constituents on absorption	156
Aguiar	Effect of excipients on chloramphenicol absorption	157
Saski	Effect of sufactants on drug absorption	158
Levy and Angelino	Intestinal hydrolysis of aspirin	159
Strahl and Barr	Glycine conjugation of benzoic acid	160
Feldman and Gibaldi	Binding of phenol red	161

The method is relatively reproducible and extremely easy to perform. Consequently, it is often used for the first exploratory experiments on the absorption of new candidate drugs (Table 12). In addition, it can readily determine if an absorption process is active or passive, and its uses have included the measurement of the effect of excipients and buffers on absorption, intestinal metabolism of drugs, the identification of absorption sites, and the intestinal binding of compounds (Table 12).

The major disadvantage of this technique, however, is that the intestinal section is removed from its blood supply so that the drug has to cross intestinal musculature as well as the mucosa (148). In addition, eversion of the intestinal segment alters its permeability characteristics, as shown by an increased permeability of phenol red (162). These limitations must, therefore, be considered when interpreting data from these studies.

3.2 Closed Loop

Since one of the major criticisms of the everted intestinal sac method is that the preparation has been removed from its normal blood supply, various in-situ techniques have been devised. Levine and Pelikan (163) described a relatively simple technique in which the small intestine of rats is exposed while the animal is under light anesthesia and a length of intestine (approximately 10 cm) is isolated by ligation, taking care not to occlude any of the major blood vessels. A solution of the drug (about 0.5 ml) is injected through the proximal ligature and the isolated loop is replaced in the peritoneal cavity. The animal is then closed and allowed to recover from the anesthetic. At a selected time, the animal is killed, and the concentration of drug within the loop and, if desired, in the blood, is measured. The method appears to be successful, and Nightingale et al. (164) used this technique to determine the effect of bile flow on the absorption of sulfadiazine. The method has also been modified to examine the disappearance of compounds from several loops within the same rat (165).

Perhaps a more popular technique is that described by Doluisio et al (43) in which rats are anesthetized with urethane, and, after exposure of the small intestine, two L-shaped cannulae are inserted into the duodenal and ileal ends of the intestinal segment to be studied. The other end of each of the cannulae is connected to a syringe via a three-way stopcock. The intestinal lumen is washed by flushing with buffer prior to the introduction of the drug solution. To sample, the intestinal contents are pumped into one of the syringes and a small aliquot is removed for drug analysis. The method can be further modified by simultaneously sampling blood, either by a cannula introduced into the jugular vein or by a tail bleeding technique. This overcomes one criticism of this technique—using the disappearance of drug from the intestine as a reflection of its appearance in the systemic circulation. Other criticisms encountered with the Doluisio method are the failure to correct for water flux and, as discussed previously, the possible effect of the anesthetic on the absorption kinetics of drug, by either altering blood flow or changing the permeability of the intestinal wall.

3.3 Perfused Loop

This method was first described by Schanker et al. (166) when measuring the disappearance of drug from the lumen of a rat's small intestine following a single pass of a drug solution through an intestinal segment at a constant rate. The method has subsequently been adapted to permit recycling of the drug solution.

The animal is again maintained under anesthesia with its inherent disadvantages; the small intestine is exposed and cannulated with polythene cannulae at the duodenal and ileal ends. The former is attached to an infusion pump and, after replacing the intestinal loop into the peritoneal cavity and closing the incision, the loop is washed and the drug solution is perfused at a rate of 1.5 ml minute^{-1}. Samples are collected at the ileal end for the determination of the drug concentration. Corrections should be made for water flux using a nonabsorbable marker.

Although this technique has found extensive use (39, 167, 168), the flow rate for the perfusion is critical, and can interfere with the absorption process.

3.4 Isolated Intestinal Loop with Complete Mesenteric Collection

This is one of the most useful of the in-situ methods utilizing small rodents, since by making a complete mesenteric blood collection with a concomitant infusion of blood the effect of anesthesia upon blood flow can be largely overcome. In addition, information about the absorbed products can also be obtained before they reach the liver.

The method, or variations, was described by a number of investigators (61, 169, 170). The animal is anesthetized and the loop of intestine to be examined is cannulated so that it can be perfused with the drug solutions (for rats a perfusion rate of 0.1 ml minute^{-1} is used). Alternatively, a closed loop technique can be used, the loop then being isolated by ligation. The hepatic portal vein from the loop is cannulated and all the mesenteric blood is continuously collected and weighed. The amount of blood lost is then

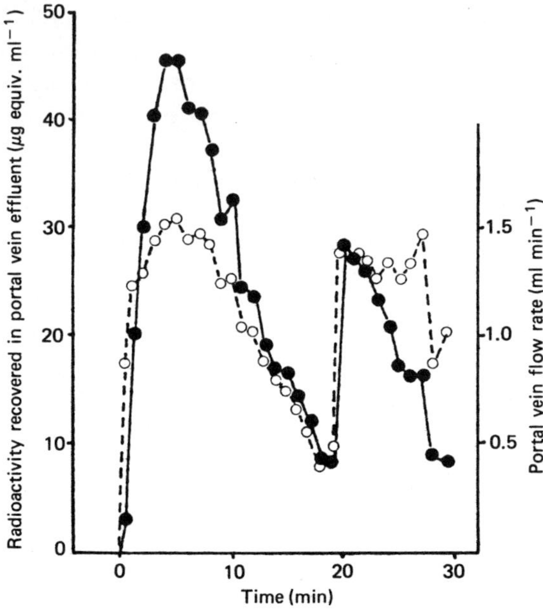

Figure 18. The effect of blood flow (○) on the absorption of intraduodenally administered isoxepac (●) as measured from total mesenteric blood collection.

replaced by infusion, via the renal vein, using blood from donor animals. Furthermore, the rate of infusion of donor blood can be used to control blood flow, thus allowing the effects of blood flow changes upon the absorption of a drug to be studied (Figure 18). With the relatively large volume of mesenteric blood collected, it is also possible to examine for metabolites of new candidate drugs to determine if microbial or intestinal wall metabolism has occurred.

3.5 Thiry-Vella Loops

Unlike the other in-situ methods presented, the Thiry-Vella loop is a chronic preparation using unanesthetized dog and, as such, is the most sophisticated technique, requiring a high degree of surgical expertise.

As originally described by Thiry (171) and Vella (172), a loop of the small intestine of dog is isolated with its blood, nerve, and lymph supply intact, and both the proximal and distal ends of the isolated segment are exteriorized through the abdominal wall. The full details of the operative procedure are given by Markowitz et al. (173). Since the animals normally survive for very long periods after surgery, and since the loop maintains its normal physiology, it is possible to use the dogs repetitively for testing the absorption and bioavailability of numerous candidate drugs administered either as solution or in other dosage forms. The drug is introduced into the loop and samples of the loop contents are removed at different times to measure the drug's disappearance. Corrections for water flux are made using a nonabsorbed marker. In addition, the drug can be administered intravenously and the absolute bioavailability determined.

The Thiry-Vella loop preparation has been evaluated in the author's laboratories with extremely encouraging results. Isoxepac was used as a test compound, and the kinetics were determined in a dog fitted with a jejunal Thiry-Vella loop after oral administration, intravenous administration, and administration directly into the loop. The plasma levels after oral dosing and administration into the loop compared very favorably (Figure 19), as did the absorption rate constants when calculated using the percent unabsorbed–time plots described by Wagner and Nelson (174) (half-life 6.6 and 7.1 min, respectively). Although no correction was made for water flux, the half-life of disappearance of isoxepac from the loop was in the same order (12.1 min) as that calculated from blood level data (Figure 20).

Taylor et al. (175) described the successful use of this technique for examining the absorption of practolol and propanolol from both jejunal and ileal loops and concluded that for these drugs the dog intestinal loop provides a more detailed and realistic model for in-vivo absorption than the in-situ preparations using rat. A similar conclusion was reached by Sample et al. (176) when studying the absorption of acetaminophen.

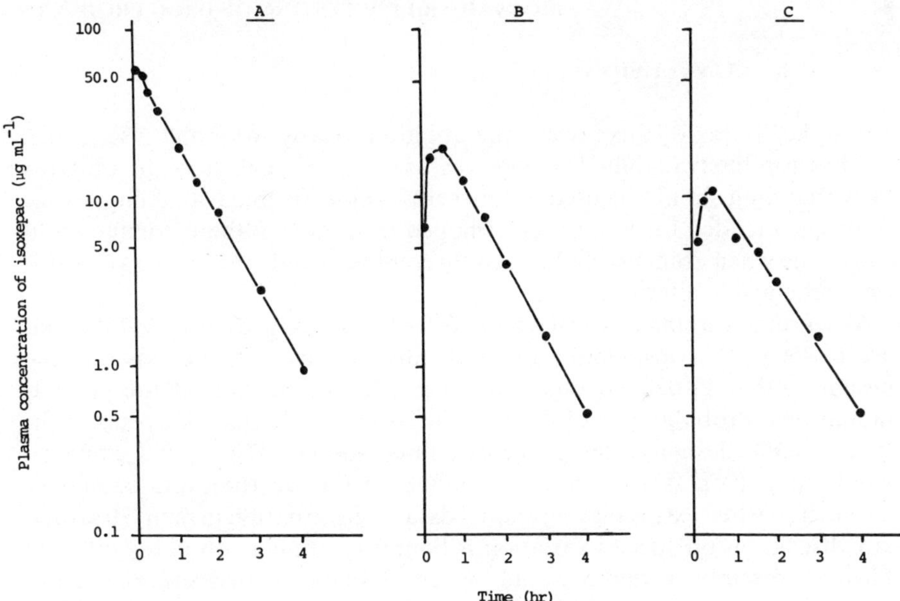

Figure 19. The plasma profiles of isoxepac when administered intravenously (*a*), orally (*b*) and directly into an intestinal loop (*c*) of a dog fitted with a Thiry-Vella loop.

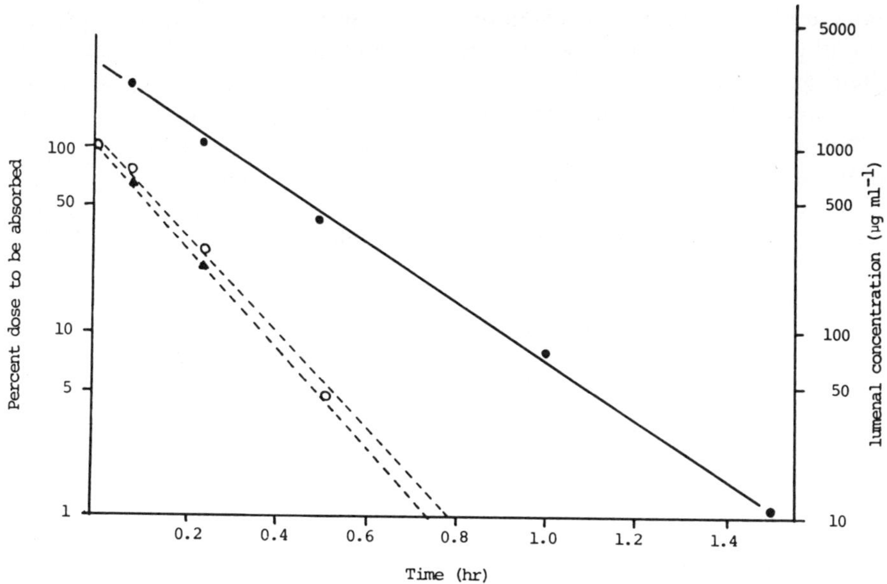

Figure 20. A comparison between oral absorption of isoxepac (○) and absorption from an intestinal loop (▲), both determined by the Wagner-Nelson method, and with the direct measurement of the disappearance of isoxepac from the intestinal loop (●) of a dog fitted with a Thiry-Vella loop.

4. CONCLUSION

At the beginning of this review, the question of why we should use animal models for bioavailability testing was asked. Although it is the author's view that man should be used, whenever possible, for bioavailability testing of drugs intended for human use, I hoped to show that there are numerous occasions when animals can be usefully employed and may even provide the only practicable alternative.

When undertaking any in-vivo bioavailability study, especially if animals are to be used, considerable thought must be given to the experimental design, with well-defined objectives and a full realization of the possible limitations. Probably one of the most important and difficult aspects of the experimental design is the choice of animal species. Thus, great emphasis has been put on factors that both influence this decision and should be considered when extrapolating animal data to the situation in man. However, any discussion on species variation is bound to impinge on many different scientific disciplines, and it would be very difficult to cover every aspect of this diverse subject. Consequently, the discussion has been orientated to bioavailability of orally administered drugs, neglecting many of the other important routes of administration, such as that of topically applied drugs.

The in-vitro and in-situ models for absorption studies have and will continue to play an important role in the determination of absorption mechanisms of candidate drugs. Also, because of their relative simplicity, they have often become incorporated into the routine screening procedures of drug discovery programs. Furthermore, if these techniques are employed in conjunction with in-vivo bioavailability studies, they can provide valuable information leading to the rational design of new dosage formulations. If this information is obtained early enough, it could prevent frustrating delays in the drug's development during subsequent clinical trials.

ACKNOWLEDGMENTS

I am grateful for the invaluable help and advice given by my colleagues, especially Dr. P. Johnson, Dr. C. Macdonald, Dr. L. Stevens, Mr. A. Pidgen, and Mr. A. Steward. I also thank Mrs. Anne Taylor for so ably typing this manuscript.

REFERENCES

1. W. H. Barr. *Drug Inf. Bull.* **3**:27 (1969).
2. G. Levy and R. Gelber. *Drug. Inf. Bull.* **3**:82 (1969).

3. S. Riegelman. *Drug. Inf. Bull.* **3**:59 (1969).

4. J. G. Wagner. Generic Equivalence and Inequivalence of Oral Products. In *Biopharmaceutics and Relevant Pharmacokinetics*, 1st ed, Drug Intelligence Publication, Hamilton, Illinois 1971.

5. G. W. Brice and H. F. Hammer. *J. Am. Med. Assoc.* **208**:1189 (1969).

6. G. Levy. *Am. J. Hosp. Pharm.* **17**:756 (1960).

7. G. H. Schneller. *Drug Inf. Bull.* **3**:100 (1969).

8. A. B. Varley. *J. Am. Med. Assoc.* **206**:1745 (1968).

9. T. R. D. Shaw, M. R. Howard, and J. Haner. *Br. Heart J.* **1**:695 (1974).

10. S. Riegelman, M. Rowland, and L. Z. Benet. *J. Pharmacokin. Biopharm.* **1**:83 (1975).

11. F. Leitner, D. R. Chisholm, Y. H. Tsai, G. E. Wright, R. G. Degeris, and K. E. Price. *Antimicrob. Agents Chemother.* **7**:306 (1975).

12. J. P. Clayton, M. Cole, S. W. Elson, H. Ferres, J. C. Hanson, L. W. Mizen, and R. Sutherland. *J. Med. Chem.* **19**:1385 (1976).

13. A. Tsuji, E. Miyamoto, I. Kagami, and J. Yamana. *J. Pharm. Sci.* **67**:1701 (1978).

14. E. J. Ariens. *Molecular Pharmacology*, Vol. 1, Academic Press New York, 1964.

15. C. F. George, T. Fenyvesi, and C. T. Dollery. Pharmacological Effects of Propranolol in Relation to Plasma levels. In D. S. Davies, and B. N. C. Prichard (eds.), *Biological Effects of Drugs in Relation to Their Plasma Concentrations*, A British Pharmacological Society Symposium, Macmillan, London, 1973, p. 123.

16. M. F. Cuthbert, and R. F. Collins. *Br. J. Clin. Pharmacol.* **2**:49 (1975).

17. W. Rupp, and P. Hajdú. In (ed.), H. J. Dengler. *Symposium on Pharmacological and Clinical Significance of Pharmacokinetics*, F. K. Schattauer Verlay, Stuttgart, 1970, p. 105.

18. D. E. Smith, and L. Z. Benet. *Pharmacology* **19**:301 (1979).

19. R. Amrein, J. P. Cano, D. Hartmann, W. H. Ziegler, and R. Dubuis. Sleep Research. In R. G. Priest, and A. Fletscher (eds.), *Northern European Symposium Basle, September 26–27th 978*, M.T.P. Press, 1978, p. 83.

20. G. T. Stewart. *Postgrad. Med. J.* **40**:160 (1964) (supplement).

21. L. McCurdy. *Arzneim. Forsch./Drug Res.* **30**:(1) 895 (1980).

22. S. Freir. *Acta Allergol.* **32**:109 (1977).

23. D. A. Smith and A. N. Fisher. *J. Pharm. Pharmacol.* (1980), in press.

24. M. J. Ashton, B. Clark, K. M. Jones, G. F. Moss, M. G. Neale, and J. T. Ritchie. *Appl. Toxicol. Pharmacol.* **26**:319 (1973).

25. W. H. Barr. *Pharmacology* **8**:55 (1972).

26. T. R. Bates and M. Gibaldi. Gastrointestinal absorption. In J. Swarbrick (ed.), *Current Concepts in the Pharmaceutical Sciences: Biopharmaceutics*, Lea and Febiger, Philadelphia, 1970, p. 57.

27. S. A. Kaplan and M. L. Jack. *In vitro*, *in situ* and *in vivo* Models in Bioavailability Assessment. In J. Blanchard, R. J. Sawchuck, and B. B. Brodie (eds.), *Principles and Perspectives in Drug Bioavailability*, S. Karger, Basel, 1979, p. 156.

28. B. E. Cabana. *Psychopharmacol. Bull.* **12**:51 (1976).

29. B. E. Cabana and L. W. Dittert. *J. Pharmacokin. Biopharm.* **3**:143 (1975).

30. L. W. Dittert, H. J. Adams, F. Alexander, C. W. Chong, T. Ellison and J. V. Swintosky. *J. Pharm. Sci.* **57**:1146 (1968).

31. C. H. Nightingale and M. Gibaldi. *J. Pharm. Sci.* **60**:1360 (1971).

32. S. H. Yalkowsky, T. G. Slunick, and G. L. Flynn. *J. Pharm. Sci.* **63**:691 (1974).

33. P. J. Cascella and S. Feldman. *J. Pharm. Sci.* **68**:401 (1979).

34. R. A. Upton. *J. Pharm. Sci.* **64**:112 (1975).

35. R. J. Brown and C. B. Breckenridge. *Biochem. Med.* **13**:280 (1975).

36. R. M. J. Ings. *Arch. Int. Pharmacodyn.* **242**:180 (1979).

37. L. S. Schanker, P. A. Shore, B. B. Brodie, and C. A. M. Hogben. *J. Pharmacol. Exp. Ther.* **120**:528 (1957).

38. P. A. Shore, B. B. Brodie, and C. A. M. Hogben. *J. Pharmacol. Exp. Ther.* **119**:361 (1957).

39. C. A. M. Hogben, D. J. Tocco, B. B. Brodie, and L. S. Schanker. *Pharmacol. Exp. Ther.* **125**:275 (1959).

40. W. G. Crouthamel, G. H. Tan, L. W. Dittert, and J. T. Doluisio. *J. Pharm. Sci.* **60**:1160 (1971).

41. H. W. Smith. *Pathol. Bact.* **89**:95 (1965).

42. W. G. Crouthamel, C. R. Abolin, J. Hsieh, and J. K. Lim. *J. Pharm. Sci.* **64**:1726 (1975).

43. J. T. Doluisio, N. F. Billups, L. W. Dittert, E. T. Sugita, and J. V. Swintosky. *J. Pharm. Sci.* **58**:1196 (1969).

44. W. L. Chiou, S. Riegelman, and J. R. Amberg. *Chem. Pharm. Bull.* **17**:2170 (1969).

45. J. M. Fromson, H. P. A. Illing, R. M. J. Ings, K. I. Johnson, P. Johnson, J. Ostrowski, E. Schraven, and A. Steward. *Arzneim. Forsch. Drug Res.* **31**(1):337 (1981).

46. A. C. Anderson. Digestive System. In A. C. Anderson and L. S. Good (eds.), *The Beagle as an Experimental Dog*, The Iowa State University Press, Ames, 1970, p. 226.

47. H. J. Rogers, F. R. House, P. J. Morrison, and I. D. Bradbrook. *Br. J. Clin. Pharmacol.* **6**:493 (1978).

48. C. R. Garcia. *Dissertation Abstracts International B* **38**:602 (1977).

49. D. Winne. *Naunyn-Schmiedeberg's Arch. Pharmacol.* **304**:175 (1978).

50. V. L. Sallee and J. M. Dietschy. *J. Lipid Res.* **14**:475 (1973).

51. F. A. Wilson and J. M. Dietschy. *Biochem. Biophys. Acta* **363**:112 (1974).

52. A. M. Hoyumpa, S. Nichols, S. Schenker, and F. A. Wilson. *Biochem. Biophys. Acta* **436**:438 (1976).

53. H. Westergadd and J. M. Dietschy. *Clin. Res.* **20**:736 (1972).

54. H. Westergaad and J. M. Dietschy. *J. Clin. Invest.* **54**:718 (1974).

55. E. S. Debnam and R. J. Levin. *J. Physiol. (London)* **252**:681 (1975).

56. N. W. Read, R. J. Levin, and C. D. Holdsworth. *Gut* **17**:387 (1976).

57. N. W. Read, C. D. Holdsworth, and R. J. Levin. *Eur. J. Clin. Invest.* **6**:314 (1976).

58. N. W. Read, D. C. Barber, R. J. Levin, and C. D. Holdsworth. *Gut* **18**:865 (1977).

59. L. Ther and D. Winne. *Ann. Rev. Pharmacol.* **11**:57 (1971).

60. D. Winne. *Pharmacology* **21**:1 (1980).

61. H. Oehsenfahrt and D. Winne. *Life Sci.* **7**:493 (1968).

62. W. H. Barr and S. Riegelman. *J. Pharm. Sci.* **59**:154 (1970).

63. A. Haass, H. Lüllmann, and T. Peters. *Eur. J. Pharmacol.* **19**:366 (1972).

64. D. Winne and J. Remischovsky. *Arch. Pharmakol.* **270**:22 (1971).

65. J. D. Myers. *J. Clin. Invest.* **29**;1421 (1950).

66. A. Blalock and M. F. Mason. *Am. J. Physiol.* **117**:328 (1936).

67. S. W. White, J. P. Chalmers, R. Hilder and P. I. Korner. *Aust. J. Exp. Biol. Med. Sci.* **45**:453 (1967).

68. J. H. Birnie and J. Grayson. *J. Physiol. (London)* **116**:189 (1952).

69. R. P. Forsyth, A. S. Nies, F. Wyler, J. Neutze, and K. L. Melmon. *J. Appl. Physiol.* **52**:736 (1968).

70. B. S. Drasar, A. G. Renwick, and R. T. Williams. *Biochem. J.* **129**:881 (1972).

71. M. J. Hill and B. S. Drasar. *Biochem. J.* **104**:55P (1964).

72. R. R. Scheline. *Acta Pharmacol. Toxicol.* **26**:189 (1968).

73. R. M. J. Ings, J. A. McFadzean, and W. E. Ormerod. *Biochem. Pharmacol.* **23**:1421 (1974).

74. G. N. Smith and C. S. Worrell. *Arch. Biochem. Biophys.* **24**:216 (1949).

75. R. R. Scheline and B. Longberg. *Acta Pharmacol. Toxicol.* **23**:1 (1965).

76. R. R. Scheline. *J. Pharm. Sci.* **57**:2021 (1968).

77. R. R. Scheline. Excepta Medica International Congress No. 254. Toxicological Problems of Drug Combinations Proceedings, XII Meeting of the European Society for the Study of Drug Toxicity, Berlin, 1971.

78. A. G. Renwick. Microbial Metabolism of Drugs. In D. V. Parke and R. L. Smiths (eds.), *Drug Metabolism from Microbe to Man*, Taylor and Francis Ltd, London, 1977, p. 169.

79. H. G. Boxenbaum, I. Berkersky, M. L. Jack, and S. A. Kaplan. *Drug. Metab. Rev.* **9**:259 (1979).

80. B. B. Brodie. *Clin. Pharmacol. Ther.* **3**:374 (1962).

81. L. B. Mellett. *Prog. Drug. Res.* **13**:136 (1969).

82. R. T. Williams. Species Variations in Drug Biotransformation. In B. N. La Du, H. G. Mandel, and E. L. Way (eds.), *Fundamentals of Drug Metabolism and Drug Disposition*, Williams and Wilkins Co., Baltimore 1972, p. 187.

83. D. V. Parke. Comparative Metabolism. In *The Biochemistry of Foreign Compounds*, Pergamon Press, Oxford, 1974, p. 117.

84. J. R. Gillette. The problems of Species Variations; Problems and Opportunities. In D. V. Parke and R. L. Smith (eds.), *Drug Metabolism from Microbe to Man*, Taylor and Francis Ltd., London, 1977, p. 147.

85. R. L. Smith and J. Caldwell. Drug Metabolism in Non-human Primates. In D. V. Parke and R. L. Smith (eds.), *Drug Metabolism from Microbe to Man*, Taylor and Francis Ltd., London, 1977, p. 331.

86. B. B. Brodie and W. D. Reid. *Fed. Proc.* **26**:1062 (1967).

87. B. Stripp and J. R. Gillette. *J. Pharm. Sci.* **61**:1682 (1972).

88. R. T. Williams. *Fed. Proc.* **26**:1029 (1967).

89. J. J. Miller, G. M. Powell, A. H. Olavesen, and C. G. Curtis. *Xenobiotica* **4**:285 (1974).

90. J. J. Miller, G. M. Powell, A. H. Olavesen, and C. G. Curtis. *Biochem. Soc. Trans.* **1**:1163 (1973).

91. J. J. Miller, G. M. Powell, A. H. Olavesen, and C. G. Curtis. *Toxicol. Appl. Pharmacol.* **38**:47 (1976).

92. K. C. Lechman and A. M. Anaclerio. *1st Int. Pharmacol. Meet.* **6**:91 (1961).

93. J. W. Bridges and R. T. Williams. *Biochem. J.* **87**:14P (1963).

94. R. H. Adamson, J. W. Bridges, M. R. Kibby, S. R. Walker, and R. T. Williams. *Biochem. J.* **118**:41 (1970).

95. L. G. Dring, R. L. Smith, and R. T. Williams. *J. Pharm. Pharmacol.* **18**:402 (1966).

96. L. G. Dring. Ph.D. Thesis, University of London, 1968.

97. L. G. Dring, R. L. Smith, and R. T. Williams. *Biochem. J.* **109**:10P (1968).

98. J. B. Keenaghan, and R. N. Boyes. *J. Pharmacol. Exp. Ther.* **180**:454 (1972).

99. J. Thomas and P. Meffin. *J. Med. Chem.* **15**:1046 (1972).

100. H. M. Kellner, C. Baeder, O. Christ, W. Heptner, I. Honke, and R. M. J. Ings. *Br. J. Clin. Pharmacol.* **4**:109S (1977).

101. D. E. Aultz, G. C. Helsley, D. Hoffman, A. R. MacFadden, H. B. Lassman, and J. C. Wilker. *J. Med. Chem.* **20**:66 (1976).

102. H. B. Lassman, R. E. Kirby, J. C. Wilker, A. R. MacFadden, D. E. Aultz, D. Hoffman, G. C. Helsley, and W. J. Novick. *Arch. Int. Pharmacodyn. Ther.* **227**:142 (1977).

103. H. P. A. Illing and J. M. Fromson. *Drug Metab. Disposition* **6**:510 (1978).

104. R. L. Smith. *Proc. Drug. Res.* **9**:299 (1966).

105. G. L. Plaa. Biliary and Other Routes of Excretion of Drugs. In B. N. Lu Du, H. G. Mandel, and E. L. Way (eds.), *Fundamentals of Drug Metabolism and Drug Disposition*, The Williams and Wilkins Co., Baltimore, 1972, p. 131.

106. R. L. Smith. *The Excretory Function of Bile*, Chapman and Hall, London, 1973.

107. D. E. Rollins and C. D. Klassen. *Clin. Pharmacokin.* **4**:368 (1979).

108. A. J. Levi, Z. Gatmuitan, and I. M. Arias. *J. Clin. Invest.* **48**:2156 (1969).

109. H. Reyes, A. J. Levi, Z. Gatmuitan, and I. M. Arias. *Proc. Natl. Acad. Sci. (Washington)* **64**:168 (1969).

110. R. W. Brauer. *J.A.M.A.* **169**:1462 (1959).

111. L. S. Schanker. Alimentary Canal. In *Handbook of Physiology*, Vol. 5, American Physiological Society, Washington, D.C., 1968, p. 2433.

112. A. G. Clark, P. C. Hirom, P. Millburn, and R. L. Smith. *J. Pharm. Pharmacol.* **23**:150 (1971).

113. P. C. Hirom. Ph.D. Thesis, University of London, 1970.

113. P. C. Hirom, P. Millburn, R. L. Smith, and R. T. Williams. *Biochem. J.* **129**:1071 (1972).

114. B. G. Katzung and F. H. Meyers. *J. Pharmacol. Exp. Ther.* **149**:257 (1965).

115. R. L. Smith. In W. N. Aldridge (ed.), *Mechanisms of Toxicity*, Macmillan, London, 1971, p. 229.

116. L. G. Ladomerg, A. J. Ryan, and S. E. Wright. *J. Pharm. Pharmacol.* **19**:388 (1967).

117. W. A. Colburn, P. C. Hirom, R. J. Parker, and P. Millburn. *Drug Metab. Disposition* **7**:100 (1979).

118. B. E. Dahlström and L. K. Paalzow. *J. Pharmacokin. Biopharm.* **6**:505 (1978).

119. K. S. Pang and J. R. Gillette. *J. Pharmacokin. Biopharm.* **6**:355 (1978).

120. R. M. J. Ings, J. A. McFadzean, and W. E. Ormerod. *Xenobiotica* **5**:223 (1975).

121. R. J. Roberts, S. L. Schriver, and G. L. Plaa. *Biochem. Pharmacol.* **17**:1261 (1968).

122. R. R. Scheline. *J. Pharm. Pharmacol.* **17**:52 (1965).

123. P. Johnson and P. A. Rising. *Xenobiotica* **8**:27 (1978).

124. F. Herrera, D. R. Kemp, M. Tsukamoto, E. R. Woodward, and L. R. Dagstadt. *J. Appl. Physiol.* **25**:207 (1968).

125. J. Meszaros, F. Nimmerfall, J. Rosenthabr, and H. Weber. *Eur. J. Pharmacol.* **32**:233 (1975).

126. F. H. Dost. *Klin. Wochenschr.* **36**:655 (1958).

127. P. K. Wilkinson, A. J. Sedman, E. Sakmar, D. R. Kay, and J. G. Wayner. *J. Pharmacokin. Biopharm.* **5**:207 (1977).

128. S. Lam and W. L. Chiou. *J. Pharmacokin. Biopharm.* **7**:227 (1979).

129. N. P. Chau. *J. Pharmacokin. Biopharm.* **4** (1976).

130. R. Runkel, E. Forchielli, H. Sevelius, M. Chaplin, and E. Segre. *Clin. Pharmacol. Ther.* **15**:261 (1974).

131. M. Kekki, R. J. K. Julkunen, and B. Wahlström. *Naunyn-Schmiedeberg's Arch. Pharmacol.* **297**:61 (1977).

132. P. J. McNamara, J. T. Slattery, M. Gibaldi, and G. Levy. *J. Pharmacokin. Biopharm.* **7**:397 (1979).

133. J. G. Wagner. Nonlinear pharmacokinetics. In *Fundamentals of Clinical Pharmacokinetics*, Drug Intelligence Publications, Inc., Hamilton, 1975, p. 247.

134. W. J. Westlake. The Design and Analysis of Comparative Blood-Level Trials. In J. Swarbrick (ed.), *Current Concepts in the Pharmaceutical Sciences. Dosage Form Design and Bioavailability*, Lea and Febiger, Philadelphia, 1973, p. 149.

135. W. R. Draper and H. Smith. In *Applied Regression Analysis*, John Wiley & Sons, Inc., New York, 1966, p. 1.

136. J. C. K. Loo, M. Rowe, and I. J. McGiliveray. *J. Pharm. Sci.* **64**:1727 (1975).

137. J. F. Nash, L. D. Bechtel, L. R. Lowary, B. E. Rodda, and H. A. Rose. *Drug Dev. Comm.* **1**:443 (1975).

138. J. F. Nash, R. F. Childers, L. R. Lowary, and H. A. Rose. *Drug Dev. Comm.* **1**:459 (1975).

139. J. D. Baggot, T. M. Ladden, and T. E. Powers. *Can. J. Comp. Med.* **40**:310 (1976).

140. S. Cotler, A. Holazo, H. G. Boxembaum, and S. A. Kaplan. *J. Pharm. Sci.* **65**:822 (1976).

141. D. C. Bloedow and W. L. Hayton. *J. Pharm. Sci.* **65**:328 (1976).

142. M. Marvola, M. L. Tuomela, M. Komulainen, M. Inkinen, and J. Pirgola. *Acta Pharm. Suec.* **15**:218 (1978).

143. J. Maeda, H. Takenaka, Y. Yamahira, and T. Noguchi. *J. Pharm. Sci.* **68**:1286 (1979).

144. T. H. Wilson and G. Wiseman. *J. Physiol.* **123**:116 (1954).

145. R. K. Crane and T. H. Wilson. *J. Appl. Physiol.* **12**:145 (1958).

146. S. A. Kaplan and S. Colter. *J. Pharm. Sci.* **61**:1361 (1972).

147. D. M. Matthews and J. L. Bell. *J. Physiol. (London)* **148**:67P (1959).

148. D. Perrier and M. Gibaldi. *J. Pharm. Sci.* **62**:1486 (1973).

149. Z. T. Chowhan and A. A. Amaro. *J. Pharm. Sci.* **66**:1249 (1977).

150. C. Dixon and L. W. Mizen. *J. Physiol.* **269**:549 (1977).

151. K. Miyazaki, O. Oyino, M. Nakano, and T. Arita. *Chem. Pharm. Bull.* **25**:246 (1977).

152. S. C. Penzotti and J. W. Poole. *J. Pharm. Sci.* **63**:1803 (1974).

153. G. Wiseman. *J. Physiol.* **133**:626 (1956).

154. L. S. Schanker and D. J. Tocco. *J. Pharmacol. Exp. Ther.* **128**:115 (1960).

155. R. Reuning and G. Levy. *J. Pharm. Sci.* **57**:1342 (1968).

156. L. Z. Benet, J. M. Orr, R. H. Turner, and H. J. Webb. *J. Pharm. Sci.* **60**:234 (1971).

157. A. J. Aguiar. *Drug. Inform. Bull.* **3**:17 (1969).

158. W. Saski. *J. Pharm. Sci.* **57**:836 (1968).

159. G. Levy and N. J. Angelino. *J. Pharm. Sci.* **57**:1449 (1968).

160. N. Strahl and W. H. Barr. *J. Pharm. Sci.* **60**:278 (1971).

161. S. Feldman and M. Gibaldi. *J. Pharm. Sci.* **58**:967 (1969).

162. S. Feldman, M. Salvino, and M. Gibaldi. *J. Pharm. Sci.* **59**:905 (1970).

163. R. R. Levine and E. W. Pelikan. *J. Pharmacol. Exp. Ther.* **131**:319 (1961).

164. C. H. Nightingale, J. E. Axelson, and M. Gibaldi. *J. Pharm. Sci.* **60**:145 (1971).

165. S. Feldman, M. Salvino, and M. Gibaldi. *J. Pharm. Sci.* **59**:705 (1970).

166. L. S. Schanker, D. J. Tocco, B. B. Brodie, and C. A. M. Hogben. *J. Pharmacol. Exp. Ther.* **123**:81 (1958).

167. T. Koizami, T. Areta, and K. Kakemi. *Chem. Pharm. Bull.* **12**:421 (1964).

168. A. Tsuji, E. Nakashima, T. Asano, R. Nakashima, and T. Yamana, *J. Pharm. Pharmacol.* **31**:718 (1979).

169. W. H. Barr and S. Riegelman, *J. Pharm. Sci.* **59**:164 (1970).

170. P. V. Kasture, S. S. Didolkar, and K. Dorle. *Ind. J. Phar.* **35**:18 (1973).

171. L. Thiry. *S.B. Akad. Wiss Wien. (Mathem.-Naturw. Cl 1)* **50**:77 (1864).

172. L. Vella. *Thiere* **13**:40 (1888).

173. J. Markowitz, J. Archibald, and H. G. Downie. In *Experimental Surgery*, 5th ed., Williams and Wilkins, Baltimore, 1964, p. 143.

174. J. G. Wagner and E. Nelson. *J. Pharm. Sci.* **52**:610 (1963).

175. D. C. Taylor, R. U. Grundy, and B. E. Loveday. *J. Pharm. Pharmacol.* **29**:51P (1977).

176. R. G. Sample, G. V. Rossi, and E. W. Packman. *J. Pharm. Sci.* **57**:795 (1968).

177. E. J. Mroszczak and S. Riegelman. *J. Pharmacokin. Biopharm.* **3**:303 (1975).

CHAPTER 3

In-Vitro Drug Product Dissolution Testing: Correlation of Results to In-Vivo Drug Bioavailability Parameters

BERNARD E. CABANA

Division of Biopharmaceutics
Food and Drug Administration
Rockville, Maryland

CONTENTS

Although dissolution rate testing was initially conceived in the early 1960s and adopted in USP XVIII in 1970 as a tool to assure product quality and uniformity, it has since taken on new significance. As a result of research on digoxin and other drugs, dissolution testing has been demonstrated as a tool for both assuring bioequivalence among generic drug products and identifying drug formulations which, because of their pH dependence, place certain patient populations at risk.

1. BIOEQUIVALENCE REQUIREMENTS

In 1977 the Food and Drug Administration (FDA) published two separate regulations dealing with issues of drug bioequivalence of multisource generic drug products and drug bioavailability involving new drug entities (1). Bioequivalence requirements may be established for any drug that meets certain criteria, as listed below:

1. Documented therapeutic failure.
2. Documented bioinequivalence.
3. Narrow therapeutic ratio.
4. Medical determination of serious adverse effect in the treatment or prevention of a serious disease or condition.
5. Physicochemical evidence:
   a. Low solubility.
   b. Poor dissolution rate.
   c. Particle size/surface area.
   d. Physical structural characteristics (e.g., polymorphic forms).
   e. High ratio of excipients to active drug.
6. Pharmacokinetic evidence:
   a. Localized absorption.
   b. Inherently poor absorption.
   c. First-pass metabolism.
   d. Rapid drug clearance.
   e. Drug instability in GI tract.
   f. Dose-dependent kinetics.

Bioequivalence requirements may consist of either in-vivo studies in humans or animals or in-vitro tests. Drugs meeting the first three criteria require in-vivo bioavailability testing to satisfy the bioequivalence requirement, unless an in-vitro bioequivalence standard (based on in-vitro/in-vivo correlative data) is established.

The FDA bioavailability/bioequivalency regulations rely on in-vitro dissolution rate studies to assure lot-to-lot bioequivalence. The necessity for this approach stems from three sources. First, a brief review of the literature and NDA files in the fall of 1973 revealed that poor dissolution accounted for about 80–90% of documented bioinequivalence. Second, experience with certified antibiotics (e.g., oxytetracycline and tetracycline) revealed that a single bioavailability study could not assure lot-to-lot bioequivalence; rather, discriminating dissolution standards must be established. For example, poor bioavailability of certain tetracycline hydrochloride products was associated with poor dissolution rate performance (2). Third, in-vitro/in-vivo correlations have been obtained for many drugs with potential bioequivalence problems. It has been observed that poorly dissolving solid oral dosage forms are generally associated with poor bioavailability.

Dissolution tests must be discriminatory and reproducible. In-vitro/in-vivo correlations can usually be achieved from such tests if the proper dissolution medium (e.g., water, acid, or buffer) is selected and the degree of agitation is sufficiently mild to permit discrimination among drug products and among lots.

2. IN-VITRO/IN-VIVO CORRELATIONS FOR SPECIFIC DRUGS

Before specific examples of in-vitro/in-vivo correlations are discussed, it should be noted that there are two correlations upon which the FDA relies to establish in-vitro bioequivalence standards. The first type concerns the statistical correlations of in-vivo parameters (e.g., peak plasma concentration, area under the plasma level-time curve) versus dissolution rate. The second type deals with an association of in-vivo data with a minimum dissolution rate. An example of the latter is the findings of Slywka et al. (3), who demonstrated that all sulfisoxazole products that passed the USP dissolution specification were bioequivalent, even though no statistical correlation was shown with any in-vivo parameters.

2.1 Prednisone

Dissolution studies for 10 lots of 5 mg prednisone tablets, using the USP rotating basket method, are shown in Figure 1. The dissolution rates of the

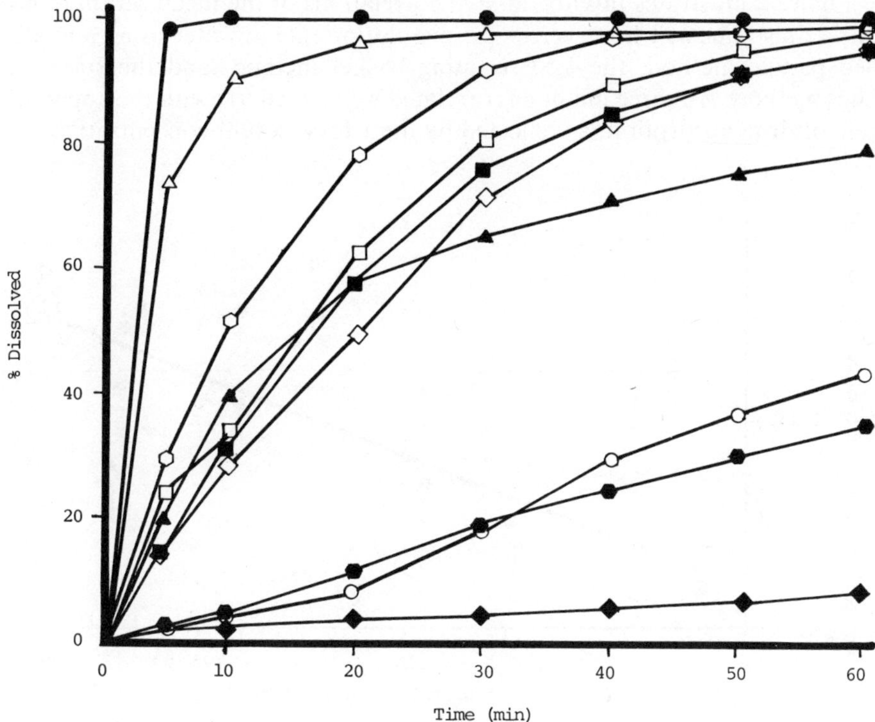

Figure 1. Dissolution profiles for 10 lots of prednisone 5 mg tablets in the USP rotating basket.

tablets varied widely, ranging from less than 10% at 1 hour for the Danbury product to 100% at 10 minutes for the Schering product. On the basis of these findings, it was anticipated that bioavailability differences would exist among these drug products. Bioavailability and dissolution studies were undertaken using the Schering or Upjohn products as a reference standard in randomized three- or four-way crossover studies. A completed report of the studies, including a novel approach to in-vitro/in-vivo correlation, was published by Wagner et al. (4, 5).

Despite the wide differences in dissolution rate profiles among the prednisone tablets, no significant variations were noted in the total area of the serum level-time curves. However, a significant difference in "apparent" rate of drug absorption was found, as reflected by the half-time to reach peak concentration. The "apparent" rate of drug absorption, as well as differences in variances associated with each drug product, were directly correlated to the dissolution rates obtained by the spinning filter method of dissolution testing (6). (See Chapter 5 for a discussion of dissolution testing methods.)

Figure 2 illustrates in-vitro/in-vivo correlations of the mean serum levels of prednisolone at 1 hour versus the dissolution rate in water using a modified paddle method, the USP rotating basket method, and the spinning filter method. All three methods correlated well ($p < 0.01$) with the apparent rate of drug absorption, as reflected by the 1-hour serum concentrations of

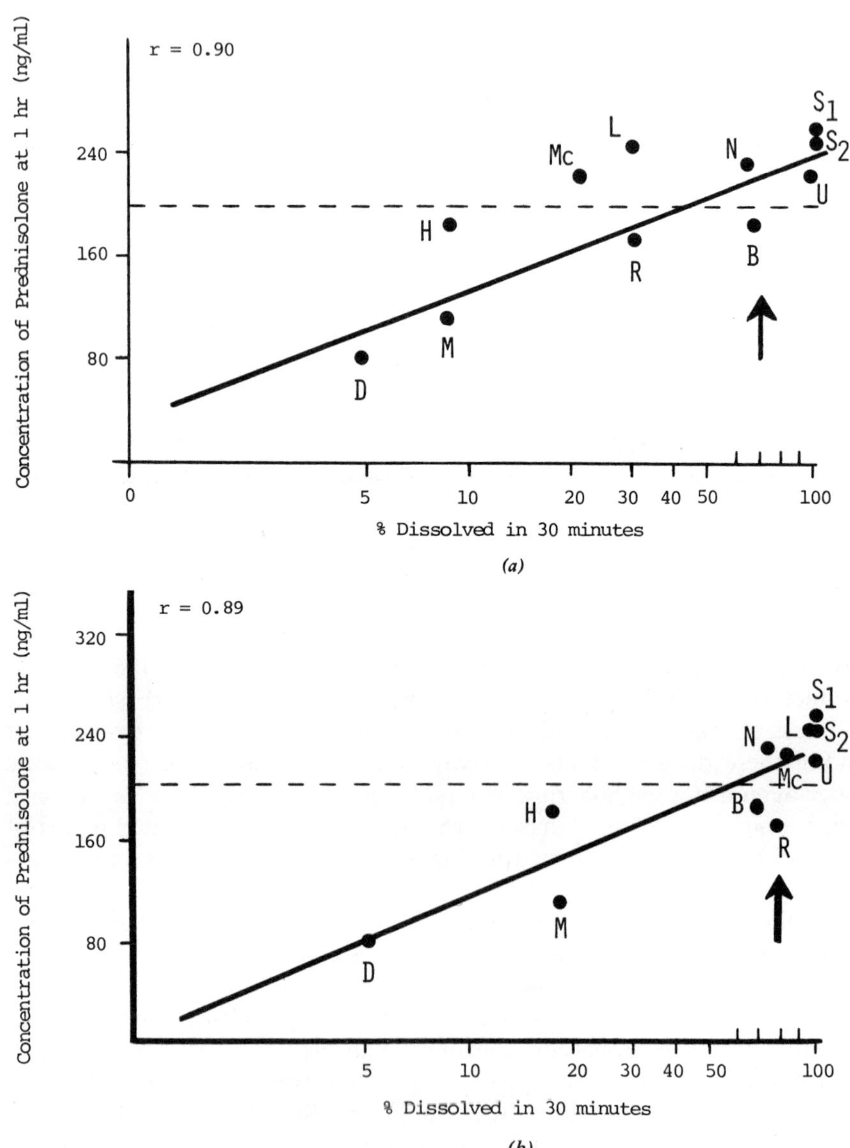

(a)

(b)

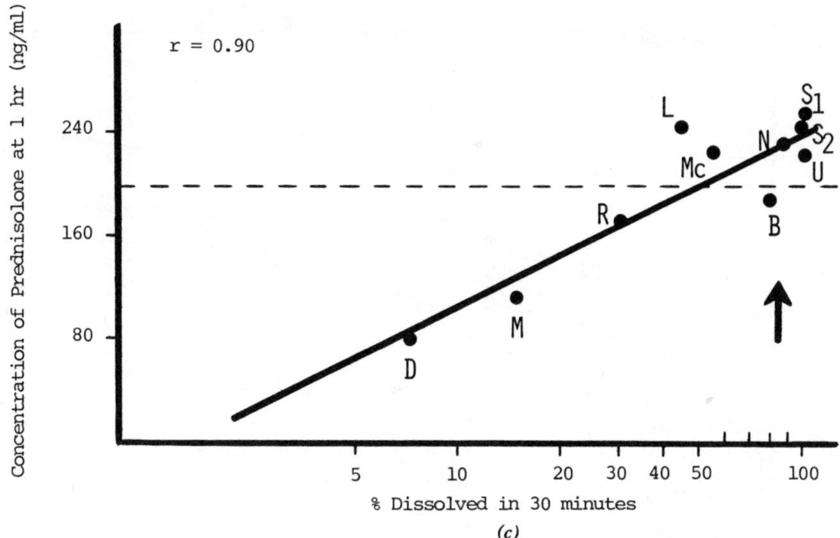

Figure 2. In-vitro/in-vivo correlation of prednisolone tablets for three different dissolution procedures. (*a*) Paddle method (1000 ml H_2O, 50 rpm, 37°C). (*b*) USP rotating basket method (900 ml H_2O, 100 rpm, 37°C). (*c*) Spinning filter method (1000 ml H_2O, 400 rpm, 37°C).

prednisolone. (The 1-hour serum level was chosen as a parameter because it corresponds closely to the peak concentration obtained with the Schering reference product, but nevertheless occurs during the absorptive phase of the drug.)

As shown in Figure 2*b*, the USP rotating basket method failed to discriminate certain poorly bioavailable products (e.g., Rexall's product, when run in 900 ml of water). The USP method does not appear to discriminate as well as the paddle method or the spinning filter method (Figure 2*a* and *c*). However, similar dissolution rate specifications would be required by the three methods to assure bioequivalency—that is, 80% dissolved in 30 minutes.

2.2 Digitoxin

Six lots of 0.1 and 0.2 mg digitoxin tablets from various manufacturers were tested using the USP dissolution test described for digoxin (7). The results are shown in Figure 3. Both the rate and extent of dissolution vary widely among these products. It is particularly noteworthy that several products failed to totally dissolve even after 2 hours of testing. On that basis alone, one could anticipate differences in bioavailability. (All of these products were selected prior to inclusion of the dissolution rate specification for digitoxin in USP XIX first supplement in 1975.)

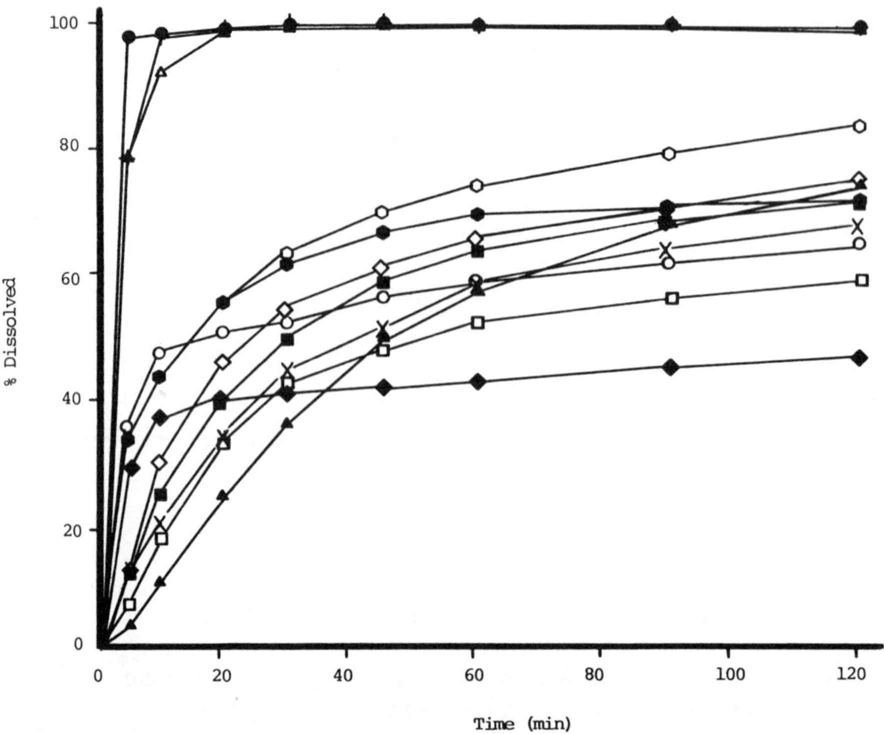

Figure 3. Dissolution profiles for six 0.1 mg and six 0.2 mg digitoxin tablets in the USP rotating basket.

The bioavailability studies revealed that rapidly dissolving digitoxin products (e.g., Parke-Davis and Wyeth) could achieve the same rate and extent of absorption as a digitoxin solution (Figure 4). The studies further disclosed that the rate of absorption, peak concentration, and total bioavailability were directly related to the dissolution rate using either the USP basket or paddle method.

Figures 5 and 6 show the peak plasma digitoxin concentrations and the percent bioavailability, respectively, versus the percent of drug dissolved in 30 and 60 minutes using the USP rotating basket. By inspection, it can be seen that slowly dissolving digitoxin products failed to achieve adequate peak serum levels relative to the standard. Peak concentrations of 6 ng/ml were generally achieved with drug products that dissolved less than 60% in 30 minutes, whereas products that dissolved greater than 85% in 30 minutes achieved peak concentration of 10–12 ng/ml. Products dissolving less than 60% in 30 minutes and 85% in 1 hour were usually less than 80% bioavailable

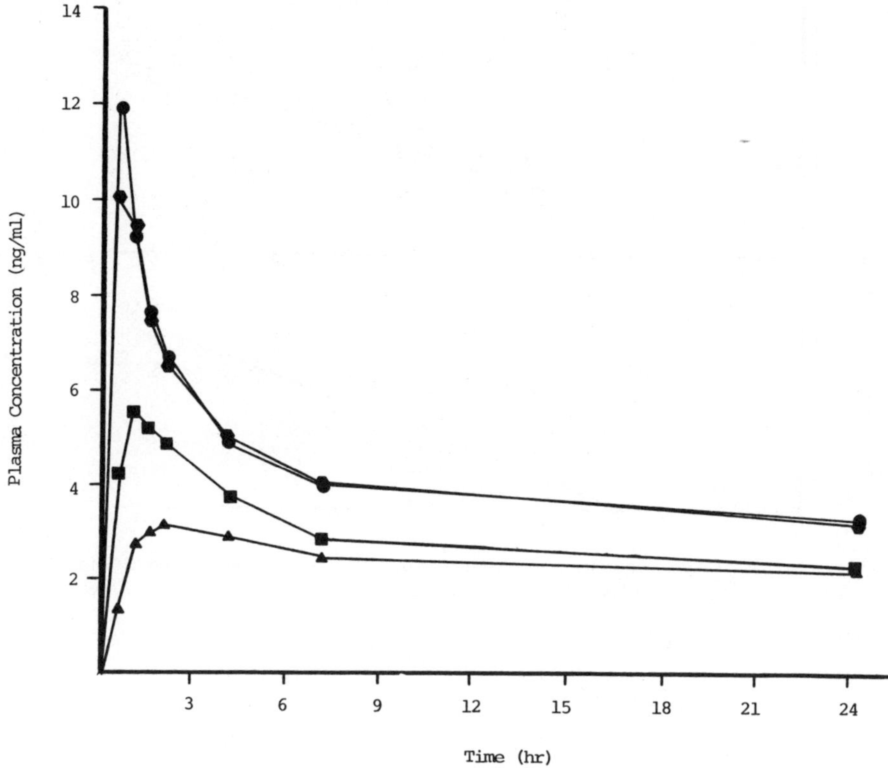

Figure 4. Bioavailability profiles for three digitoxin tablets, as compared with a solution. (●): solution; (⬣): 0.2 mg Wyeth tablet; (▲): 0.2 mg Kasco-Afco tablet; (■): 0.2 mg Rondex tablet.

relative to the reference standard. Digitoxin products dissolving less than 50% in 30 minutes were associated with 60% bioavailability relative to the reference standard (Figure 6).

On the basis of the bioavailability findings, the FDA imposed a dual dissolution requirement on digitoxin products: not less than 60% dissolved at 30 minutes and not less than 85% dissolved at 60 minutes. The initial points were deemed necessary to assure total bioavailability. The latter specification was required because several digitoxin drug products failed to dissolve totally, even after 2 hours of testing.

To further substantiate the findings, six additional lots of digitoxin tablets were selected, based on the new dissolution specification. These lots were chosen for bioavailability studies to be performed since they were borderline of 60% dissolved at 30 minutes but failed to meet the upper limit of 85% at

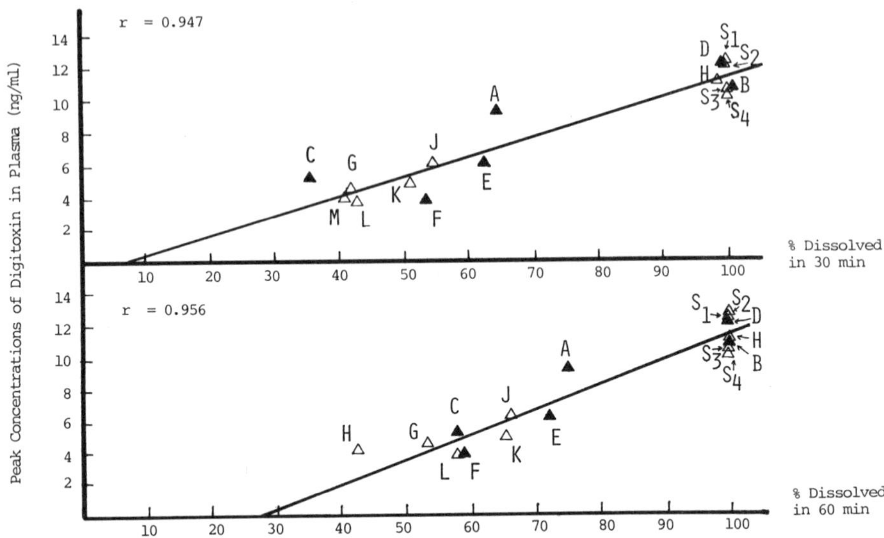

Figure 5. In-vitro/in-vivo correlation for digitoxin tablets. Dissolution tests performed in the USP rotating basket with 500 ml 0.6% HCl, 120 rpm, 37°C. (△): 0.1 mg tablets; (▲): 0.2 mg tablets.

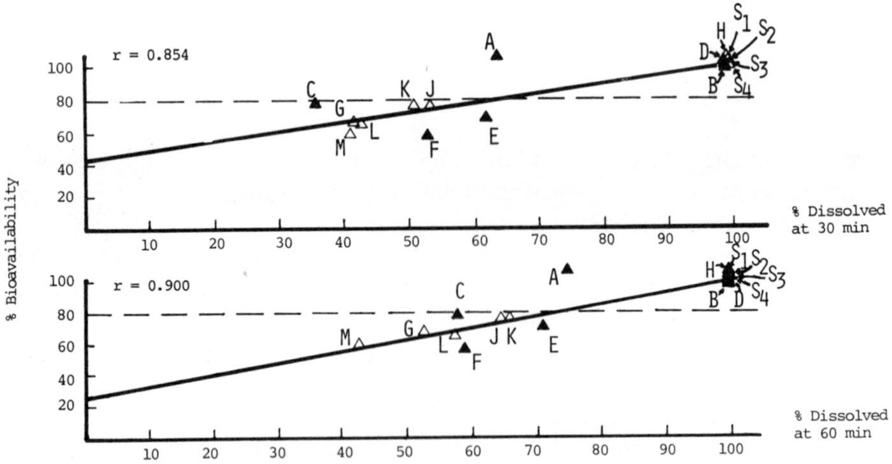

Figure 6. In-vitro/in-vivo correlation for digitoxin tablets. Dissolution tests performed in the USP rotating basket with 500 ml 0.6% HCl, 120 rpm, 37°C. (△): 0.1 mg tablets; (▲): 0.2 mg tablets.

1 hour. When these products were tested, an excellent correlation was obtained with the peak concentrations (C_{max}) (Figure 7). A few of these products, nevertheless, were bioequivalent in terms of extent of absorption (Figure 8).

Digitoxin products dissolving less than 80% in 1 hour are associated with a failure rate of greater than 25%; that is, more than 25% of subjects tested failed to achieve an acceptable level of absorption relative to the oral solution. Employing such correlative data, the FDA developed a statistical approach that allows computation of the probability of accepting a poor product (PA) and rejecting a good product (PR) based on the individual tablet dissolution and bioavailability data. Accepting the USP dissolution specification of 60% at 30 minutes and 85% at 1 hour, and given an acceptable relative bioavailability level of 75%, the probabilities of accepting a poor product and reject-

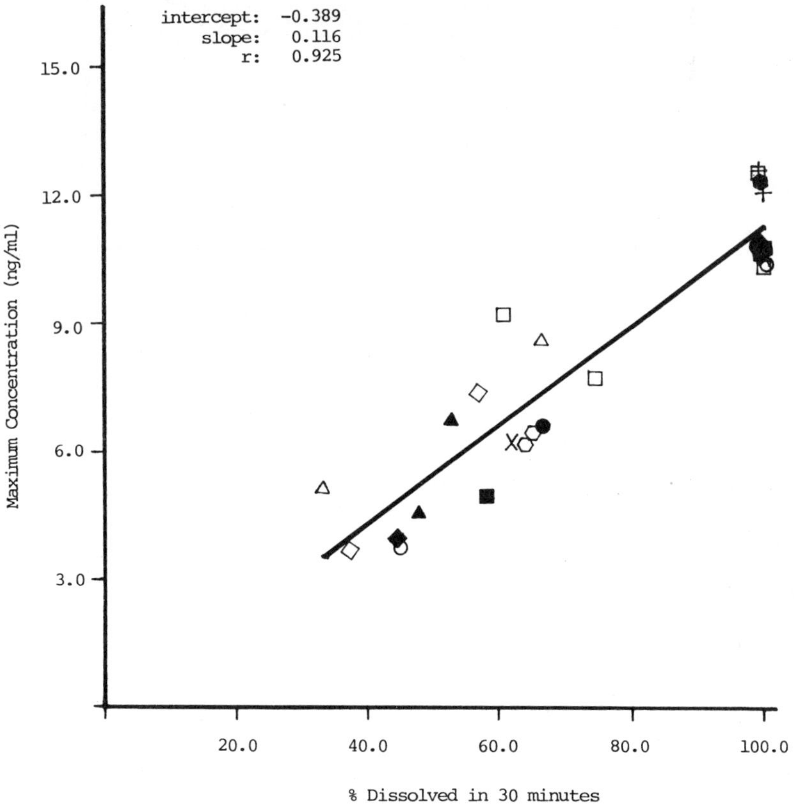

Figure 7. In-vitro/in-vivo correlations for 0.1 and 0.2 mg digitoxin tablets. Dissolution tests performed in the USP rotating basket, 500 ml 0.6% HCl, 120 rpm, 37°C.

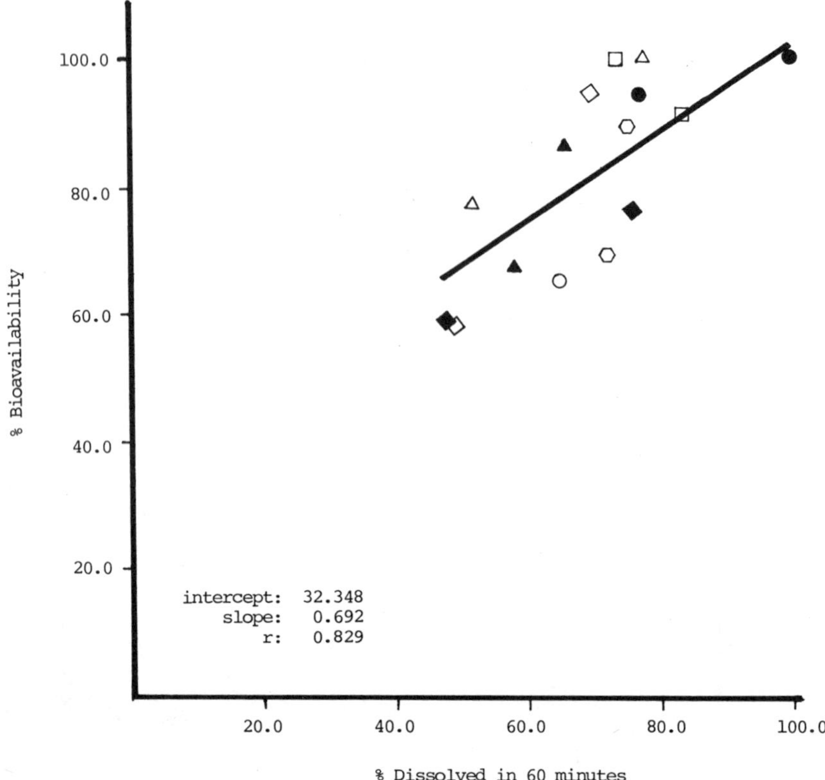

Figure 8. In-vitro/in-vivo correlation of 0.1 and 0.2 mg digitoxin tablets. Dissolution tests performed in the USP rotating basket with 500 ml 0.6% HCl, 120 rpm, and 37°C.

ing a good product based on these specifications are PA = 0.04 and PR = 0.10. The FDA is currently refining these statistical techniques by varying the decision rule so as to minimize the total risk involved in setting dissolution standards. Products dissolving less than 60% in 1 hour are associated with failure rates of greater than 50%, and at times nearly approaching 80–90%.

2.3 Tetracycline Hydrochloride

The importance of dissolution medium selection and degree of agitation in the development of an in-vitro bioequivalence standard cannot be overlooked. This is best illustrated by findings on tetracycline hydrochloride capsules and tablets (8, 9). Preliminary dissolution rate studies of tetracycline hydrochloride capsules performed in water and in pH 6.0 buffer, using a three-blade paddle method, indicated significant differences in dissolution rate profiles. Similarly, in-vitro studies involving 25 brands of tetracycline hydrochloride 250 mg capsules, using the rotating basket, revealed large differences in dissolution rate profiles, ranging between 7 and 100% at 30 minutes (Figure 9). Using the rotating basket at 50 rpm, with water as the dissolution medium, four of the products dissolved less than 40% in 30 minutes and were anticipated to be bioinequivalent relative to the reference standard. In reality, only one of these products failed to be bioavailable and, therefore, no correlation could be established.

The conditions initially employed (i.e., USP rotating basket at 50 rpm) tend to overdiscriminate among the products. Subsequent dissolution using the spinning filter at 300 rpm (a condition resulting in slightly greater agitation) showed that, with the exception of one product, all products dissolved greater than 50% at 30 minutes and 75% at 60 minutes. Even in the absence of a statistical correlation, one could utilize these findings to establish a

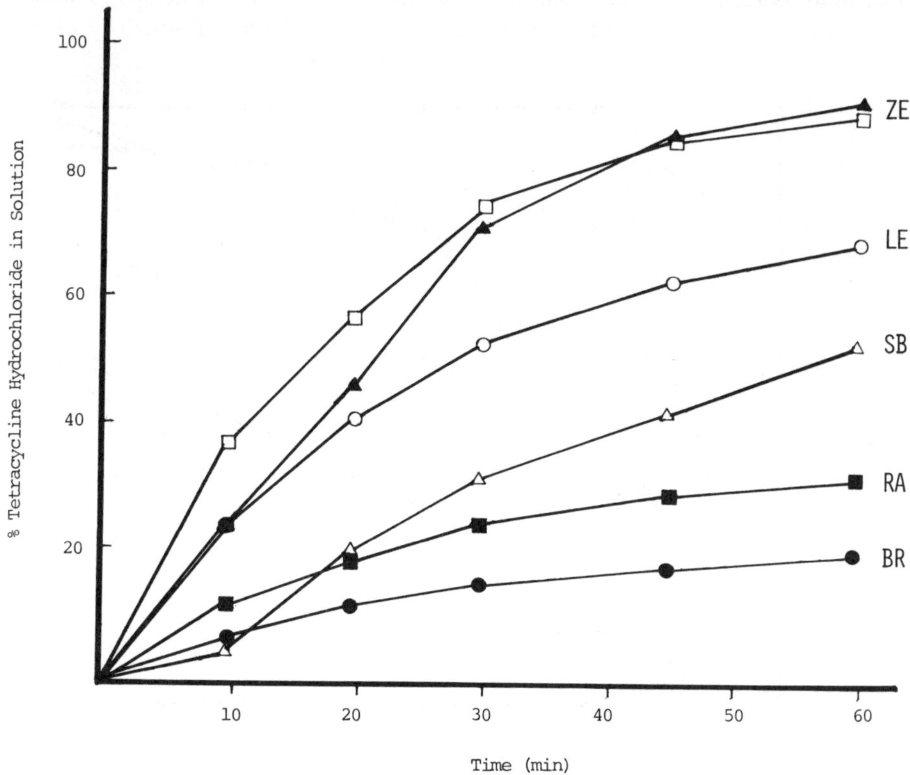

Figure 9. Dissolution profiles of 500 mg tetracycline hydrochloride capsules in the USP rotating basket with distilled water, 50 rpm, and 37°C.

dissolution specification for tetracycline hydrochloride capsules since all bioavailable products dissolved greater than 75% in 60 minutes.

2.4 Phenytoin Sodium

In-vitro/in-vivo correlations have been obtained with several medicinally important drugs. Phenytoin sodium in capsule form is perhaps one of the most critical drugs currently under study. Figure 10 illustrates the dissolution profile of phenytoin sodium products that underwent bioavailability testing (10, 11). It can be readily seen that the dissolution profiles of these products, using the USP rotating basket method, differ significantly in terms of both rate and extent of dissolution, with 3 products dissolving only approximately 60% in 1 hour.

The differences in dissolution profiles of phenytoin products manifests itself in a significant variation in rate but not extent of bioavailability. An excellent correlation was obtained relating the time to peak (t_{max}) and peak levels (C_{max}) to dissolution rate at 30 and 60 minutes (Figures 11 and

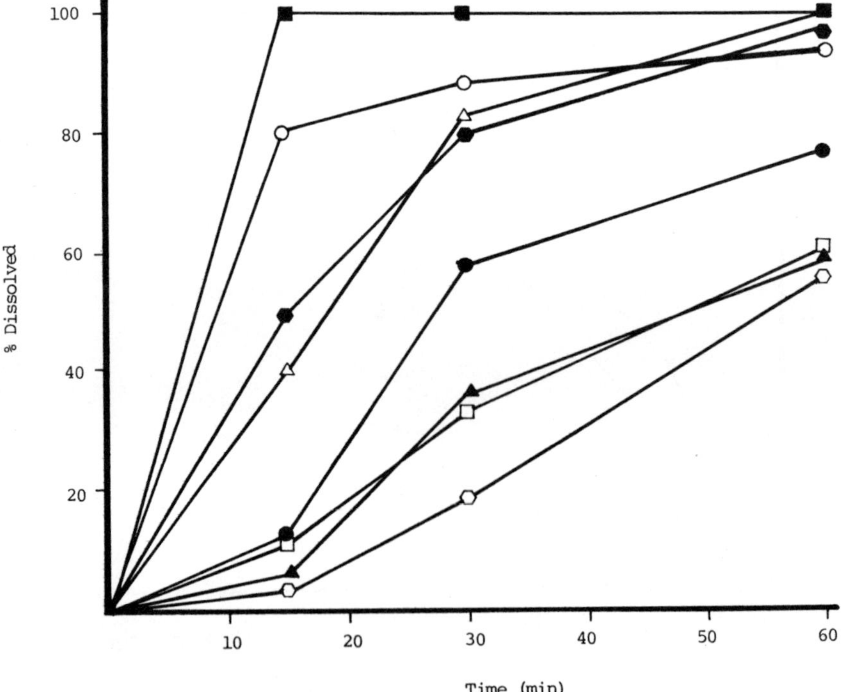

Figure 10. Dissolution profiles of phenytoin sodium capsules in the USP rotating basket.

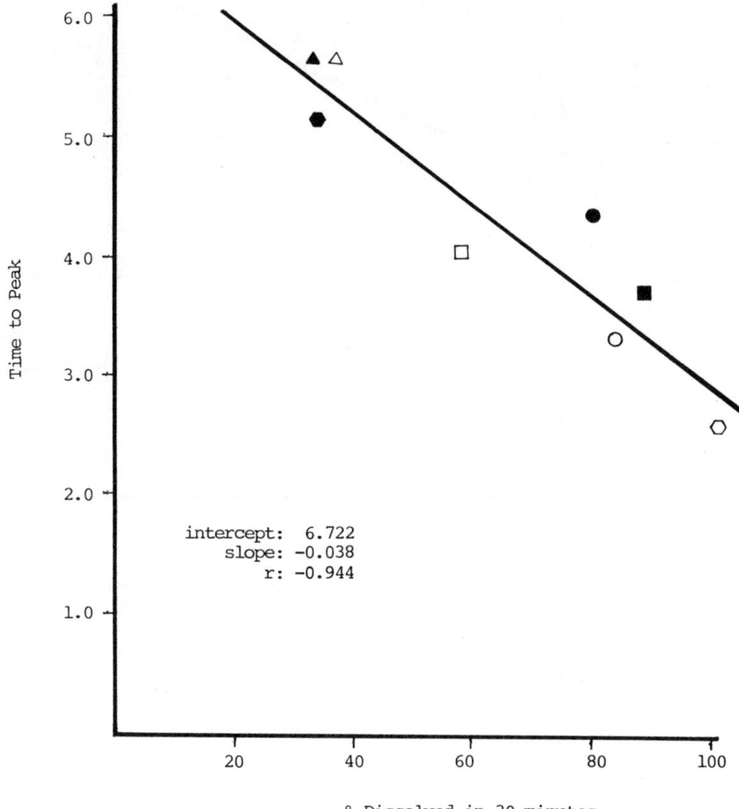

Figure 11. In-vitro/in-vivo correlation of t_{max} versus percentage dissolved in 30 minutes for 100 mg phenytoin sodium capsules. Dissolution tests performed in the USP rotating basket.

12). A similar correlation was also obtained using the spinning filter method at 300 rpm (Figures 13 and 14). The paddle method failed to perform as well with this drug.

2.5 Aminophylline

The FDA's dissolution approach is not limited to immediate release dosage forms, but has been applied to slow release dosage forms of phenytoin, controlled release dosage forms of papaverine, and enteric coated preparations of aminophylline.

Figure 15 illustrates the use of a dissolution rate test for aminophylline and its enteric coated products (12). It can be observed that the plain amino-

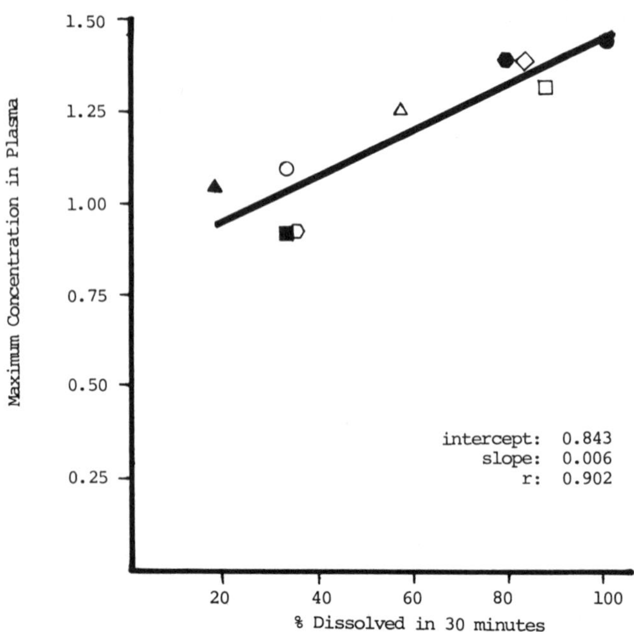

Figure 12. In-vitro/in-vivo correlation of C_{max} versus percentage dissolved in 30 minutes for 100 mg phenytoin sodium capsules. Dissolution tests performed in the USP rotating basket.

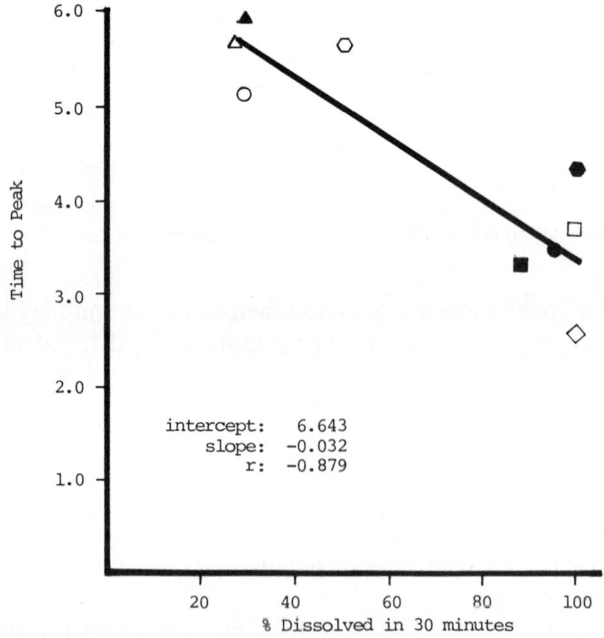

Figure 13. In-vitro/in-vivo correlation of t_{max} versus percentage dissolved in 30 minutes for 100 mg phenytoin sodium capsules. Dissolution tests performed by the spinning filter method.

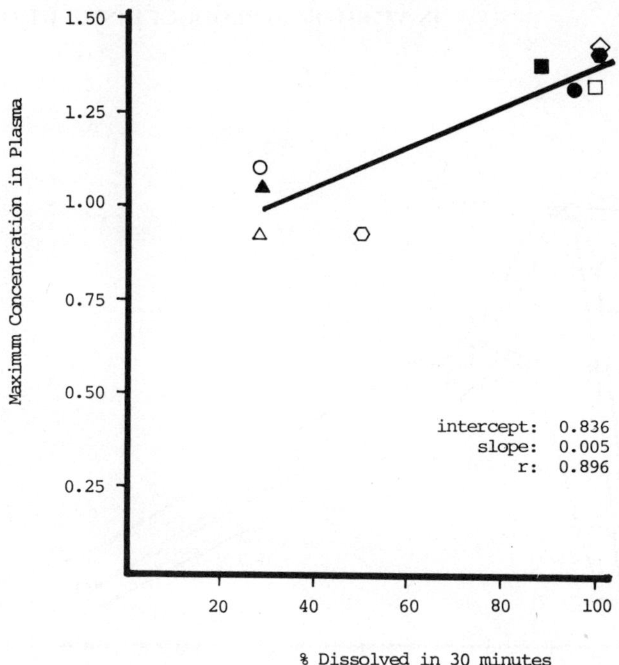

Figure 14. In-vitro/in-vivo correlation of C_{max} versus percentage dissolved in 30 minutes for 100 mg phenytoin sodium capsules. Dissolution tests performed by the spinning filter method.

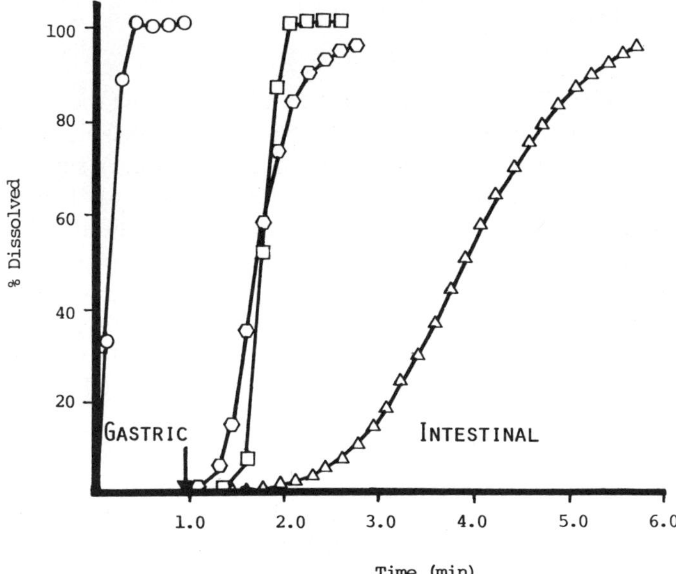

Figure 15. Dissolution profile of aminophylline uncoated (○) and enteric coated (□, ⬡, △) tablets.

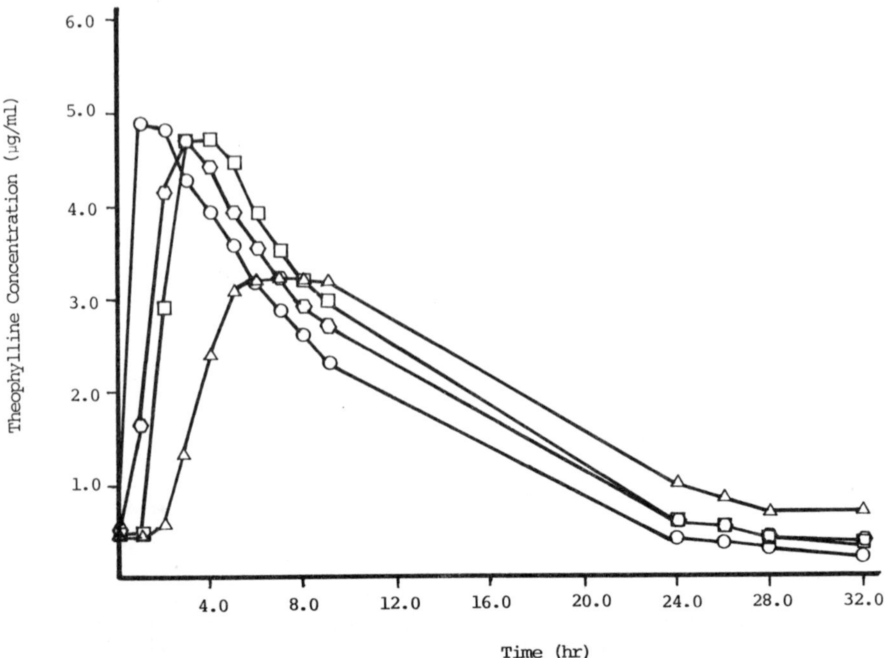

Figure 16. Bioavailability profile of aminophylline uncoated (○) and enteric coated (□, ⬡, △) tablets.

phylline tablet readily dissolves in gastric juice, but that the enteric coated products require simulated intestinal fluid (pH 7.2) for dissolution. One such product requires 5–6 hours to achieve total dissolution. A similar bioavailability profile is obtained with these products (Figure 16). The two enteric products that readily dissolved in simulated intestinal fluid achieved peak levels similar to the plain aminophylline, but the time to peak was shifted about 1–2 hours. However, the slowly dissolving enteric product achieved significantly lower levels at 5–8 hours after oral administration. From such data, it may be possible to arrive at a dissolution standard for aminophylline products that assures product performance and lot-to-lot bioequivalence.

2.6 Papaverine Hydrochloride

The use of different solvent media in dissolution testing often allows anomalies to surface. This is best illustrated by findings on papaverine hydrochloride using the NF XIV rotating bottle method, which calls for a change in pH conditions over a 7-hour period (Figure 17). Regardless of the total dissolution rate achieved by individual products, the bulk of the dissolution

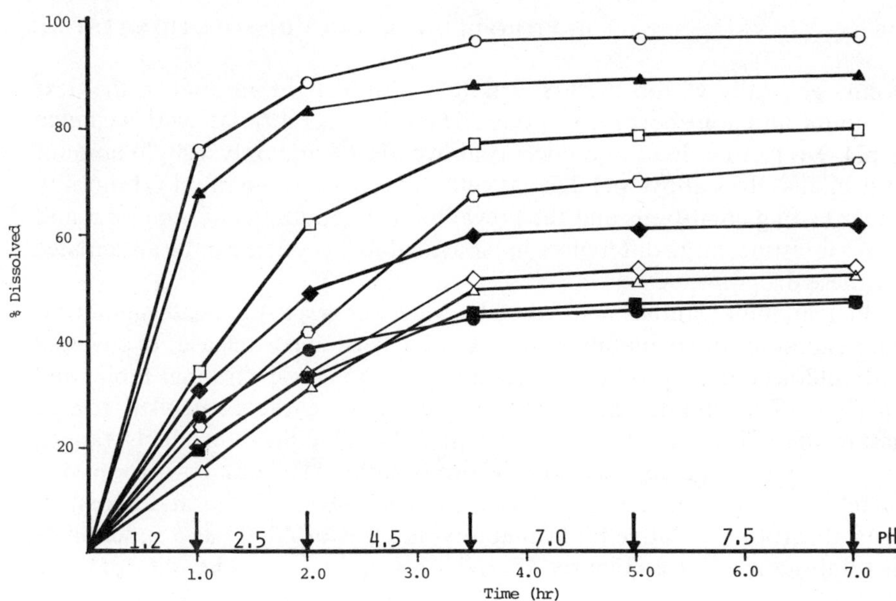

Figure 17. Dissolution profile of papaverine hydrochloride 150 mg sustained release capsules and tablets utilizing the NF XIV rotating bottle method.

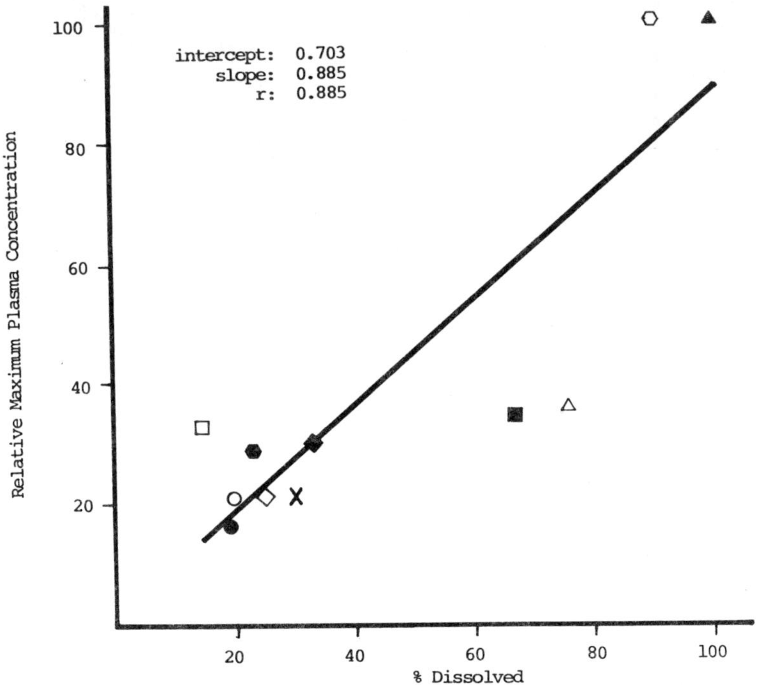

Figure 18. In-vitro/in-vivo correlation of C_{max} versus percentage dissolved in pH 1.2 dissolution medium for papaverine HCl.

occurs generally within the first 2 hours, with a slight amount in the next 1.5 hours, and none beyond 3.5 hours. These findings correlate with a change in pH. No further dissolution occurs above pH 4.5 and only a slight amount of drug dissolves above pH 2.5. Therefore, because of the rapid GI motility under fasting conditions and the prevailing pH conditions of the upper and lower intestine, large differences in bioavailability profiles can be anticipated for these drug products.

Bioavailability studies performed by Meyer et al. (13) indicate significant differences in bioavailability among nine sustained release papaverine hydrochloride drug products when compared to a conventional tablet and an elixir. The findings also failed to substantiate the controlled release nature of such drug products. Bioavailabilities of these products ranged from 19 to 64% in comparison to the oral solution. The best in-vitro/in-vivo correlation was obtained by relating the peak levels (C_{max}) and extent of drug absorption (relative bioavailability in terms of AUC) as a function of dissolution at pH 1.2 (Figures 18 and 19, respectively). The data indicate

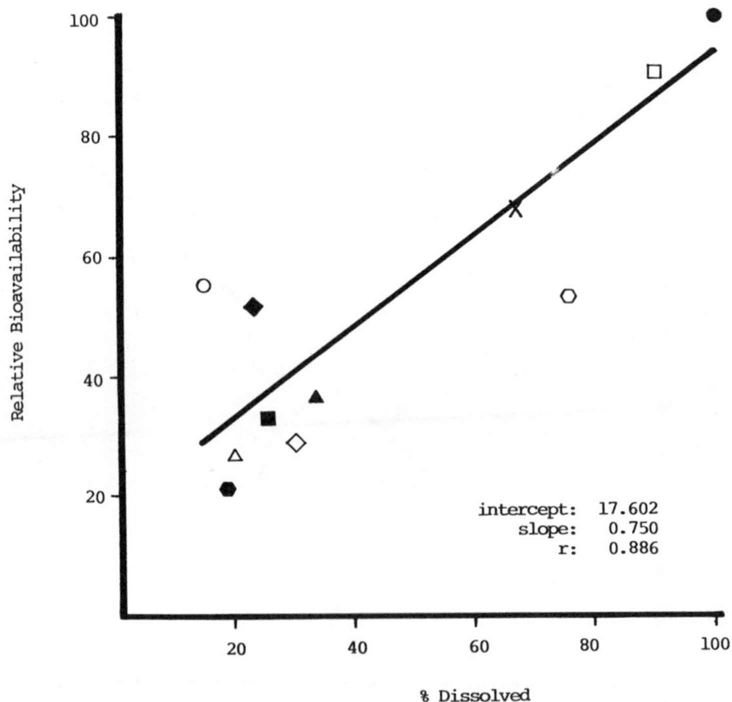

Figure 19. In-vitro/in-vivo correlation of relative bioavailability (in terms of AUC) versus percentage dissolved in pH 1.2 dissolution medium for papaverine HCl.

that the relative bioavailability of papaverine hydrochloride products is directly related to dissolution obtained during the first hour at gastric pH, and the correlation progressively worsens as the pH of the dissolution medium increases.

REFERENCES

1. Bioavailability and bioequivalence requirements. *Fed. Regist.* Part 320, **42**(5):1624 (January 7, 1977).
2. K. A. DeSante, A. R. DiSanto, D. J. Chodos, and R. G. Stoll. Antibiotic batch certification and bioequivalence. *JAMA* **232**:1349 (1975).
3. G. W. A. Slywka, A. P. Melikian, A. B. Straughn, P. L. Whyatt, and M. C. Meyer. Bioavailability of 11 sulfisoxazole products in humans. *J. Pharm. Sci.* **65**:1494 (1976).
4. T. J. Sullivan, E. Sakmar, K. S. Albert, D. C. Blair, and J. G. Wagner. In-vitro and in-vivo availability of commercial prednisone tablets. *J. Pharm. Sci.* **64**(10):1723 (1975).
5. T. J. Sullivan, E. Sakmar, and J. G. Wagner. Comparative bioavailability: A new type of in-vitro/in-vivo correlation exemplified by prednisone. *J. Pharmacok. Biopharm.* **4**(2):173 (1976).
6. V. K. Prasad, J. P. Hunt, B. E. Cabana, and J. G. Wagner. Establishment of Bioequivalency of 5 mg Prednisone and Prednisolone Tablets—Revised In-Vitro Dissolution Specification. Presented at the APhA Academy of Pharmaceutical Sciences 23rd Meeting, Phoenix, 14 November 1977.
7. J. H. Wood. Bioequivalency Establishment of Marketed Digitoxin Products. Presented at APhA Academy of Pharmaceutical Sciences 23rd Meeting, Phoenix, 16 November 1977.
8. V. P. Shah, J. Hunt, V. K. Prasad, and B. E. Cabana. In-Vitro/In-Vivo Correlation of Tetracycline Hydrochloride Capsules—Part II. Bioequivalence Establishment. Presented at APhA Academy of Pharmaceutical Sciences 22nd Meeting, New York, 18 May 1977.
9. S. V. Dighe, B. E. Cabana, and V. K. Prasad. In-Vitro/In-Vivo Correlation of Tetracycline Hydrochloride Tablets and Capsules—Part III. Bioequivalence Establishment. Presented at APhA Academy of Pharmaceutical Sciences 22nd Meeting, New York, 18 May 1977.
10. A. P. Melikian, A. B. Straughn, G. W. A. Slywka, P. L. Whyatt, and M. C. Meyer. Bioavailability of 11 Phenytoin products. *J. Pharmacokin. Biopharm.* **5**:133 (1977).
11. V. P. Shah, V. K. Prasad, T. Alston, B. E. Cabana, R. P. Gural, and M. C. Meyer. Phenytoin, Part I: In-vitro/in-vivo correlations for 100 mg sodium phenytoin capsules. *J. Pharm. Sci.* (in press).
12. R. A. Upton, J. F. Thurcelin, J. R. Powell Jr., L. Sansom, T. W. Guentert, P. E. Coates, P. Ravencroft, V. P. Shah, B. E. Cabana, and S. Riegelman. Absorption From Some Commercial Sustained and Enteric Release Preparations of Theophylline. Presented at the APhA Academy of Pharmaceutical Sciences 24th Meeting, Montreal, 14–20 May 1978.
13. W. H. Pitlick, B. E. Cabana, and M. C. Meyer. Absorption Kinetics and Bioavailability of 9 Sustained-Release Papaverine Products. Presented at the American Pharmaceutical Association Meeting, Kansas City, November 1979.

CHAPTER 4

Computational Conversion of In-Vitro Drug Dissolution Data Into In-Vivo Drug Response Versus Time Profiles

DANIEL B. TUEY

PharmaControl Corporation
Englewood Cliffs, New Jersey

CONTENTS

An ideal in-vitro dissolution test procedure is one providing data that is predictive of the performance of an oral dosage form when administered to human subjects. This biorelevance criteria is commonly addressed through attempts to identify some dependent parameter of the in-vitro test (such as the amount of drug dissolved within a specified time interval or the time to dissolve a specified amount) that correlates with one or more in-vivo characteristics (such as the peak or time-to-peak blood level, the area under the blood concentration versus time curve, the maximum excretion rate, or the amount of drug excreted in a specified time interval). Such univariate, single-point correlations of in-vitro drug dissolution behavior with in-vivo bioavailability parameters are arbitrarily and heuristically determined, and are frequently the result of fortuitous observation.

Single-point representations can obscure much of the information otherwise available from dissolution and blood level or excretion versus time profiles. An optimal test procedure would provide predictive descriptions of the entire time course of a drug product's in-vivo behavior from its in-vitro dissolution profile. An innovative, apparatus-based BioPredictor® method that attains this goal is described in a subsequent chapter. The topic of this chapter is a method utilizing a mathematical transform analog of the convolution integral representation of linear system response.

Linear systems analysis and numerical convolution-deconvolution methods have been described by several authors (1–5). Previous approaches, however, relied on the use of either explicit analytic solution representations of *a priori* (e.g., drug specific) model functions, classical time-domain algorithms, or expensive special-purpose computer devices. The transform technique described here was developed as a user-friendly, interactive, general purpose computer software package, which can be run on inexpensive microcomputers and provides for the desired computational conversion of in-vitro drug dissolution data into predicted in-vivo drug response versus time profiles (6).

In the following sections we first review the theoretical basis and mathematical assumptions of the transform algorithm as applied to physical systems. We then describe the computational restrictions necessary to obtain an operational procedure. Finally, we outline the computational steps involved in numerically converting in-vitro dissolution data into predicted in-vivo bioavailability profiles. Following this, two examples are presented. The chapter concludes with an outline of some additional applications of this methodology.

1. THEORETICAL BASIS

The response $Q_B(t)$ of a linear, time-invariant system $G(t)$ to an input $Q_D(t)$ can be expressed by the convolution integral

$$Q_B(t) = \int_0^t G(t-T)Q_D(T)dT \tag{1}$$

The expression $G(t-T)$ denotes the impulse response of the system and indicates that it is time-invariant; that is, it is a function only of the elapsed time of observation since the occurrence of the pulse. Thus, the shape of the response to an input applied at any instant depends only on the shape of the input, and not on the time of application. Equation 1 can be interpreted as the limiting case ($\Delta T \rightarrow 0$) of a summation of the system's response to a succession of pulses, the envelop of which comprises $Q_D(t)$. If $Q_D(T)$ is the magnitude of the pulse at time T, and ΔT is its duration, the discrete version of equation 1 is

$$Q_B(t) = \sum_{T=0}^{t} G(t-T)Q_D(T)\Delta T \tag{2}$$

The important observation is that once the impulse response of the system has been determined, the response to an arbitrary input is also known.

The present application of linear systems theory is exemplified in Figure 1. The input function $Q_D(t)$ is shown as a cumulative in-vitro drug dissolution profile, but could alternatively be a dissolution rate curve $\dot{A}(t)$. Similarly, the output response $Q_B(t)$ is depicted as a plasma drug concentration versus time profile, but could just as easily be a drug or metabolite in-vivo excretion curve or a pharmacologic response intensity profile. The only necessary

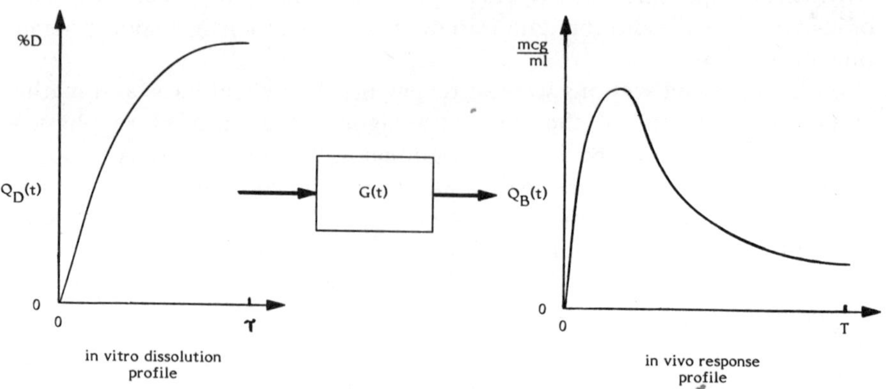

Figure 1. Linear systems theory representation of input–output response profile transformation.

condition is that the net result of all of the kinetic processes encompassed by the weighting, or transfer function $G(t)$, is linear in the region of interest or can be approximated as being linear.

In-vivo, both the preabsorption dynamics of the drug's release from its dosage forms and the subsequent systemic absorption into the blood, as well as its disposition and elimination from the body, must be dose independent and nonsaturable. In practice, it may be sufficient that the in-vivo system approximates linearity over the range of difference seen between the dosage forms tested. However, it is not necessary that the in-vivo bioavailability of the drug be rate limited only by its dissolution from its dosage forms, but that the in-vivo absorption, as well as any presystemic metabolism of the drug in the gut lumen, wall, or liver, is linear and describable by proportional rate constants that are time invariant. In other words, drug absorption occurring by site specific, facilitated, or active transport, as well as the involvement of saturable metabolic processes, could vitiate the approach, depending upon the magnitude of the effects.

The in-vitro time course of dissolution rates or extents of release of the drug from its dosage form can theoretically have any type of kinetic behavior, provided that the apparatus and conditions of the in-vitro dissolution test are such that the experimentally recorded drug dissolution rate or extent versus time profiles are direct reflections of drug release into the dissolution media or are consistently related to it by first- or higher-order lag times. In situations where a drug dissolves so slowly that its dissolution time exceeds its transit time in the GI tract, in-vitro dissolution curves run to completion predict a greater in-vivo bioavailability than would actually be observed. Conceivably, this result could be approximately corrected for by truncating in-vitro dissolution experiments after a time in-vitro known to exceed a correspondingly proportional time in-vivo at which further absorption of the drug no longer proceeds. The other extreme of instantaneous drug release, accomplished by administering a solution of the drug, merely represents an impulse input to the GI contents and poses no theoretical difficulties.

The specific application of equation 1 to assess the bioequivalence of various dosage forms presumes that all of the relevant in-vitro and in-vivo kinetic processes are qualitatively the same for all of the dosage formulations being tested. Thus, if G_1 and G_2 are the respective transfer functions for two different dosage forms it is assumed that

$$G_1(t-T)=G_2(t-T) \tag{3}$$

The physical interpretation of equation 3 is that no specific chemical or biochemical effects are operative with any dosage form being tested that are not operative with the rest. The operation of such biologically specific factors can be introduced if the drug forms soluble, nonabsorbable complexes with excipients in the formulations, or if such excipients alter the barrier properties of the gastrointestinal mucosa through which the drug must pass to be systemically absorbed. Such biological occurrences obviously could not be easily detected, or taken into account by in-vitro testing results, unless they consistently occurred in all dosage forms.

Prediction of the time course of in-vivo bioavailability from in-vitro dissolution test data, using the convolution integral equation 1, is conceptually straightforward. In theory, all that is necessary is to identify the impulse response weighting function $G(t-T)$ for a set of reference in-vitro dissolution data and corresponding in-vivo response data. Once the weighting function has been determined, subsequent convolution with dissolution results from test dosage forms will predict the in-vivo bioavailability profiles expected if those test doses had been given to the same panel of subjects who received the reference doses. In practice, numerical algorithms for evaluating convolution–deconvolution integrals tend to be inherently computationally unstable and can cause serious computational difficulties. Several methods have been proposed to circumvent these operational realization problems. Approximation techniques (5, 7), special-purpose computers (8), and a variety of analytic expressions corresponding to explicit functional forms associated with pre-specified *a priori* model systems have been employed with varying degrees of success. However, a more robust solution to weighting function convolution–deconvolution realization difficulties in the time-domain is to use the equivalent transfer function representation of equation 1 in the complex frequency domain. As represented in Figure 2, the computationally difficult convolution–deconvolution step in the time-domain corresponds to the much simpler complex multiplication–division operations in transform space. Examples of the versatility of this approach, in which a Fast Fourier Transform algorithm is used, are described below.

Another important practical consideration is that in contrast to transfer function identification of a deterministic engineering system, in human bioavailability studies nondeterministic population effects are inevitable in both the in-vitro dissolution data for individual doses and dosage forms and the in-vivo response profiles from different subjects and panels of subjects. Although optimized dissolution testing methods are always to be preferred, the predictive estimates of in-vivo drug product performance, obtained by the methods and apparatus commonly used, may conceivably be improved and expanded through the incorporation of data from an increasing number of dosage formulations into a population transfer function as such additional data become available. For this purpose, the in-vitro data must always be obtained using the same dissolution test conditions; however, in-vivo data would generally be obtained with different panels of human subjects. One approach is to combine transfer functions obtained for different drug formulations into an average.

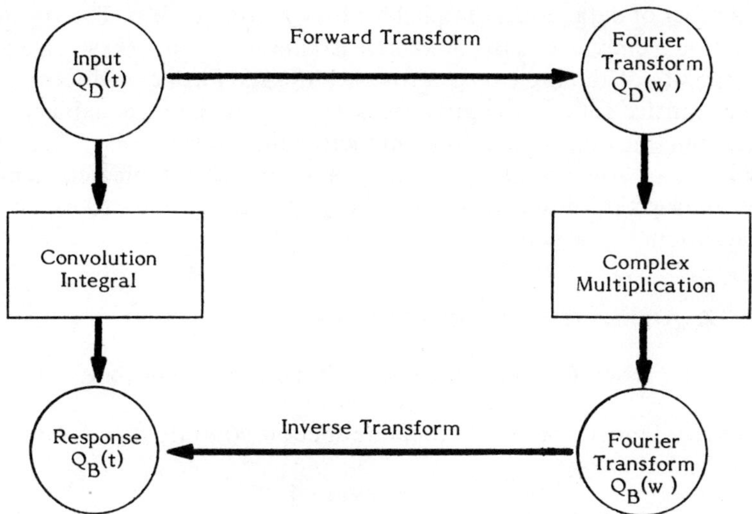

Figure 2. Transform relationships in the time and the frequency domain.

For example, an average function obtained for three tablets A, C, and D would likely predict the plasma level curves for other dose treatments resembling A, C, and D. However, each individual dosage form transfer function would not be expected to produce predictions with equal fidelity. Therefore, it is reasonable to weight the contribution of each individual transfer function on the basis of its predictive capability. Such a weighted average transfer function for different formulations could be defined by equation 4,

$$\overline{G}(w) = \sum_{i=1}^{N} W_i G_i(w) \tag{4}$$

where W_i $(\sum_{i=1}^{N} W_i = 1)$ respresents the weight factors for the transfer functions derived from data observed for each ith drug formulation. A weighting scheme that might be used to obtain the W_i values could be based on the ability of the ith transfer function to predict the plasma curves observed for the other $N-1$ dosage forms contributing to the average, as expressed by

$$W_i = \frac{\sum_{j=1 \neq i}^{N-1} \sum_{q=1}^{K} (P_{\text{pred}} - P_{\text{obs}})_q^2}{\sum_{i=1}^{N} \sum_{j=\neq i}^{N-1} \sum_{q=1}^{K} (P_{\text{pred}} - P_{\text{obs}})_q^2} \tag{5}$$

where P_{pred} and P_{obs} represent computationally predicted and observed data points corresponding to the qth sampling time, respectively, and K is the total number of data points sampled for the ith dosage form. The W_i defined by equation 5 emphasizes the predictive capability of each $G_i(w)$. Weighting for variability of the in-vivo data for each dosage form contributing to the average transfer function is attenuated by the predictive capability of the transfer function and is, therefore, implicit in the value of each W_i. By using this scheme or some alternative, transfer functions for predicting in-vivo temporal drug response behavior can be continuously updated as new data from additional dosage forms become available.

2. OPERATIONAL PROCEDURES

2.1 Discrete Finite Fast Fourier Transform Algorithms

The Fourier Transform of a P-domain function $x(p)$ into a U-domain function $y(u)$ is defined as

$$y(u) = \int_{-\infty}^{\infty} x(p)e^{-i2\pi pu}\,dp \tag{6}$$

The Inverse Fourier Transformation from u to p is defined as

$$x(p) = \int_{-\infty}^{\infty} y(u)e^{i2\pi pu}\,du \tag{7}$$

If p represents time (i.e., let $p=t$), so that $x=x(t)$ is a time domain function, then u represents frequency (i.e., let $u=f$) and $y=y(f)$ is the (complex) frequency domain spectrum of $x(t)$. In terms of radian frequency, $w=2\pi f$ and

$$e^{\pm wt} = \cos wt \pm i \sin wt, \; i=\sqrt{-1} \tag{8}$$

is called the *kernel* of the transform.

We can write the Discrete Fourier Transform of a sampled time domain function as

$$y(w) = \sum_{n=-\infty}^{n=+\infty} x(n\Delta t)\, e^{-i(n\Delta t)w} \tag{9}$$

where n is an integer (counter) in the t-domain, and Δt is the time between samples (i.e., sampling period, assumed equi-spaced for simplicity). Equation 9 contains the infinite series $x(n\Delta t)$, and any practical application requires that we replace the infinite summation with a finite, time-limited representation. Therefore, setting $0 \leqslant n \leqslant N-1$, equation 9 becomes

$$y(w) \approx \sum_{n=0}^{n=N-1} x(n\Delta t)e^{-i(n\Delta t)w}$$

$$= x(0) + x(\Delta t)e^{-i(\Delta t)w} + \cdots + [(N-1)\Delta t]e^{-i(N-1)\Delta tw} \tag{10}$$

with $T=(N-1)\Delta t$ (i.e., the "time window" is $[0, T]$ and there are N samples).

The second approximation needed is to limit w to some finite set of discrete frequencies, for example, M of them. Let us take them to be equi-spaced in the frequency domain, $[0, \delta w, 2\delta w, \ldots, (M-1)\delta w]$ or $\{w_0, w_1, \ldots, w_m, \ldots, w_{M-1}\}$. Then

$$y(m\delta w)=\sum_{n=0}^{n=N-1} x(n\Delta t)e^{-i(n\Delta t)(m\delta w)}, \quad m=0, 1, 2, \ldots, M-1 \tag{11}$$

is the Discrete Finite Fourier Transform (DFFT) of $x(t)$.

From sampling theory we know that

$$\frac{(M-1)\delta w}{2\pi}<\frac{1}{2\Delta t} \tag{12}$$

or slightly more than two samples per period of the highest frequency to be resolved are required. Therefore, to minimize sampling errors we would like frequencies higher than $w_{\max}=(M-1)\delta w$ to be negligible. If $x(n\Delta t)$ represents a real-valued function, as is usually the case, and since $y(m\delta w)$ possesses both real and imaginary parts, then N points in the time domain allow us to define at most $N/2$ complex quantities in the frequency domain, so that

$$\frac{\delta w}{2\pi}=\frac{1}{T} \tag{13}$$

Except for the calculation of very coarse spectra for which N and M are small numbers, the direct numerical evaluation of equation 11 still imposes a substantial computational burden. A significant reduction in the number of calculations was realized with the discovery of the cyclically repetitive nature of the discrete transform (9). Such algorithms, known as Fast Fourier Transform (FFT) algorithms, simplify and speed up calculations of equation 11 to the extent that small, general purpose microcomputers can now routinely evaluate the DFFT of a function.

2.2 Computational Schema

The algorithms for computationally converting in-vitro dissolution data into predicted in-vivo bioavailability profiles form two distinct operational phases. The first phase consists of transfer function identification (deconvolution) operations, and the second phase consists of the predictive conversion (convolution) procedures. The former identification phase pertains to the stepwise processing of reference dosage form(s) data, as outlined symbolically below, to define a weighted average transfer function $\bar{H}(w)$ in the frequency domain where complex division is equivalent to deconvolution.

Reference dosage form(s)

Step 1. In-vitro dissolution data.

$$Q_D(t) \xrightarrow{\text{FFT}} G_D(w)$$

Step 2. In-vivo response data.

$$Q_B(t) \xrightarrow{\text{FFT}} G_B(w)$$

Step 3. Transfer function.

$$\bar{H}(w) = \frac{G_B(w)}{G_D(w)}$$

All operations are performed numerically, and no *a priori* assumptions or restrictions are imposed on either the in-vitro dissolution versus time profiles or the in-vivo bioavailability response data.

The predictive conversion phase involves the three additional steps shown below, where the primes denote a specific test dosage form, SF is a scalar normalizing scale factor to adjust for assayed drug content differences, and IFT denotes the Inverse Fourier Transform operation. Step 5 depicts complex multiplication in transform space and corresponds to convolution in the time domain.

Test dosage form(s)

Step 4. In-vitro dissolution data.

$$Q'_D(t) \xrightarrow{\text{FFT}} G'_D(w)$$

Step 5. Predicted in-vivo response transform.

$$G'_B(w) = \bar{H}(w) G'_D(w) \text{SF}'$$

Step 6. In-vitro predicted in-vivo response.

$$G'_B(w) \xrightarrow{\text{IFT}} Q'_B(t)$$

Additional steps in the actual processing of dosage form data and in the presentation of results are apparent in the examples that follow.

3. EXAMPLE: NITROFURANTOIN URINARY EXCRETION LEVELS

The computation conversion of in-vitro dissolution data into a predicted in-vivo urinary excretion profile is shown below, using a commercially available microcomputer software program.* The program is friendly in the sense that the user is guided through each step of the process with gentle interactive dialogue. Subprogram modules provide for data entry/output with error checking and correction capability, a uniform data interval generating module, the DFFT algorithm, a weighting and scale factor normalization module, statistics and graphical plot packages, and algorithms for multiple-dose predictions of in-vivo steady-state blood levels of drug.

In Figure 3, previously entered in-vitro dissolution data and in-vivo excretion data (10) for six reference dosage forms is recalled from computer storage and processed sequentially. Each dataset pair underwent a 512 point transform, and the compressed printout corresponds to Steps 1–3 of the previously described operational schema (Section 2.2). The completion message signifies that a mean system transfer function has been determined. Figure 4 is the interactive dialogue for processing a test dataset. In this example, the raw data has also been previously stored, and includes optional in-vivo excretion results for comparison to the transfer function predicted results. Figure 5 shows the convolution predicted in-vivo excretion levels compared to the actual excretion observed. Note that the in-vitro dissolution time interval of 304 minutes has been transformed into a 12 hour predicted excretion period. In this example, the slope of the linear regression line was 1.12 with 95% confidence limits of 1.03 and 1.22. The corresponding correlation coefficient was 0.996, highly significant with $t=28.5$. The program also has the ability to present these results graphically, as shown in Figures 6 and 7.

4. EXAMPLE: WARFARIN PLASMA LEVELS

The in-vivo response variable generated through the computational conversion of in-vitro dissolution data depends solely on the type of in-vivo reference data available. Thus, in the present example reference dosage form warfarin plasma level data (11) was input to the BioConverter® program to subsequently predict single, multiple, and steady state warfarin plasma levels from in-vitro warfarin dissolution results for test dosage forms. As in the previous example, Figure 8 shows that reference dosage form data has already

*BioConverter® Software Package, PharmaControl Corp., Englewood Cliffs, N.J. 07632.

```
WANT TO ENTER YOUR REFERENCE
DATA FROM A DISK(Y/N) ? Y
  DRIVE 1 OR 2 (DEFAULT=2) ?
 ENTER FILENAME ? NITROFURAN-RAWDATA

LOADED DATASET: NITROFURAN-RAWDATA  (6 DOSAGE FORMS)

  1) 6  REFERENCE DOSAGE FORMS
  2) 50 MG NOMINAL DOSE AMOUNT
  3) 13  IN VITRO SAMPLES/DOSAGE FORM
  4) 304 MINUTES, LAST IN VITRO SAMPLE
  5) IN VIVO EXCRETION DATA
  6) 8  IN VIVO SAMPLES/DOSAGE FORM
  7) 12 HOURS, LAST IN VIVO SAMPLE

ANY CHANGES(Y/N) ? N
WANT TO DISPLAY THIS DATA(Y/N) ? N


ANALYZING
 REFERENCE DOSAGE FORM 1


ANALYZING
 REFERENCE DOSAGE FORM 2


ANALYZING
 REFERENCE DOSAGE FORM 3


ANALYZING
 REFERENCE DOSAGE FORM 4


ANALYZING
 REFERENCE DOSAGE FORM 5


ANALYZING
 REFERENCE DOSAGE FORM 6


DONE
```

Figure 3. Representative printout of reference data processing steps by the BioConverter® program: Nitrafurantoin excretion.

```
WANT TO ENTER YOUR TEST
DATA FROM A DISK(Y/N) ? Y

LOADED DATASET: NITROFURAN-ABC RAWDATA  (3 DOSAGE FORMS)

 TEST DOSAGE FORM 1 DATA

  1) 50.75 MG ASSAYED DOSE AMOUNT
  2) 13  IN VITRO TEST DOSE SAMPLES
  3) 304 MINUTES, LAST IN VITRO SAMPLE
  4) 8  IN VIVO TEST DOSE SAMPLES
  5) 12 HOURS, LAST IN VIVO SAMPLE

ANY CHANGES(Y/N) ? N

WANT TO DISPLAY YOUR DATA
FOR TEST DOSAGE FORM 1 (Y/N) ? Y


IN VITRO DISSOLUTION DATA
FOR TEST DOSAGE FORM 1

TIME(MIN)        % DISSOLVED

 TD(1)= 0          QD(1)= 0
 TD(2)= 16         QD(2)= 2.96
 TD(3)= 32         QD(3)= 20.69
 TD(4)= 48         QD(4)= 37.44
 TD(5)= 64         QD(5)= 56.16
 TD(6)= 80         QD(6)= 59.11
 TD(7)= 112        QD(7)= 62.07
 TD(8)= 144        QD(8)= 63.05
 TD(9)= 176        QD(9)= 63.05
 TD(10)= 208       QD(10)= 65.02
 TD(11)= 240       QD(11)= 67.98
 TD(12)= 272       QD(12)= 69.95
 TD(13)= 304       QD(13)= 70.94

WANT TO REENTER THIS DATA(Y/N) ? N


IN VIVO EXCRETION DATA
FOR TEST DOSAGE FORM 1

TIME(HRS)            % OF DOSE

 TB(1)= 0          QB(1)= 0
 TB(2)= 1          QB(2)= 3.33
 TB(3)= 1.5        QB(3)= 9.65
 TB(4)= 2          QB(4)= 14.88
 TB(5)= 3          QB(5)= 24.92
 TB(6)= 4          QB(6)= 30.16
 TB(7)= 6          QB(7)= 34.59
 TB(8)= 12         QB(8)= 36.38

WANT TO REENTER THIS DATA(Y/N) ? N
```

Figure 4. Example of interactive dialogue for test dosage form processing Nitrofurantoin.

```
ANALYZING
 TEST DOSAGE FORM 1

DONE

                RESULTS  04/28/82


FOR 6 DEGREES OF FREEDOM AT P = 0.05

     CRITICAL T = 2.45

SLOPE(REGRESSION COEFFICIENT) B = 1.12
  95% CONFIDENCE INTERVAL = (1.03,1.22)


                TEST DOSAGE FORM 1
                IN VIVO EXCRETION

# TIME(HRS)               % OF DOSE
                -----------------------------
                 PREDICTED(95%)      OBSERVED

1    0          1.35   (-1.09,3.41)     0
2    1          5.61   (2.9,6.89)       3.33
3    1.5        11.39  (10.41,13.57)    9.65
4    2          17.88  (16.51,19.21)    14.88
5    3          26.61  (27.73,30.52)    24.92
6    4          36.94  (33.35,36.66)    30.16
7    6          41.14  (38.02,41.93)    34.59
8    12         41.08  (39.9,44.08)     36.38

CORRELATION COEFFICIENT R = .9963
     SIGNIFICANCE LEVEL: T = 28.54


WANT A PLOT OF THESE RESULTS ? Y
```

Figure 5. Convolution predicted in-vivo Nitrofurantoin excretion response results for dosage form 1.

been entered, verified, corrected, and saved, and is simply recalled for processing. This condensed printout shows that data for test dosage form 3 has also been previously entered and stored, and that in-vivo as well as in-vitro data is available.

Figure 9 shows the in-vitro predicted in-vivo warfarin plasma profile results compared to the actual observed in-vivo values. A statistically significant ($t = 10.18$) strong correlation ($r = 0.9678$) was obtained here. Figures 10 and 11 are the graphical plots corresponding to these results. Figure 12 shows an additional feature of the program, which is the ability to predict

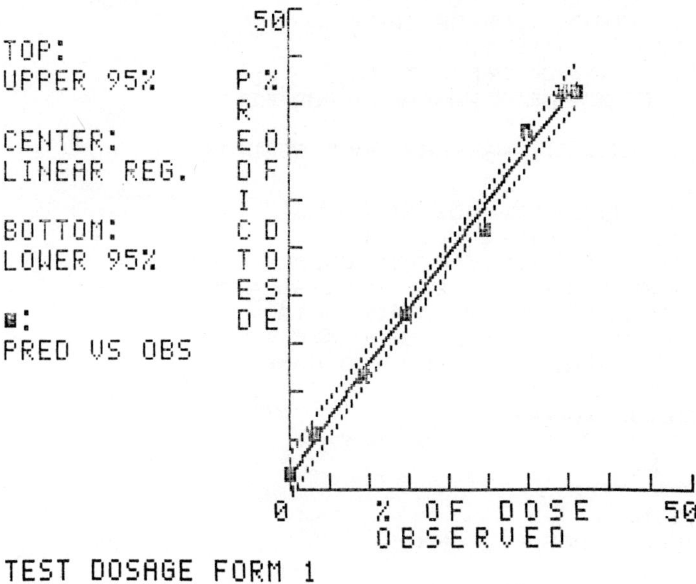

Figure 6. Regression line and 95% confidence band for predicted versus observed Nitrofurantoin excretion profile data tabulated in Figure 5.

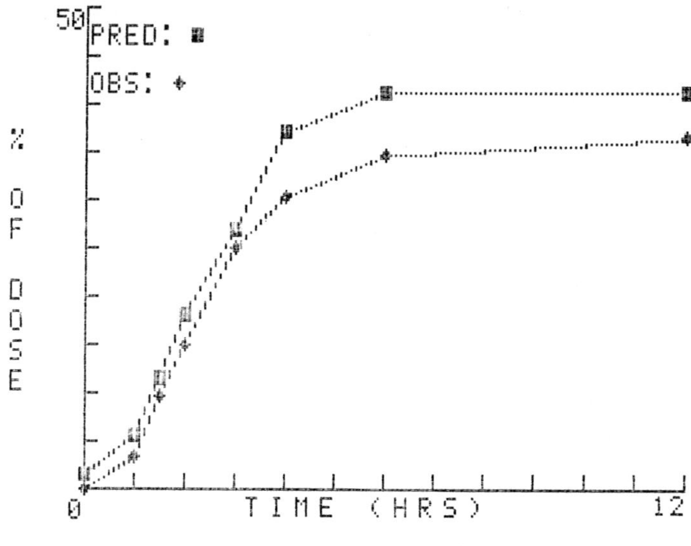

Figure 7. Predicted and observed Nitrofurantoin excretion versus time.

```
WANT TO ENTER YOUR REFERENCE
DATA FROM A DISK(Y/N) ? Y
  DRIVE 1 OR 2 (DEFAULT=2) ?
 ENTER FILENAME ? WARFARIN-ACD REFDATA

LOADED DATASET: WARFARIN-ACD REFDATA  (3 DOSAGE FORMS)

   1) 3  REFERENCE DOSAGE FORMS
   2) 10 MG NOMINAL DOSE AMOUNT
   3) 18  IN VITRO SAMPLES/DOSAGE FORM
   4) 400 MINUTES, LAST IN VITRO SAMPLE
   5) IN VIVO CONCENTRATION DATA
   6) 9  IN VIVO SAMPLES/DOSAGE FORM
   7) 96 HOURS, LAST IN VIVO SAMPLE

ANY CHANGES(Y/N) ? N
WANT TO DISPLAY THIS DATA(Y/N) ? N


ANALYZING
 REFERENCE DOSAGE FORM 1

 REFERENCE DOSAGE FORM 2

 REFERENCE DOSAGE FORM 3

DONE



WANT TO ENTER YOUR TEST
DATA FROM A DISK(Y/N) ? Y
  DRIVE 1 OR 2 (DEFAULT=2) ?
 ENTER FILENAME ? WARFARIN

LOADED DATASET: WARFARIN

TEST DOSAGE FORM 3 DATA

  1) 9.4 MG ASSAYED DOSE AMOUNT
  2) 18  IN VITRO TEST DOSE SAMPLES
  3) 400 MINUTES, LAST IN VITRO SAMPLE
  4) 9  IN VIVO TEST DOSE SAMPLES
  5) 96 HOURS, LAST IN VIVO SAMPLE

ANY CHANGES(Y/N) ? N
```

Figure 8. BioConverter® program interactive dialogue for processing Warfarin in-vitro dissolution and in-vivo blood level data.

```
ANALYZING
 TEST DOSAGE FORM 3
DONE

            RESULTS  04/28/82


FOR 7 DEGREES OF FREEDOM AT P = 0.05

    CRITICAL T = 2.36

SLOPE(REGRESSION COEFFICIENT) B = .97
  95% CONFIDENCE INTERVAL = (.75,1.19)


             TEST DOSAGE FORM 3
             IN VIVO CONCENTRATION

# TIME(HRS)         CONC(MCG/ML)
             ------------------------------
             PREDICTED(95%)        OBSERVED

1    0       0       (-.15,.15)       0
2    1       .79     (.49,.64)        .58
3    4       1.05    (.93,1.2)        1.1
4    8       .87     (.81,1.03)       .95
5    12      .81     (.73,.92)        .85
6    24      .63     (.58,.74)        .68
7    48      .44     (.4,.55)         .49
8    72      .31     (.27,.45)        .37
9    96      .2      (.15,.36)        .26

CORRELATION COEFFICIENT R = .9678
    SIGNIFICANCE LEVEL: T = 10.18
```

Figure 9. Convolution predicted in-vivo Warfarin blood concentration results for dosage form 3.

steady state plasma levels following multiple dosing for any given dose interval. In this example, after 15 daily doses plasma levels are within 99% of their predicted mean 2.4 mcg/ml value.

5. COMPUTATIONAL CONVERSION OF ARBITRARY INPUT-RESPONSE RELATIONSHIPS

Transfer functions in the complex frequency domain can, in addition to computationally converting bio-relevant in-vitro drug product dissolution data into predicted blood or excretion level versus time curves, be used as a generalized method for performing drug input–output computations. Other

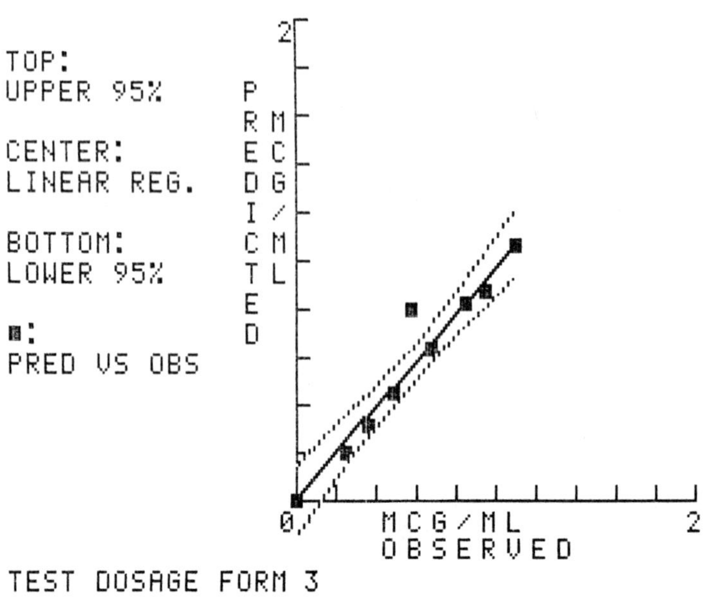

Figure 10. Regression line and 95% confidence band for predicted versus observed Warfarin blood concentration data tabulated in Figure 9.

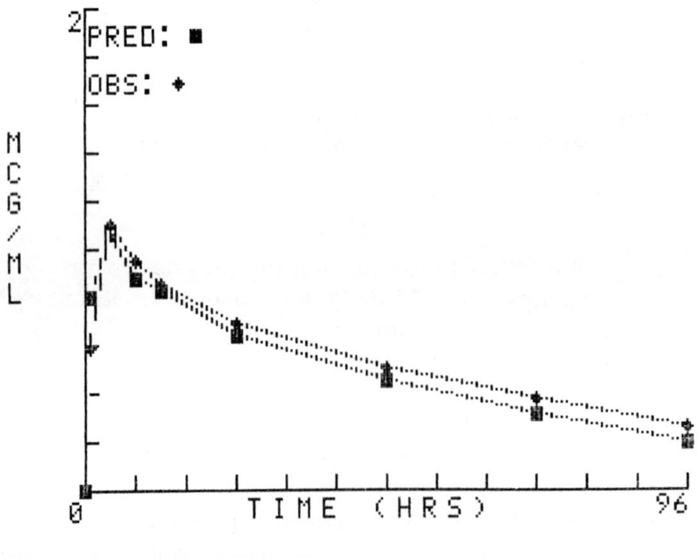

Figure 11. Predicted and observed Warfarin blood concentration versus time.

```
WANT A PREDICTION OF STEADY STATE BLOOD LEVELS ? Y
ENTER DOSE INTERVAL(HRS)? 24

DOSE       TOTAL        INTERVAL    BLOOD
 NO        TIME(HR)     TIME(HR)    LEVEL

1           0            0          0
            1            1          .791
            4            4          1.052
            8            8          .872
            12           12         .814
            24           24         .634

DOSE       TOTAL        INTERVAL    BLOOD
 NO        TIME(HR)     TIME(HR)    LEVEL

2           24           0          .634
            25           1          1.417
            28           4          1.654
            32           8          1.442
            36           12         1.352
            48           24         1.077

   .
   .
   .

DOSE       TOTAL        INTERVAL    BLOOD
 NO        TIME(HR)     TIME(HR)    LEVEL

15          336          0          1.941
            337          1          2.704
            340          4          2.882
            344          8          2.593
            348          12         2.428
            360          24         1.943

WITHIN 99% OF STEADY STATE AFTER DOSE # 15

PREDICTED MEAN S.S. BLOOD LEVEL IS 2.413 MCG/ML

PRESS <RETURN> TO CONTINUE...?
```

Figure 12. In-vitro predicted in-vivo steady state Warfarin blood concentration profile following multiple dosing.

than the general conditions of linear systems dynamics required by convolution/deconvolution theory, there are no *a priori* assumptions or dependencies on pharmacokinetic models. Therefore, this model-independent numerical transformation method has practical, noncompartmental applications in pharmacokinetics and pharmacodynamics related to drug delivery system development and optimization in general. Several practical applications of drug input/output relationships can be summarized as:

1. Drug input optimization (e.g., hypothetical time response⇄drug input).
2. Drug bioavailability input analysis (e.g., experimental time response⇄drug input).
3. Drug response analysis (e.g., known or predicted drug input⇄drug response output).

In the first application, where the drug response profile is a hypothetical, ideally sought, optimal response, the objective is to compute the optimal drug input to which it corresponds. Such computed results are useful in establishing criteria for the design of drug delivery systems and the selection of optimal drug dosage regimens. In the second application, where the drug response profile is an experimentally observed result, the corresponding input is computed to evaluate the dynamic (time domain) bioavailability behavior of the drug delivery system. Such information is useful for suggesting modifications in the formulation, design, or use of drug products that can lead to their improvement. The third use of input–output relationships is the inverse computation of drug response output from drug inputs. Such results can be applied to the prediction of time responses for a given dosage regimen or for drug delivery systems having *a priori* known inputs. The inputs may be known simply from a proposed schedule of intravenous dosing, the design of a dosage form, or the results of applying biologically relevant in-vitro drug release testing methods to drug products, as discussed above.

REFERENCES

1. L. Z. Benet and C. W. N. Chiang. The use and application of deconvolution methods in pharmacokinetics. In Abstracts of Papers Presented at the 13th National Meeting of the APhA Academy of Pharmaceutical Sciences, Vol. 2, Chicago, November 5–9, 1972, pp. 169–171.
2. V. F. Smolen. Theoretical and computational basis for drug bioavailability determinations using pharmacological data. I. General considerations and procedures. *J. Pharmacokin. Biopharm.* **4**:337 (1976).
3. V. F. Smolen. Theoretical and computational basis for drug bioavailability determinations

using pharmacological data. II. Drug input-response relationships. *J. Pharmacokin. Biopharm.* **4**:355 (1976).

4. D. J. Cutler. Numerical deconvolution by least squares: Use of prescribed input functions. *J. Pharmacokin. Biopharm.* **6**:243 (1978).
5. D. J. Cutler. Numerical deconvolution by least squares: Use of polynomials to represent the input function. *J. Pharmacokin. Biopharm.* **6**:243 (1978).
6. D. B. Tuey, R. J. Cosgrove, M. C. Meyer, and V. F. Smolen. Computational conversion of dissolution test data into in vivo response profiles. Presented at the 129th APhA Annual Meeting, Las Vegas, April 24–29, 1982.
7. D. P. Vaughan and M. Dennis. Mathematical basis and generalization of the Loo-Riegelman method for the determination of in vivo drug absorption. *J. Pharmacokin. Biopharm.* **8**:83 (1980).
8. V. F. Smolen and R. J. Erb. Predictive conversion of in vitro drug dissolution data into in vivo drug response versus time profiles exemplified for plasma levels of warfarin. *J. Pharm. Sci.* **66**:297 (1977).
9. J. W. Cooley and J. W. Tukey. An algorithm for the machine calculation of complex Fourier series. *Math. Comp.* **19**:297 (1965).
10. M. K. T. Yau and M. C. Meyer. In-vivo–in-vitro correlations with a commercial dissolution simulator I: Methenamine, Nitrofurantoin, and Chlorothiazide. *J. Pharm. Sci.* **70**:1017 (1981).
11. J. G. Wagner, P. G. Welling, K. P. Lee, and J. E. Walker. In-vivo and in-vitro availability of commercial warfarin tablets. *J. Pharm. Sci.* **60**:666 (1971).

CHAPTER 5

In-Vitro Drug Product Dissolution Testing: Apparatus and Methodologies

VICTOR F. SMOLEN

PharmaControl Corporation
Englewood Cliffs, New Jersey

LUANN BALL

Ciba-Geigy Corporation
Summit, New Jersey

CONTENTS

In formulating new dosage forms, the in-vivo drug release characteristics must be designed to achieve systemic drug bioavailability consistent with satisfactory therapeutic performance. In general, the clinical effectiveness of both old and new drug products depends not only upon the amount of drug ingested, but also upon the availability of the drug to the body. Even seemingly trivial changes in the formulation or production of drug products can greatly influence their therapeutic performance. For example, choice of mannitol-lactose versus compressible sugar as the diluent in nitrofurantoin tablets makes a significant difference in in-vitro dissolution rates, as well as urinary recovery rates, of the drug (1, 2). Changing the lubricant in a penicillin tablet can have a pronounced effect on dissolution and blood levels of the antibiotic (3). With the increasing abundance of generic drug products arising from the expiration of patents, it is important to test drug products for bioequivalency between manufacturers, testing for lot-to-lot variations within a single manufacturer's product, as well as assuring bioavailability during the course of a product's shelf life.

The most reliable means of ensuring drug product bioequivalency would be to perform human studies on all lots of drug products, but the time, cost, and human risk involved makes such extensive testing impractical. However, *not* testing all products could result in even greater risk if ineffective drug products are allowed on the market. Officials of the Food and Drug Administration are of the opinion that the development and implementation of in-vitro tests that correlate with in-vivo data (i.e., blood levels, urinary recovery rates, pharmacological response intensities, etc.) can minimize the amount of human testing required (4).

From among the various chemical and physical tests that can be performed on solid drugs, dissolution testing is the most sensitive, reliable, and rational for use in correlating or predicting in-vivo drug product bioavailability behavior (5). This can readily be seen, since before a drug can be absorbed from an orally administered dosage form it must be in solution. Disintegration or deaggregation of a tablet or capsule increases the surface area of drug exposed to gastrointestinal fluids, but it alone does not guarantee that the drug will in effect dissolve, present itself to absorption sites in a solution state, and ultimately be absorbed. Therefore, a dissolution test performed on the drug product is a better guide to its subsequent bioavailability.

For some drugs, the rate of dissolution is so rapid that the rate of appearance of drug in the blood depends on the rate of drug transfer across the gastrointestinal membrane. This is termed "absorption rate limited bioavailability." Some drugs are so rapidly absorbed, however, that the limiting step in their bioavailability is the rate at which drug is available for absorption (i.e., the dissolution rate of the drug product). This is termed "dissolution rate limited bioavailability." It is for these drugs that in-vitro dissolution testing is a most useful tool for measuring product quality.

1. THEORY OF DISSOLUTION

The first quantitative study of the dissolution process was reported in 1897 by Noyes and Whitney (6). Using water as a dissolution medium, they rotated cylinders of benzoic acid and lead chloride with constant surface area and analyzed the resulting solutions at various time intervals. They found that the rate of change of concentration of dissolved substance (dC/dt) was proportional to the difference between the saturation solubility for that substance (C_s) and the concentration existing at any time t (C). Using k as a proportionality constant, this can be expressed as:

$$\frac{dC}{dt}=k(C_s-C) \tag{1}$$

Nernst and Brunner (7) discussed the dissolution of a solid drug in an agitated liquid in terms of the film theory. It is assumed that there is a thin stagnant film of liquid of thickness h at the surface of the dissolving solid, as shown in Figure 1. The solid is believed to dissolve at an infinitely rapid rate, maintaining a saturated layer at the solid-liquid interface (at $X=0$ in Figure 1). Within the bulk medium (at a distance $X>h$ from the solid surface in Figure 1), it is thought that the agitation of the medium maintains a uniform concentration of dissolved drug. This sets up a concentration gradient throughout the stagnant film. Dissolved solid is transported through this film to the bulk medium totally by Brownian motion diffusion. Therefore, the rate of dissolution of the solid depends on the rate of solute diffusion through this layer. Mathematically this can be described by equation 2.

$$\frac{dW}{dt}=\frac{DS}{h}(C_s-C) \tag{2}$$

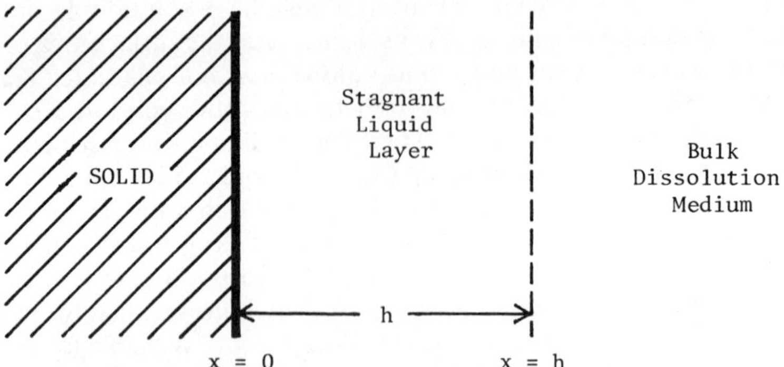

Figure 1. Schematic interpretation of the film theory of dissolution.

where D is the diffusion coefficient of the solute molecules in the medium, S is the solid surface area, h is the thickness of the diffusion layer, W is the mass of the solid, and dW/dt is the rate at which the solid dissolves.

The film theory has much support, including work done by VanName and Edgar (8) and Bosworth (9), who studied dissolution rates of certain metals in halogens and concluded the theory to be correct. However, many other workers have found cases where the film theory does not hold. One criticism is the inordinately large calculated film thicknesses (20–50 μ), considered to be unacceptable (10, 11).

Wilderman (12) challenged the fundamental assumption that equilibrium was established almost instantaneously at the solid–liquid interface. Examination of data of Nernst and Brunner showed that the "constant" D/h increased much faster with temperature than does D alone.

If the surface reaction rate is rate-limiting, then the concentration at the solid–liquid interface can be less than the solubility of the drug. This led Dankwerts (13) to suggest that turbulence within the bulk medium extends to the surface of the solid, and that there is no stagnant film or diffusion layer surrounding the solid. Rather, the layer is continuously being replaced with fresh liquid from the bulk. Molecules of solid must "solvate." The rate limiting step in this surface renewal theory is the diffusion of solvent from the bulk to the solid surface.

Dankwerts' model can be expressed mathematically as:

$$\frac{dC}{dt}=p^{1/2}D^{1/2}(C_s-C) \tag{3}$$

where p is the mean rate of production of fresh surface.

These two dissolution theories—the film theory and the surface renewal theory—are pertinent only for single, nondisintegrating particles. This is rarely the case in pharmaceutical systems. Disintegration or deaggregation of the solid dosage form results in a large number of smaller granules with a distribution of sizes. The total surface area changes during the dissolution process owing to complete dissolution of the smaller particles with time. Hixson and Crowell (14) studied the dissolution process in an agitated system where the surface area is changing. They derived a relation, known as the cube root law, based on the Noyes-Whitney equation. This expression assumes the existence of "sink conditions," meaning that the dissolution medium is less than about 10–20% saturated at any time during the test. In a monodisperse particle system the equation can be written as:

$$\sqrt[3]{W^0}-\sqrt[3]{W}=\left(\frac{\pi N\rho}{6}\right)^{1/3}\frac{2DC_s}{\mathrm{h}\rho}\,t \tag{4}$$

where W^0 is the initial weight of the particles, W is the weight of the particles at time t, N is the number of particles, and ρ is the particle density.

Goyan (15) derived a similar equation based on Dankwerts' theory.

$$\sqrt[3]{W^0}-\sqrt[3]{W}=\left[\frac{2e+b(\sqrt[3]{W^0}+\sqrt[3]{W})}{3(\sqrt[3]{W^0}+\sqrt[3]{W})}\right]t \tag{5}$$

where

$$\mathrm{e}=2DC_s\left(\frac{6\pi^2N^2}{\rho}\right)^{1/3}$$

and

$$b=(\sqrt{D_p})C_s\left(\frac{36\pi N}{\rho^2}\right)^{1/3}$$

Both cube root equations are for monodisperse particulate systems. Actual size distributions occurring in pharmaceutical systems are not this simple. Polydisperse multiparticulate dissolution kinetics has been studied on a theoretical basis (16–18), but little experimental work has been done to substantiate these theoretical treatments.

2. DISSOLUTION TEST PROCESS VARIABLES

The conditions under which an in-vitro drug product dissolution test is performed can have tremendous impact on the dissolution rate of the drug. Examination of the theoretical dissolution rate expressions (equations 2 and 3) show that D, S, h or p, C_s, and C all play a role in determining the rate of dissolution of a solid drug particle. The diffusion coefficient, D, depends on the drug molecule and the solvent in which it must diffuse; C_s also depends on the solvent. Solubility can be affected by pH, ionic strength, enzyme or surfactant concentration, or use of nonaqueous media. The concentration of dissolved drug in the bulk medium, C, varies with time and is dependent upon the amount of drug in the dosage form and the volume of dissolution medium. If a column flow-through dissolution test is used, C is also influenced by the flow rate of dissolution medium and the presence or absence of a recycle flow stream. (A recycle flow stream takes dissolution medium containing dissolved drug as it passes out of the dissolution cell and recycles it back through the cell. This will affect the sink conditions within the cell.) If C is allowed to approach C_s, the concentration gradient (C_s-C) necessary for diffusion of dissolved solid through the stagnant layer declines. Therefore, the diffusion rate decreases, resulting in a subsequent decrease in dissolution rate. To preserve an adequate dissolution rate, sink conditions should be maintained. This means that the concentration of dissolved drug in the bulk medium should be kept below 10–20% of saturation.

The surface area of dissolving drug in contact with the dissolution medium(s) depends on the state of subdivision of the solid. Generally, a tablet that disintegrates has more drug surface area than a nondisintegrating tablet. This assumes, of course, that the drug is not trapped within the granules, rendering it unavailable for dissolution. The degree of agitation in the in-vitro system can influence the disintegration or deaggregation of a solid dosage form. In some cases, the disintegrated tablet forms a mound at the bottom of the dissolution testing apparatus, reducing the *effective* surface area of drug exposed to the dissolution medium. Agitation also affects h, the thickness of the diffusion layer (film theory), or p, the mean rate of production of fresh surface (Dankwerts' theory). Increasing agitation reduces the thickness of the diffusion layer in the film theory. A thinner diffusion layer leads to a shorter path for diffusion and hence a faster dissolution rate. Increasing agitation also increases the rate of production of fresh surface in the Dankwerts theory. This leads to a faster rate of dissolution.

It is imperative in performing dissolution tests that the proper testing conditions of agitation intensity, dissolution medium composition, and solubility volume of the medium (sink conditions that determine the extent to which the medium becomes saturated with the drug) be used. These conditions, known as the dissolution test process variables, determine the rate at which the drug dissolves. Improper selection of the process variables can lead to dissolution results that mask significant differences in bioavailability between dosage forms, or are overly sensitive in detecting dissolution differences that are insignificant in-vivo.

The only good and useful dissolution test is one whose results correlate with some aspect of the drug product's in-vivo performances, such as peak blood level, time to peak, area under the blood level versus time curve, pharmacological response intensity, urinary recovery rate of the drug, etc. A knowledge of the physicochemical factors or properties of the components of the dosage form, and of the biological factors or conditions existing in the gastrointestinal tract at the drug's site of release and absorption, can be a valuable aid in the development of meaningful dissolution tests. However, it is futile and unnecessary to try to reproduce in-vitro the complex of biological factors operating in-vivo.

The composition of the dissolution medium depends, of course, on the drug product being tested. The fluid chosen should be an essentially aqueous system and should be as simple as possible. Because the solubility of many drugs is dependent upon pH, buffered solutions are often used. Distilled water, being completely unbuffered, may give results that are not reproducible, so should be used only in cases where pH changes resulting from dissolution of the dosage form do not affect the results. Additional substances, such as organic solvents, surfactants, enzymes, and so forth, should be added only if essential for the results of the test, and must have no artificial interaction with the drug substance or excipients (e.g., denaturation of starch, which could artificially prevent disintegration and dissolution of the formulation).

In testing some formulations, it may be necessary to employ stepwise pH changes. Even continuous pH variations may be essential to provide acceptable results. However, for some testing methodologies, this presents a procedural problem. The rotating bottle apparatus was once an official method for testing drug release rates from timed release drug products using stepwise changes in pH. Column flow-through devices can easily provide continuous pH change.

In-vitro dissolution tests for standard oral drug products are generally run at $37.0 \pm 0.5^\circ$C. At this temperature, excess air may come out of solution in the aqueous vehicle, producing tiny air bubbles that can affect the performance of the test in several ways. For example, air bubbles surrounding the solid drug granules reduce the effective surface area in contact with the dissolution medium and can cause smaller particles to float on the surface. Therefore, excess air should be removed from the dissolution medium before use.

The means for providing agitation depends on the apparatus used. Various methods include tumbling the dosage form in a revolving container, rotating a paddle or basket in the dissolution medium, and forcing liquid past a stationary dosage form (column flow-through devices). The agitation rate can be changed simply by changing the rate of revolution of the container, the rate of rotation of the paddle or basket, or the flow rate of the dissolution medium.

As stated earlier, the solubility volume of the medium can influence the rate of dissolution. In a batch method of dissolution testing, where the drug is dissolved in a fixed volume of liquid, as much as 20 liters of dissolution medium were used to maintain sink conditions. In some cases, an organic solvent was employed in combination with the dissolution medium to extract drug from the aqueous solvent, thus keeping the aqueous drug concentration low. Sink conditions in a flow-through system can be affected by changing the flow rate of the dissolution medium. The solubility volume can be further influenced by taking a portion of the effluent fluid and recycling it back through the dissolution cell.

3. DISSOLUTION TESTING METHODOLOGIES

Hundreds of dissolution testing methods and minor modifications have been reported in the pharmaceutical literature since dissolution of drug products became accepted as an important in-vitro testing method in the 1960s. It is not the purpose of this section to review all of these methods, but to describe only a few, including the rotating basket, rotating paddle, disintegration apparatus, rotating filter–stationary basket, rotating bottle, column flow-through, in-vivo simulative methods (e.g., Sartorius apparatus, Sartorius Filters, Inc., Hayward, California), and the feedback controlled in-vivo predictive apparatus (e.g., Biopredictor, PharmaControl Corp., Englewood Cliffs, New Jersey).

Reproducibility of results is of major importance in any dissolution testing method. The geometry of the apparatus and the testing conditions (process variables) must be carefully specified so that results may be accurately duplicated not only in the same apparatus, but also in other apparatuses in the same or other laboratories. The test must be sufficiently sensitive to be able to discriminate between dosage forms with bioavailability differences, without being overly discriminatory in detecting differences that are negligible in-vivo. The in-vitro results obtained should correlate with some characteristic of the in-vivo data.

A dissolution testing method should be flexible, so that it can be used for a wide range of drug products. Automation is also a consideration. With the increasing role of dissolution testing in industrial quality control, many man hours of work can be saved by automating the testing procedure (including sampling, change of test fluids or agitation rates, assay, and recording and processing of data).

3.1 USP Rotating Basket (Apparatus 1)

The 1980 USP XX–NF XV describes three dissolution testing procedures, using the rotating basket (apparatus 1), the rotating paddle (apparatus 2), and the disintegration apparatus (apparatus 3).

Apparatus 1 consists of a 1000 ml cylindrical vessel with a spherical bottom and a cylindrical basket rotated by a variable-speed drive (see Figure 2). The vessel, made of glass, or preferably for its uniformity, colorless transparent plastic, is immersed in a water bath to maintain the dissolution medium at $37.0 \pm 0.5°C$ throughout the test. Agitation of the medium is provided by rotation of the small 40-mesh stainless steel basket positioned 2.5 ± 0.2 cm above the inside bottom of the vessel. The dosage form being tested is placed inside the basket, which keeps floating dosage forms, such as capsules, completely submerged in the dissolution medium until disintegration occurs. Samples are withdrawn from a zone midway between the surface of the dissolution medium and the top of the basket at a point not less than 1 cm from the wall of the vessel. A volume of fresh dissolution medium equal to the sample volume is usually added.

Although this testing method is widely used, numerous problems have

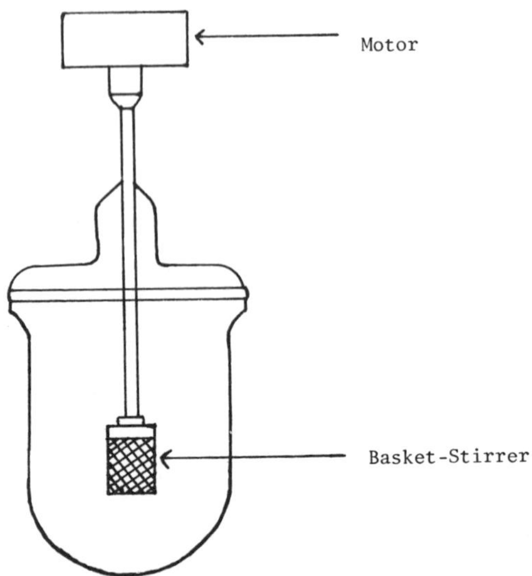

Figure 2. The rotating basket dissolution testing apparatus.

been reported. To obtain reproducible hydrodynamics of the dissolution medium, it is important that the stirring shaft be perfectly centered within the vessel. Special centering tools were developed for this purpose (19, 20). The rotating basket must be free of wobble, which could be caused by a bent shaft or a basket that is not perfectly cylindrical. The shaft or basket should be replaced if wobble is significant. The apparatus itself should not vibrate in any way. Differences in vibrational levels can lead to differences in dissolution rates at low levels of agitation (21).

At low rotational speeds, the basket might be described as a protective envelope around the tablet. Solvent must flow through the basket at a sufficient rate so as to disperse the disintegrating tablet components and sweep them through the openings of the basket screen. If this does not occur, disintegration may be impeded, resulting in unusually slow dissolution of the active drug component. Changes in stirring rate or mesh size of the basket, or addition of a stirring blade on the shaft directly above the basket, would have a minor effect on dissolution rates if this is the case (22).

3.2 Rotating Paddle (Apparatus 2)

The rotating paddle apparatus uses the same vessel as apparatus 1. A paddle is used to provide agitation rather than the basket assembly, and is positioned 2.5 ± 0.2 cm above the inside bottom of the vessel (Figure 3). The

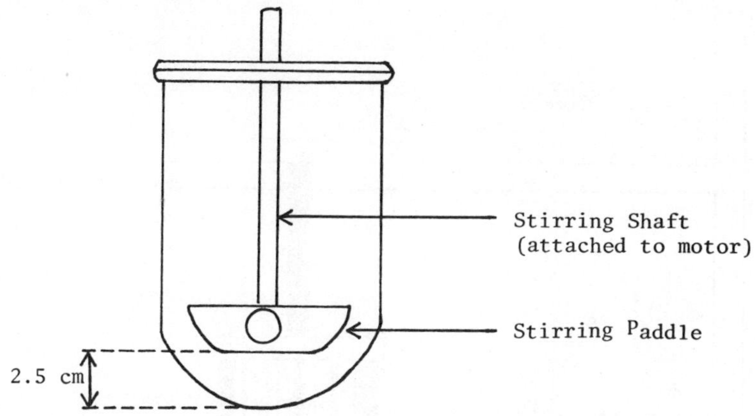

Figure 3. The rotating paddle dissolution testing apparatus.

dosage form to be tested is dropped along the side of the vessel and is allowed to sink to the bottom. Floating dosage units are held in place by a small loose piece of nonreactive material, such as a wire or glass helix, until disintegration occurs. Samples are withdrawn from a zone midway between the surface of the dissolution medium and the top of the paddle, as with apparatus 1.

It is important that the stirring shaft be centered in the vessel and free of wobble. Deviation in vessel curvature from that of a sphere can also cause bias in the dissolution results obtained (23).

3.3 Disintegration Apparatus (Apparatus 3)

The apparatus used to test tablet or capsule disintegration can also be used (with minor alterations) for dissolution testing. The apparatus (Figure 4) consists of a basket-rack assembly, which is raised and lowered at a constant frequency, in a 1000 ml beaker. The basket-rack assembly consists of six open-ended glass tubes (40-mesh stainless-steel cloth covers the lower end of the glass tubes) held in a vertical position by two plastic plates. If necessary, the upper end of the glass tube is also covered with a 40-mesh screen to prevent the dosage form from floating out of the tube assembly. The apparatus is adjusted so that, on the upward stroke, the lower portion of the glass tube remains immersed in the dissolution medium. On the downward stroke, the bottom of the basket-rack assembly descends to 1.0 ± 0.1 cm from the inside bottom surface of the vessel.

One problem with this apparatus is the agitation intensity. The basket-rack assembly is moved at a fixed rate. This rate often produces too much agitation, resulting in a test that fails to discriminate between drug products.

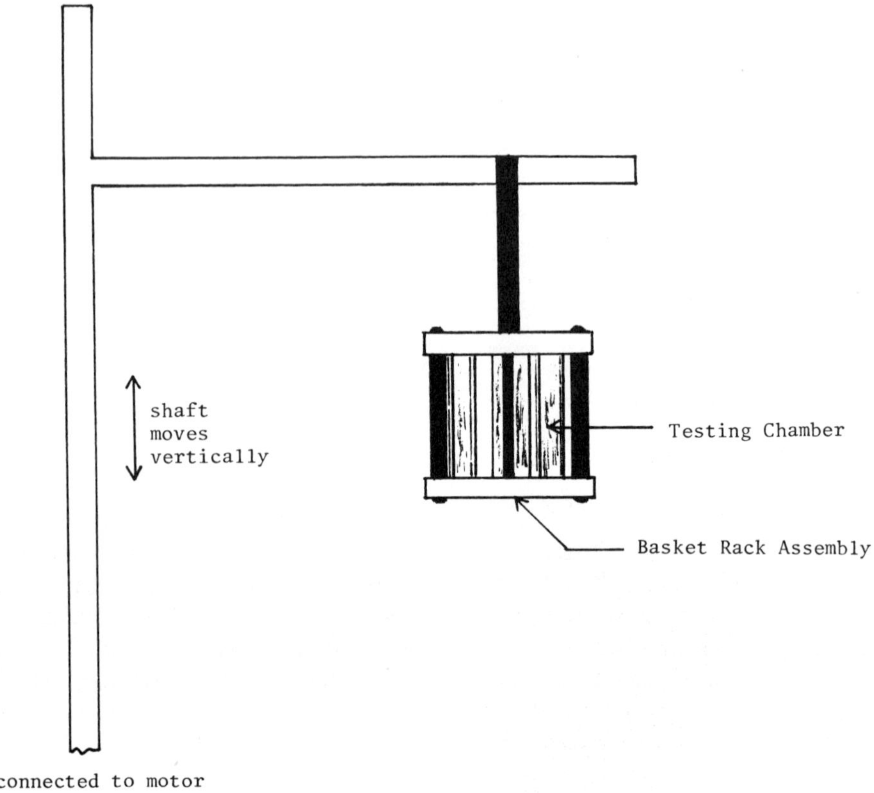

Figure 4. The disintegration testing apparatus.

3.4 Rotating Filter–Stationary Basket

This apparatus (Figure 5) features either a large or small jacketed vessel, a magnetically driven rotating filter assembly, and a stationary sample basket containing the dosage form. As with apparatus 1, the basket keeps any dosage form from floating to the surface of the dissolution medium. Unlike the rotating basket, however, rotation of the filter assembly provides agitation of the dissolution fluid and functions as an in-situ microporous non-clogging filter element for sample removal (24).

3.5 Rotating Bottle Apparatus

This apparatus (25) consists of round screw-capped bottles attached at right angles to a horizontal rotating shaft, mounted in a constant temperature bath (Figure 6). The bottle capacity can vary, but usually 90 ml is used. The

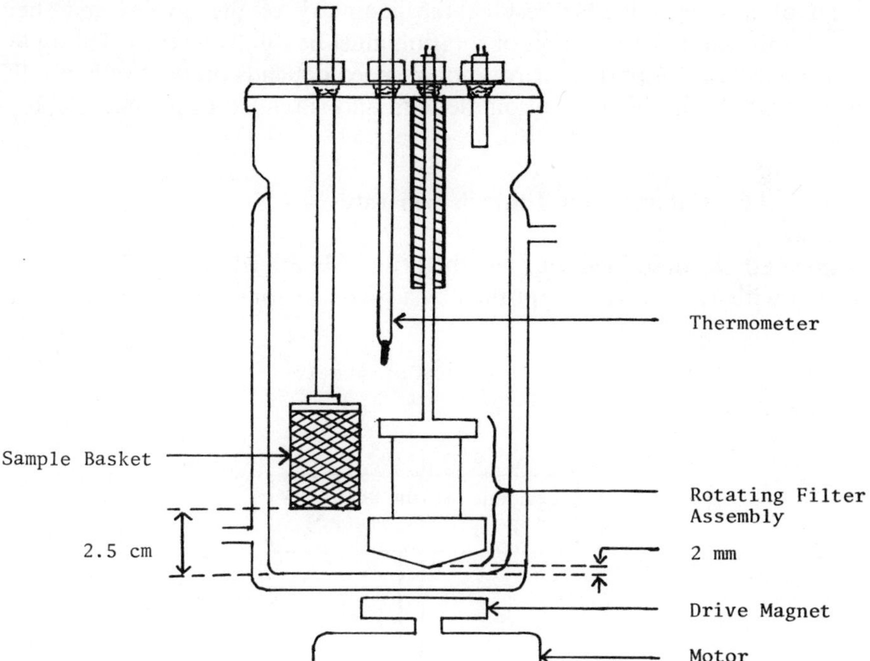

Figure 5. The rotating filter/stationary basket dissolution testing apparatus.

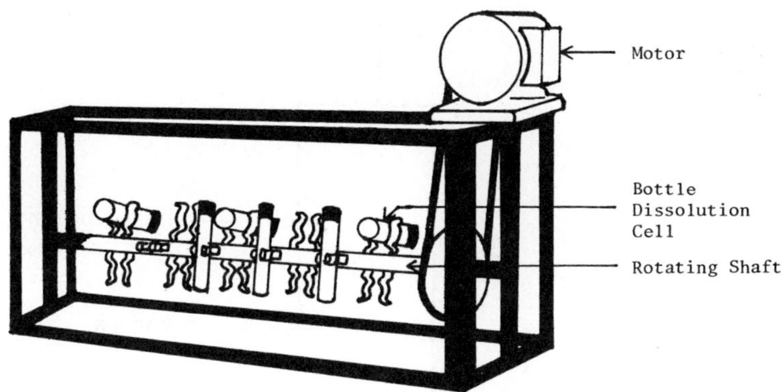

Figure 6. The rotating bottle dissolution testing apparatus.

shaft can be rotated from 6 to 50 rpm. The dosage form is placed in the bottle is dissolution medium (usually 60 ml) of increasing pH value. For example, the dosage form could be placed in pH 1.2 for 0–1 hour, then changed to pH 2.5 for 1–2 hours, followed by pH 4.5 for 2–3.5 hours, pH 7.0 for 3.5–5 hours, and pH 7.5 for 5–7 hours. This procedure was once an official method for determining release rates of drugs from timed release dosage forms.

To obtain reproducible results, the geometry of the bottles and their positioning relative to the axis of rotation must be rigidly defined. The agitation intensity for a particular rotational speed depends on the "rate of fall" of the particles in the dissolution medium and is related to the particle density.

3.6 Column Flow-Through Apparatus

In the methods described thus far, the drug is dissolved in a fixed volume of solvent with agitation accomplished by a stirrer or some rocking action. The

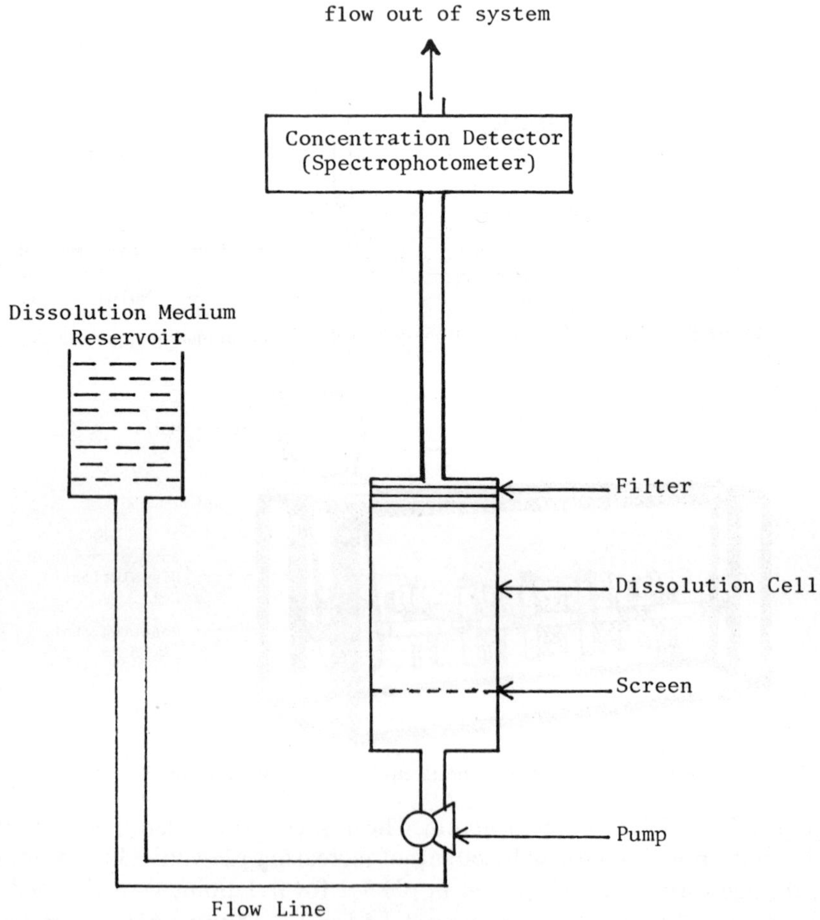

Figure 7. Schematic of a typical column flow-through dissolution testing apparatus.

liquid volume chosen depends on the solubility and dosage of the drug, with volumes ranging from 100 milliliters to 20 liters reported in the literature. In the column flow-through apparatus, the dosage form is held in a small vertical column through which dissolution medium is continually pumped upward from a reservoir at a definite rate (Figure 7). Agitation of the dissolving drug is provided by the flow rate of dissolution fluid through the cell. The eluate leaving the cell is analyzed for drug content. If desired, the effluent can be recycled back through the dissolution cell. However, to maintain sink conditions, an unlimited volume of fresh dissolution medium can be pumped through the column.

3.7 In-Vivo Simulative Methods (Sartorius Apparatus)

The Sartorius apparatus is composed of two pieces of equipment designed to be used in conjunction with one another in an effort to simulate in-vivo drug product dissolution. The absorption simulator (Figure 8) simulates passive drug transport processes that occur in-vivo from the gastrointestinal tract to the plasma across a lipoidal mucosal barrier (26). The solubility simulator (Figure 9) simulates drug dissolution and the subsequent absorption of the drug into the plasma as the drug passes through the gastrointestinal tract (27). The pH of the medium is changed to mimic passage of the drug from the stomach to the intestine.

The dissolution process in-vivo most likely takes place from particles adhering near the mucosal surface. Therefore, the pathway for diffusion to the site of absorption is very short. The drug molecules are absorbed almost instantly into what is, for all practical purposes, a perfect sink—the body fluids (28). Samples are removed from the solubility simulator at a rate dependent upon the absorption rate constant, in an attempt to maintain sink conditions in-vitro.

3.8 In-Vivo Predictive Methods (BioPredictor)

Most in-vitro/in-vivo correlations reported in the literature relate only univariate characteristics of the drug product's behavior in the form of a single point correlation. These correlations are made after the fact, with arbitrarily selected in-vitro and in-vivo parameters, and the results can be misleading. For example, digoxin tablets often fractionate in-vitro, leading to a rapid initial dissolution rate (29). However, this does not necessarily mean that the rest of the tablet releases drug similarly. Therefore, a correlation such as amount of drug dissolved in 30 minutes versus peak blood levels could be misleading.

A better approach is to predict the time course of in-vivo response from an

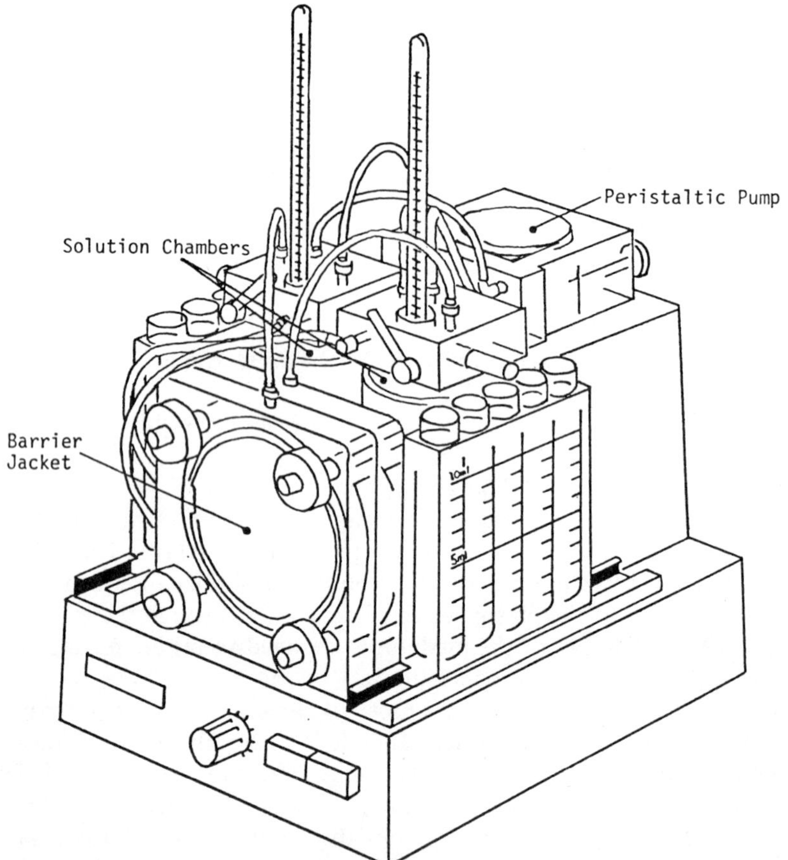

Figure 8. The Sartorius absorption simulator.

in-vitro dissolution test. Two such methods have been reported in the literature (30, 31). The first is a mathematical approach utilizing dissolution results from any standard in-vitro procedure and transforming this data into a predicted bioavailability profile by means of a transfer function relationship. This concept is discussed further in Chapter 4. The second approach employs an apparatus-based methodology, known as the BioPredictor, which predicts the time course of in-vivo drug response in the form of a dissolution rate versus time profile. The dissolution test process variables, such as dissolution medium composition, agitation intensity, or solubility volume (sink conditions) are automatically and continually changed throughout the in-vitro test to produce a dissolution rate profile that simulates a scaled in-vivo response profile for a reference dosage form. When a test dosage

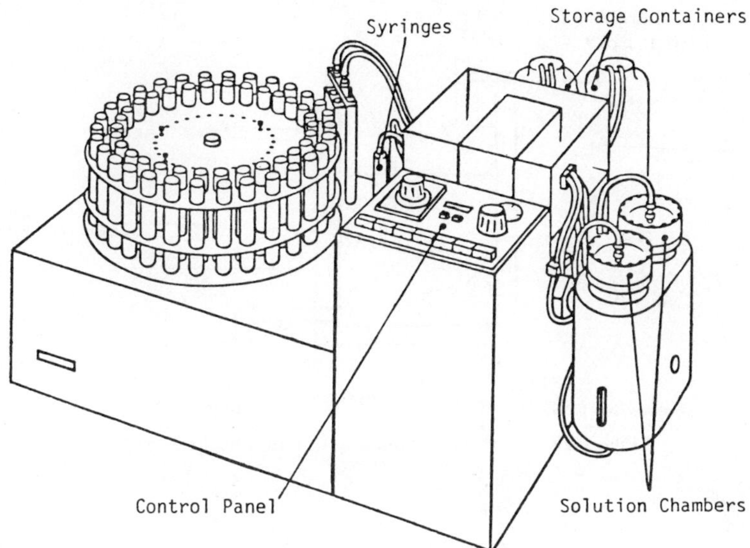

Figure 9. The Sartorius solubility simulator.

form is exposed to the same time-varying dissolution process variables, the resultant dissolution rate profile is the in-vitro predicted in-vivo response profile for that dosage form (32–34).

The time-varying dissolution process variables are determined by classical process control methods. Engineers have been automatically controlling chemical processes for decades. Control was originally performed by human operators who observed the process and many any necessary adjustments in certain parameters to obtain the proper output. Later, the control function was performed by analog computers. With recent technical advances, microprocessors and minicomputers are becoming economically feasible for use as controllers.

The concept of process control is best described by an illustrative example (35). Consider the case of a heat exchanger, shown in Figure 10. Liquid at temperature T_i flows into a well-stirred steam jacketed tank at a rate dm/dt. The temperature of liquid leaving the tank is the same as that in the tank (T_o) and is dependent upon T_i, dm/dt, and the amount of steam. Determining how changes in these parameters affect the process is called system analysis.

Assume that the desired temperature of liquid leaving the tank is T_r (the set point). To maintain this temperature, the actual temperature (T_o) must be measured and compared with the desired value. The magnitude of this difference ($T_r - T_o$), known as the error signal, determines the magnitude

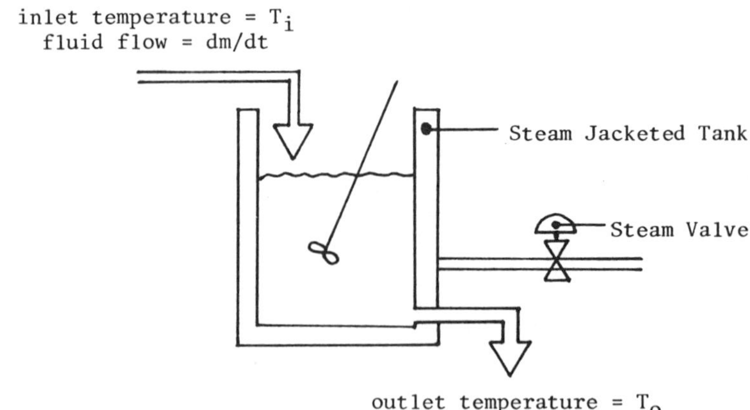

Figure 10. Schematic representation of a heat exchanger.

of the changes to be made in the controllable parameters T_i, dm/dt, and steam pressure. It is the function of the controller to determine these magnitudes.

There are four major types of classical controllers, based on the way in which the error signal is manipulated. The first and simplest is proportional (P) control. It produces an output signal proportional to the error signal, ε, as expressed in equation 6.

$$p = K_c\varepsilon + p_s \tag{6}$$

where p is the output signal, K_c is the gain, ε is the error (set point − measured variable), and p_s is a constant (the desired signal value when $\varepsilon = 0$).

Proportional-integral control (PI) adds a term that is proportional to the integral of the error, as seen in equation 7.

$$p = K_c\varepsilon + \frac{K_c}{\tau_I}\int_o^t \varepsilon dt + p_s \tag{7}$$

where τ_I is the integral time in minutes.

The controller can include a term proportional to the derivative of the error, as in the case of PD or proportional-derivative control.

$$\mathrm{p} = K_c\varepsilon + \tau_D K_c \frac{d\varepsilon}{dt} + p_s \tag{8}$$

where τ_D is the derivative time in minutes.

Equations 7 and 8 can be combined to yield the relationship for proportional-integral-derivative (PID) control.

$$p = K_c \varepsilon + \frac{K_c}{\tau_I} \int_o^t \varepsilon \, dt + K_c \tau_D \frac{d\varepsilon}{dt} + p_s \tag{9}$$

Addition of integral or derivative control does more than lengthen the control algorithm. Figure 11 shows the results of adding a step disturbance to a system. If the system is not controlled (curve A), the disturbance creates a new steady state value in the measured variable. With control, the system eventually takes action to maintain the controlled variable at its steady state set point value. With proportional action alone (curve B) the system is able to limit the rise of the controlled variable and bring it to a new steady state value. The difference between this new value and the initial set point value is known as the offset. Addition of integral action (curve C) eliminates the offset, but the behavior of the system is quite oscillatory. Proportional-integral-derivative control shows a definite improvement in the response of the system. The deviation of the controlled variable is eliminated more quickly and with a minimum of oscillation (curve D).

Selection of the proper control depends on its application. Proportional control is cheapest and easiest to implement. If no offset is tolerable, integral action should be added. Derivative action could be added if excessive oscillation needs to be eliminated; however, the addition of each mode makes the controller more expensive and more difficult to adjust. In general, the simplest method for achieving adequate control is the one that should be used.

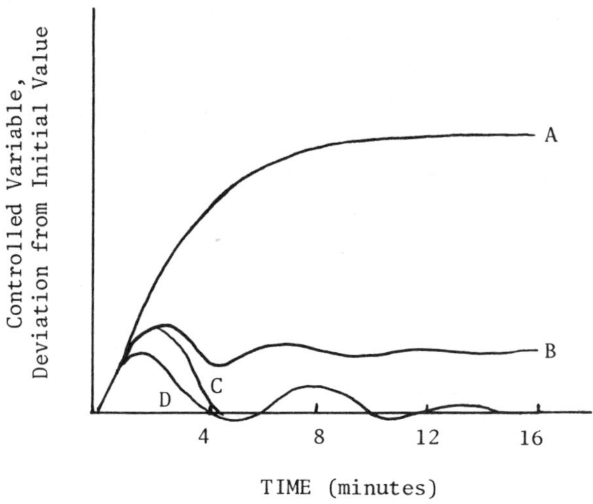

Figure 11. System response to a step disturbance for (*A*) no control, (*B*) proportional control, (*C*) proportional-integral control, and (*D*) proportional-integral-derivative control.

The BioPredictor's time-varying dissolution process variables are determined by operating the apparatus in the closed-loop feedback controlled mode (Figure 12) to produce an in-vitro dissolution rate profile that simulates an average in-vivo profile (blood levels, urinary recovery rates, pharmacological response intensities, etc.) for a reference dosage form. The in-vivo data, obtained from a panel of human subjects, is programmed into the digital computer controller as a variable set point. The error signal is generated by comparing the measured in-vitro drug concentration with the time and amplitude scaled in-vivo data at discrete times during the closed-loop dissolution test. The control algorithm operates on each error signal to generate a new set of process variables (total flow rate, dissolution medium composition, agitation intensity, and solubility volume) that will bring the in-vitro concentration to the desired in-vivo set point value. Test drug products are run simultaneously in the open-loop mode. Open-loop dissolution testing (Figure 13) consists merely of using the time-varying process variables generated during the closed-loop study to do a dissolution test on another dosage form of the same drug. The in-vitro dissolution rate profile produced is a prediction of the average in-vivo profile for that test dosage form in a panel of human subjects.

The BioPredictor feedback control system utilizes four PID controllers

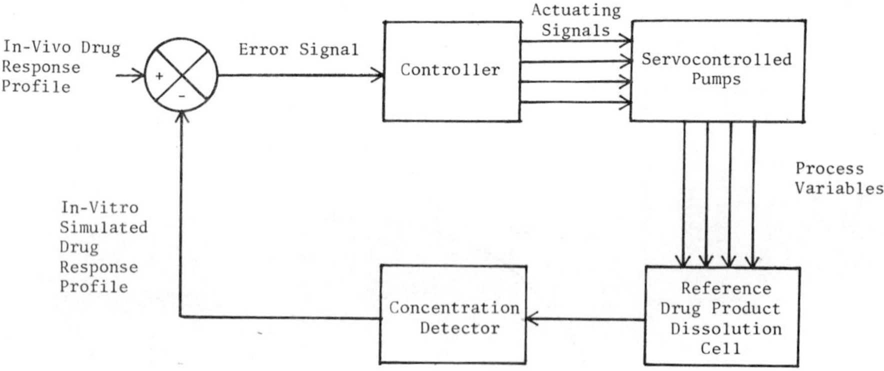

Figure 12. Operation scheme for the BioPredictor in the closed loop mode.

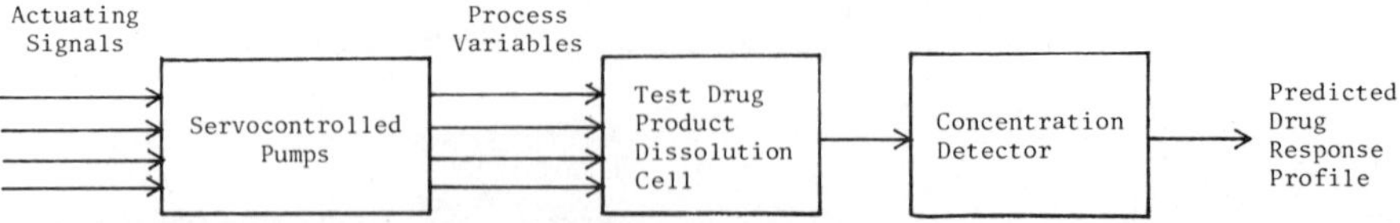

Figure 13. Operation scheme for the BioPredictor in the open loop mode.

corresponding to each of the four controlled process variables. The controllers are automatically adjusted for optimal performance, utilizing a random input modeling and self-tuning approach involving the generation of pseudo-random binary signals (PRBS), and cross-power spectral density analysis to accomplish dynamic model identification and tuning of each control loop in simultaneous operation with the other three. This assures that the feedback control of the process variables is maintained adaptively optimal. The control system can be periodically and automatically retuned during a dissolution test, as needed to compensate for changes in the dynamics of drug release from a complex dosage form. For example, the immediate mechanism of drug release may be by dissolution of a priming dose contained in a tablet matrix itself, followed by permeation of the drug across membranes coated onto beads that are also compressed into the tablet.

The BioPredictor approach to in-vitro predicted bioavailability provides the most rational and rigorous means of establishing in-vitro bioequivalency requirements. In addition to being used in quality control, such methods, when successfully applied, can also provide an optimized in-vitro alternative to the expensive and time-consuming human testing generally required to develop drug product formulations possessing optimally sought controlled drug release dynamics and a maximum therapeutic utility. However, judgment and caution must be exercised with regard to the limitations and applications of in-vitro dissolution testing for in-vivo bioavailability.

ACKNOWLEDGMENTS

The authors thank Ms. Susan Koet and Ms. Judy Cherevka for typing the manuscript and Ms. Velinda McClellan for her assistance with the illustrations.

REFERENCES

1. R. W. Mendes, S. Z. Masih, and R. R. Kanumuri. Effect of formulation and process variables on bioequivalency of nitrofurantoin I: Preliminary studies. *J. Pharm. Sci.* **67**(11): 1613 (1978).
2. R. W. Mendes, S. Z. Masih, and R. R. Kanumuri. Effect of formulation and process variables on bioequivalency of nitrofurantoin II: In-vivo/In-vitro correlation. *J. Pharm. Sci.* **67**(11):1616 (1978).
3. J. W. Poole. Some experiences in the evaluation of formulation variables on drug availability. *Drug Inf. Bull.* **3**(1):8 (1969).
4. The acceptability of in-vitro data as evidence of bioequivalence. *Fed. Regist.* **42**(5):1627 (1977).

5. V. F. Smolen. In-vitro drug product bioequivalency requirements: What can they become? *Pharm. Tech.* **1**:27 (1977).
6. A. A. Noyes and W. R. Whitney. The rate of solution of solid substances in their own solutions. *J. Am. Chem. Soc.* **19**:930 (1897).
7. W. Nernst and E. Brunner. Theorie der reaktionsgeschwindigkeit in heterogenen systemen. *Z. Phys. Chem.* **47**:52 (1904).
8. R. Van Name and G. Edgar. On the velocities of certain reactions between metals and dissolved halogens. *Am. J. Sci.* **29**:237 (1910).
9. R. G. VanName and R. S. Bosworth. On the rates of solution of certain metals in dissolved iodine, and their relation to the diffusion theory. *Am. J. Sci.* **32**:207 (1911).
10. E. L. Parrott, D. E. Wurster, and T. Higuchi. Investigation of drug release from solids. I. Some factors influencing the dissolution rate. *J. Am. Pharm. Assoc. Sci. Ed.* **44**:269 (1955).
11. W. E. Hamlin, E. Nelson, B. E. Ballard, and J. G. Wagner. Loss of sensitivity in distinguishing real differences in dissolution rates due to increasing intensity of agitation. *J. Pharm Sci.* **51**:432 (1962).
12. M. Wilderman. Uber die geschwindigkeit molecularer und chemisches reactionen in heterogenen systemen. *Z. Phys. Chem.* **66**:445 (1909).
13. P. V. Dankwerts. Significance of liquid-film coefficients in gas absorption. *Ind. Eng. Chem.* **43**:1460 (1951).
14. A. Hixson and J. H. Crowell. Dependence of reaction velocity upon surface and agitation. I. Theoretical considerations. *Ind. Eng. Chem.* **23**:923 (1931).
15. J. E. Goyan. Dissolution rate studies III. Penetration model for describing dissolution of a multicompartment system. *J. Pharm. Sci.* **54**:645 (1965).
16. W. I. Higuchi and E. N. Hiestand. Dissolution rates of finely divided drug powders. I. Effects of distribution of particle size in a diffusion-controlled process. *J. Pharm. Sci.* **52**:67 (1963).
17. J. T. Carstensen and M. N. Musa. Dissolution rate patterns of log-normally distributed powders. *J. Pharm. Sci.* **61**:223 (1972).
18. D. Brooks. Dissolution profile of log-normal powders: exact expression. *J. Pharm. Sci.* **62**:795 (1973).
19. D. Cox, C. Douglas, W. Furman, R. Kirchhoefer, J. Myrick, and C. Wells. Guidelines for dissolution testing. *Pharm. Tech.* **2**:41 (1978).
20. A. Serino. Centering tool for dissolution vessels. *J. Pharm. Sci.* **71**(6):725 (1982).
21. W. Beyer and D. Smith. Unexpected variable in the USP-NF rotating basket dissolution test. *J. Pharm. Sci.* **60**(3):496 (1971).
22. G. Haringer, B. Poulsen, and R. Havemeyer. Variation on the USP-NF rotating basket dissolution apparatus and a new device for dissolution rate studies of solid dosage forms. *J. Pharm. Sci.* **62**(1):130 (1973).
23. D. Cox, C. Wells, W. Furman, T. Savage, and A. King. Systemic error associated with apparatus 2 of the USP dissolution test. II. Effects of deviations in vessel curvature from that of a sphere. *J. Pharm. Sci.* **71**(4):395 (1982).
24. A. Shah, C. Peot, and J. Ochs. Design and evaluation of a rotating filter–stationary basket in-vitro dissolution test apparatus. I: Fixed fluid volume system. *J. Pharm. Sci.* **62**(4):671 (1973).
25. J. Souder and W. Ellenbogen. Laboratory control of dextro amphetamine sulfate sustained release capsules. *Drug. Stand.* **26**:77 (1958).

26. H. Stricker. Drug absorption in the gastrointestinal tract II. *Drugs Made in Germany* **16**:80 (1973).

27. H. Stricker. In-Vitro Studies on the Dissolution and Absorption Behavior of Orally Administered Drugs and the Connection to Their Bioavailability. In P. B. Deasy and R. F. Timoney (eds.), *The Quality Control of Medicines*, Elsevier Scientific Publishing Co., New York, 1976, p. 253.

28. J. Tingstad and S. Riegelman. Dissolution rate studies I: Design and evaluation of a continuous flow apparatus. *J. Pharm. Sci.* **59**:692 (1970).

29. L. Nyberg, K. Anderson, and A. Bertler. Bioavailability of digoxin from tablets. III. Availability of digoxin in man from preparations with different dissolution rates. *Acta Pharm. Suec.* **11**(5):471 (1974).

30. V. F. Smolen and W. A. Weigand. Optimally predictive in-vitro drug dissolution testing for in-vivo bioavailability. *J. Pharm. Sci.* **65**:1718 (1976).

31. V. F. Smolen and R. J. Erb. The predictive conversion of in-vitro drug dissolution data into in-vivo drug response versus time profiles exemplified for plasma levels of warfarin. *J. Pharm. Sci.* **66**:297 (1977).

32. V. F. Smolen. In-vitro drug product bioequivalency requirements: What can they become? *Pharm. Tech.* **1**(4):26 (1977).

33. V. F. Smolen. Bioavailability and pharmacokinetic analysis of drug responding systems. *Annu. Rev. Pharmacol. Toxicol.* **18**:495 (1978).

34. V. F. Smolen, L. Ball, and M. Scheffler. Predicting the time course of in-vivo bioavailability from in-vitro dissolution tests: control systems engineering approaches. *Pharm. Tech.* **3**(6):88 (1979).

35. D. R. Coughanowr and L. B. Koppel. *Process Systems Analysis and Control*, McGraw-Hill, New York, 1965, p. 1.

CHAPTER 6

Pharmacokinetic Considerations in Drug Studies

JEROME SKELLY

Deputy Director
Division of Biopharmaceutics
Food and Drug Administration
Rockville, Maryland

KEITH ROTENBERG

Pennwalt Corporation
Rochester, New York
Formerly, Supervisory Reviewer
Pharmacokinetics Branch, FDA

CONTENTS

Drug bioavailability and bioequivalence studies submitted to the Food and Drug Administration vary widely, not only in the complexity and quality of science, but also in the clarity and completeness of the data presented. Most pharmacokinetic scientists today would readily agree that pharmacokinetic studies on highly-cleared, short half-life drugs are more complex than a study on a long half-life drug excreted unmetabolized. They would also agree on the quality (or lack) of the data obtained from such studies. Nevertheless, on the basis of our experience in FDA, there has been great disparity in the completeness of the information submitted to FDA and in the clarity with which it is presented.

There are a number of reasons for this situation. The most obvious is that the requirements for pharmacokinetic data submission and review were promulgated only as late as July 7, 1977. Even today, NDA Form 356H neither explicitly details what data must be submitted nor specifies the proper format for such submission. Although the IND–NDA rewrite and the revised regulations that will issue as a result address these issues, a number of considerations involving data and calculations take place in submission preparation. It is the author's intention in this chapter to present considerations for facilitating the preparation of that information, which when followed, would provide the quickest, most facile review by FDA.

All "New Drug Applications" containing the required pharmacokinetic data are reviewed by an FDA pharmacokineticist. Given that each application is reviewed on the basis of a clearly enunciated priority system, which favors new chemical entities involving drugs offering significant therapeutic gain, and that the FDA traditionally has a large backlog, those presenting data for review are well-advised to consider the clear presentation of data in a single concise biopharmaceutic package. The more the reviewer has to "dig" into different volumes of data to locate information he views important in conducting his audit and in the preparation of the clinical pharmacokinetic portion of the labeling, the greater is the likelihood that delays will occur. If necessary information cannot be located in an application and a non-approvable letter is sent, a lengthy delay in drug application approval could occur, because the new application amendment containing that information might be given a new priority, based on the importance of the submission and the date the amendment arrives at the FDA.

Consider, for example, how much better prepared FDA pharmacokineticists would be to initiate their audit of a new drug, if they had at their fingertips background information concerning the proposed indications for use, therapeutic ratio and metabolism, and the drug's solubility in the physiological fluids of interest. Having to obtain such information by searching into a number of volumes, physically located in different sections of the National Center, requires considerable time and effort on the part of reviewer. Consider, as an alternative, the ease with which this same reviewer could approach an NDA review, when the many studies submitted are clearly identified as "early pharmacokinetic using nonspecific assay," "pilot," "definitive pharmacokinetic," "dose response," or "bioequivalence for development of a new dosage form" versus studies not so identified, where the reviewer must try to determine the significance of each to his evaluation. The considerations that follow should likewise be viewed by the impact they will have in facilitating the biopharmaceutic evaluation of the NDA review, rather than as minimum federal requirements.

1. ELEMENTS NECESSARY FOR BIOPHARMACEUTIC REVIEW

The utilization of elements such as those listed below would provide the reviewer with an organized, comprehensive document enabling efficient and effective review.

1. *Summary*
   a. Background
   b. Labeling
   c. Clinical pharmacology
   d. Drug metabolism and preclinical pharmacology
   e. Chemistry
2. *Biopharmaceutics*
   a. Background
   b. Bioavailability/bioequivalence
   c. Dose proportionality
   d. Statistics
   e. Pharmacokinetics/modeling

1.1 Summary

At the time of NDA submission, no one knows more about the drug than the firm that has invested the time and resources to study it. Because of agency personnel changes, as well as alterations in review priorities, a firm cannot be assured that the scientist who reviewed information submitted under the IND mechanism will necessarily review the information in its NDA. Therefore, we recommend that the biopharmaceutic portion of the NDA be organized as though a new reviewer, unfamiliar with the drug, will review it. We suggest the best way to bring such a reviewer "up to speed" is to provide a summary. An appropriately written summary section could enable the reviewer to acquire the basic information concerning the class of drug, indications for use, pharmacology, therapeutic ratio, and essential physical chemistry—as well as the drug's absorption, distribution, metabolism, and elimination. When the information provided is insufficient, the reviewers must attempt to obtain and review other volumes of the NDA, thereby prolonging the deliberative process.

1.1.1 *Background*

A clear free-flowing discussion giving the salient history pertaining to the drug's marketing outside of the United States, its adverse reactions, and drug/drug interactions (if any) may well satisfy the reviewer's concern in those areas, enabling him to focus his attention toward studies with unresolved questions. For instance, when a drug has been marketed for several years overseas and used in accordance with proposed application labeling without toxic manifestations, rigorous dose response data would seem to be unnecessary. In the absence of such knowledge, however, the pharmacokinetic reviewer would be interested in it.

Where such information is not available, one paragraph could provide the necessary chronic and acute toxicity data necessary for the reviewer. If information relative to the therapeutic index is lacking, summary LD_{50} data under the various routes of administration should be reported. The routes of administration for which approval is sought for marketing (including the dosage strength) should be given.

1.1.2 *Labeling*

A copy of the proposed text of the labeling provided to the pharmacokineticist will alert and orient him not only to the intended use of the drug, but also to the possible targeted subpopulations (e.g., pediatrics, geriatrics, premenopausal females, etc.). In addition, he will be aware of possible side effects and adverse reactions. This information will serve the purpose of quickly orienting the reviewer.

1.1.3 *Clinical Pharmacology*

Knowledge of the pharmacologic class to which a drug belongs and its potential clinical benefit is important. Where possible, data indicating the time of onset of the effect, the time of maximum effect, and the duration of activity should be described. Since biliary recycling can occur for any drug having an affinity for bile, any such occurrence in animal or human studies should be discussed. This information provides valuable reviewer insight, even though such studies were not performed to meet the bioavailability requirement.

The maximum plasma concentration and time to reach that concentration (C_{max}, T_{max}), especially when they vary as a function of dose or in different patient populations, are important pieces of information for the reviewer.

When other therapeutic agents are commonly used in conjunction with the drug being evaluated, drug interaction studies may be required. Interactions, such as alteration of the effects of one or more drugs by another substance, could result in either a diminution of therapeutic efficacy or an increase in drug activity, including possible toxic drug reactions. When known or suspected, they are an important portion of the summary. The concurrent or sequential administration of two or more agents possessing similar pharmacologic actions or side effects may likewise give rise to drug interactions by the additive or synergistic effect of these properties. The administration of a sympathomimetic amine (e.g., amphetamine) with an adrenergic sensitizer (e.g., imipramine) can produce additive or synergistic effects that may be dangerous. The administration of one drug with the potential to alter the basic mechanism of action of another drug may also result not from a simple additive effect, but rather as a result of drug induced changes in the patient. For example, thiazide diuretics, by producing potassium loss, can predispose patients to toxic reactions from cardiac glycosides, which affect ionic transfer in cardiac cells.

Drug interaction phenomena could be pharmacodynamic or pharmacokinetic in origin. Where they are pharmacokinetic, all or any of the various pharmacokinetic processes (absorption, distribution, metabolism, or elimination) could be influenced by administration of another drug. The most critical case would be that involving drugs with a narrow therapeutic index. When displacement of one drug by another from tissue and binding sites occurs, displacement is important to data interpretation, and protein binding information is clearly necessary.

Drug–drug interaction study information will be expected by the reviewer, when such drugs have a high likelihood of being administered together. Studies will be required in which one drug has a demonstrable clinical effect on another. In each of the above instances, presence of data, or adequate explanation as to why it is not necessary, will give the reviewers the information they need to arrive at an intelligent decision. If the reviewer feels that such data should be present to determine the drug's clinical relevance, but finds that it is not, delays will occur while he tries to locate it or requests it via a letter informing the applicant that this is one of the deficiencies resulting in an FDA determination of nonapprovability.

1.1.4 *Drug Metabolism and Preclinical Pharmacology*

In conducting their evaluation, the reviewing pharmacokineticists will be interested in the drug's major active metabolites. These should be identified and quantitated where possible in blood and urine. If they account for a significant portion of the administered dose, pharmacokinetic interaction of the metabolites should be reported. The finding that a major metabolite is active and has a long half-life may suggest a potential for metabolite accumulation following multiple dosing of the drug. In this case, the labeling must reflect the fact that a long half-life active metabolite is present, which may require additional patient monitoring if the dosing regimen is changed.

Although many details of drug biotransformation are necessarily based upon observations in animals, the mechanisms in man are often similar. As this chapter is being written, important discussions are under way in academia, the government, and especially the pharmaceutical industry concerning this area. Such studies performed for toxicological reasons often contain data regarding urinary recovery of parent drug and major metabolites. Radiolabeled drugs are often employed in early preclinical and Phase I clinical studies, since this study method offers an opportunity to obtain material balance as well as early pharmacokinetic information on new drug entities, for example, biological half-life, tissue distribution, and urinary excretion data. Characterization of the drug's metabolic profile will alert the reviewer to the type of data he should seek in conducting his review. When full characterization is not possible, discussion as to why it is not will keep the reviewer from trying to locate the data in other volumes or requesting it in a nonapprovable letter.

We strongly recommended that preliminary human drug metabolism studies be undertaken during the course of tolerance studies. The effort made to identify and quantitate the presence of parent drug and major metabolites should be reported. Obtaining a material balance and defining the pharmacokinetic profile of major metabolites (particularly if the metabolite is suspected to possess pharmacological activity) cannot but strengthen the clinical pharmacokinetic labeling. In certain instances, such findings may suggest the potential for drug metabolite accumulation during multiple dose regimen, or indicate a significant difference in metabolic rate, enterohepatic recycling, or renal tubular reabsorption, all of which must be considered in other clinical studies.

Information concerning the distribution of drug or metabolite(s) (e.g., blood brain barrier, placental drug transfer, etc.) from animal studies and pharmacokinetic modeling studies are of immense importance to some dosage forms and for certain patient populations. The route(s) by which the drug is removed from the body is of fundamental importance in the evaluation of pharmacokinetic data. A discussion of this in relation to drug concentration and metabolism is critical to the evaluation. Data on the relationship of dose to pharmacological effect (when known), especially the intensity of the pharmacological response from increasing doses, is of great value. The relationship between chemical structure and pharmacological activity and between the concentration of drug in blood and successful clinical therapy (MEC), also provides worthwhile information to the reviewer.

1.1.5 *Chemistry*

In their review of the chemistry section, the pharmacokineticists will be interested in both the bulk drug and the drug product. For most drug products, the bulk drug is the active ingredient and the drug product is a finished dosage form, such as tablet, capsule, or solution. (For some, the active ingredient is the drug product as well.) In the former group, the reviewer is concerned with the influence of the formulation on the therapeutic activity of drug product. This involves consideration of the chemical and physical properties of the drug and its dosage formulations, as well as the biological effects observed after administration. It should not be shocking, therefore, that the reviewer would be interested in information such as that listed below.

Bulk Drug	Drug Product
Description	Dissolution
Structure	Formulation
pK_a	Stability
Equilibrium solubility	pH/Solubility profile
pH/Solubility profile	Content uniformity
Stability	Assay methods
Crystal form	In-vitro
pH of a solution	In-vivo
Particle size	
Surface area and density	

Obviously, all of this information will not be pertinent to all products. However, to the extent that it is provided, the easier or more difficult it will be for the reviewer to determine the potential for absorption problems, the likelihood for first pass effect, and so forth. The more information he has, the less chance that the reviewer will go to alternative sources to obtain additional background information on the drugs of this class, which nearly always delays the completion of the review.

Specification of physical-chemical parameters that prevent the formulation of a particular dosage form will alert the reviewer to certain data that requires review and at the same time alleviate the need for other data. For example, very low aqueous solubility could negate use of an aqueous solution, necessitating a suspension in bioavailability studies.

A profile of the solubility of the drug substance as a function of pH (between pH 2.0 and 10) is highly desirable for those drugs whose solubility varies as a function of pH, but it is rarely necessary for water soluble drugs. If the drug has low solubility in aqueous media having physiological significance, then solubility in aqueous ethanol and/or partition coefficient should be given. This information could additionally be used to support the dissolution procedure employed by the manufacturer to provide assurance of lot-to-lot bioequivalence consistency, once bioavailability has been determined.

The pH solubility profile can also be used to determine if there is a drug excipient interaction when compared to the bulk drug. This information becomes important if the product is pH dependent (as opposed to pH independent formulations, which dissolve in the gastrointestinal tract). If the formulation is pH dependent and requires an acidic pH for solution and absorption, the achlorhydric patient population should be either considered by exception in the clinical pharmacokinetic portion of the labeling, or by ancillary data provided to establish the absorption of drug in that subpopulation.

Polymorphism and particle size information are not routinely submitted in an NDA. Nevertheless, their availability for the first FDA evaluation will probably speed approval of future reformulations and affect the type of studies required for such approval. Requests for formulation changes range from total reformulation, including substitution of water insoluble excipients for water soluble ones, to minor changes, wherein a minute amount of one coloring agent is exchanged for another. In the first case, in-vivo study data will be required, whereas (unless there are special circumstances) the latter would not require such data. Consider the pharmacokineticist's position, however, when reviewing formulation changes lying between these extreme examples. Having available information on particle size and/or the existence (or lack) of polymorphism may provide the additional information wherein the reviewer would permit the change on the basis of dissolution data alone.

Chemists outside the Division of Biopharmaceutics are primarily concerned with drug stability problems; an indication of such problems in the presence of light, pH, heat, and moisture, as part of the overall summary, is important to the pharmacokineticist's evaluation of the formulation and its effect in physiological fluids. If polymorphism is present and affects drug bioavailability, the polymorphs should be identified and characterized. Obviously, if bioavailability is significantly affected, then the processes the firm proposes to control the ratio of polymorphs present should be reported.

Information and controls on particle size, surface area, and density will certainly be reviewed. However, summary information reported in the Biopharmaceutics portion of the application will facilitate the application review where special conditions are employed (e.g., if a buffered dissolution media was employed, or if surfactants are employed either in the formulation or in the dissolution media). When dissolution is performed under conditions other than those reflective of in-vivo bioavailability, such as dissolution in an organic solvent or under conditions of high shear, or is not supported by the characteristics of the bulk drug or drug product, the reviewer will want an explanation. The necessity for a reviewer to request additional information or clarification of information almost always results in drug approval delay.

Since drug bioavailability varies with changes in formulation, each ingredient of the drug product must be identified, along with the amount contained per dosage unit. Reproducible in-vitro content uniformity determinations and reproducible dissolution data can be especially convincing in explaining that the variability in observed clinical studies is attributible to intra/inter-subject variation.

1.2 Biopharmaceutics

Although the aforementioned information submitted in summary form will aid the pharmacokineticist's review of the application, the following information should be submitted in detail.

1.2.1 *Background*

This section should allow the reviewer to assess progress of the drug investigation and to determine its status at the time of NDA filing. It is important that all bioavailability, bioequivalence, dose response, and pharmacokinetic studies, including those completed under IND's, be listed in this background section. Pharmacokinetic studies carefully conducted in the early developmental stages provide assurance of known drug delivery during pivotol clinical studies, and should prevent reformulations during the Phase III clinical studies because of poor drug absorption. Since early studies usually employ assays lacking in specificity or precision, less weight should be given to the data obtained, but considerable emphasis should be placed on the data obtained from carefully conducted studies using precise, specific assays. Table 1 is an example of one method of quickly informing the reviewer of the kinds of relevant studies conducted and will allow the reviewer to quickly locate those essential to application approval. Note that the table includes two important areas of evaluation by the firm: type of study and firm's conclusion. If a study conducted during the drug's early developmental stages, using a nonspecific assay, was intended primarily to obtain some indication of the drug's pharmacokinetic parameters, it would be important for the reviewer to know that, lest he spend precious hours of review time to determine that a particular study was unimportant. However, reports of such studies may be important, because they may support one or more marginal studies in the NDA.

We suggest that all submission dates be listed in chronological order, followed by the study number, the type of study, (e.g., pharmacokinetic, bioavailability, dose proportionality, bioequivalence, etc.), a short description of the objective of the study (e.g., a comparison between a tablet vs. solution, tablet vs. capsule, or a dose proportionality study using a solution in a three-way crossover design, etc.), the strength of the products tested, the batch number used in the critical bioavailability studies, indication as to whether the same batch was used in any pivotal clinical studies, and the number of subjects in the study. Such information allows the reviewer to quickly determine whether this should be considered as a pilot study or as something requiring definitive analysis. When the IND or NDA number (which indicates where this information can be located) is accompanied by the firm's conclusions regarding the study and the Agency's response (including the date of correspondence), the reviewer can quickly determine the need for additional review. In the absence of this information, the reviewer will make these determinations on his own; including such a table will result in a quicker and more perceptive review of the application.

The types of studies that could be performed are listed below.

1. Bioequivalence study(ies) generally provide for:
   a. An in-vivo comparison of dosage form(s) used in pivotal clinical study(ies) to the proposed marketed dosage form(s).
   b. An in-vivo comparison of the proposed marketed dosage form(s) (i.e., multiple strengths).
   c. An in-vivo comparison of a proposed generic form to an approved marketed form and/or a solution.
2. Bioavailability study(ies) generally provide for comparison of a proposed marketed dosage form(s) to a reference(s) product (e.g.,

Table 1. Background

Submission date	Study number	Type of study	Dosage form(s) (narrative)	Strength	Batch number	Number of subjects	IND or NDA #	Firm's conclusion	Agency's response and date
12/15/76	BA054	PK	Solution, 50 mg dose	10 mg/ml	ALB186A	6	IND	1st-order kinetics	Acceptable 6/1/77
6/28/78	A01025	BA	Tablet versus solution, crossover, 50 mg dose	50 mg tablets 10 mg/ml	L21465A ALB187A	12	IND	95% bioavailable	Acceptable 12/2/78
3/14/79	D4532	DP	25, 50, 100 mg solution, three-way crossover	10 mg/ml	ALB200A	18	IND	dose proportional	Drug is not dose proportional between 25 and 50 mg Need additional study for labeling. 7/19/79
1/15/80	92	BE	Tablet versus capsule, 50 mg dose	50 mg tablets 50 mg capsules	L21465C Z1564C	18	IND	bioequivalent	Awaiting response

evaluation of a solid dosage form to a reference solution, an intravenous solution, and/or other routes of administration).

3. Dose proportionality study(ies) provide for a determination of the linearity of in-vivo response over the dosing range proposed in labeling.
4. Dissolution of solid oral dosage form(s) studies provide for:
   a. Dissolution profiles of all solid dosage form(s) used in pivotal clinical studies.
   b. Dissolution profiles of all solid dosage strength(s) and forms proposed for marketing.
   c. Evaluation of (a) and (b) with respect to similarity and/or deviations from the proposed marketed product.

Other additional studies conducted during drug development include:

1. *Multiple dose studies.* Studies conducted to demonstrate that steady state drug plasma and/or other biological fluid concentrations can be predicted from single dose.
2. *Nonlinear kinetic studies.* Steady state studies conducted to describe the effects of nonlinear kinetics in the body at steady state where single dose studies indicate the possibility of Michaelis–Menten kinetics.
3. *Specific patient populations/diseased state studies.* Studies conducted in a particular patient population, whether a disease state or an age group (e.g., pediatrics, geriatrics). For instance, the effect of renal disease (i.e., reduced glomerular filtration rate) should be described for drugs extensively cleared by the kidney.
4. *Effect of food.* Studies conducted to support labeling claims concerning administration with food.
5. *Drug–drug interaction studies.* Studies conducted where drugs are indicated for coadministration to a significant portion of the population. (Time dependent kinetics, such as induction and clearance changes, fall under 1 and 2 above.)
6. *Drug comparability study.* Study similar to bioequivalence study, except that the purpose is to demonstrate the lack of equivalence of two formulations.

The assay methods for all dissolution testing should be described, as well as appropriate validation of the assay method. Since the drug and/or metabolite concentrations in biological fluids are the basis of drug bioavailability, the analytical method used to determine these concentrations in the definitive in-vivo studies should be described giving, where necessary, data establishing the assay sensitivity, specificity, linearity, and reproducibility. When more than one assay was employed, a statement could be advanced that Assay #1 was used in in-vivo studies 1 through 5, whereas Assay #2 was used in in-vivo studies numbered 6 through 10, and so forth. If there are differences in specificity, sensitivity, reproducibility, and linearity between the assays, a comparison of similarities as well as differences would obviously save the reviewer time he/she would otherwise spend trying to make such comparisons.

1.2.2 *Bioavailability/Bioequivalence Studies*

The type of bioequivalence study varies depending upon such factors as:

1. The date that the original product was first marketed.
2. Whether an in-vivo test was required on the basis of the following six criteria:
    a. Clinical evidence that such drug products do not give comparable therapeutic effects.
    b. Biopharmaceutic evidence that such drug products are not bioequivalent.
    c. Evidence that the drug products exhibit a narrow therapeutic ratio.
    d. Medical determination that a lack of bioequivalence would have an adverse effect on the treatment or prevention of a serious disease or condition.
    e. Physical chemical evidence that:
        i. The drug has low solubility in water (less than 5 mg/ml), or if dissolution in the stomach is critical to absorption, the volume of gastric fluid required to dissolve the recommended dose far exceeds the volume of fluids present in the stomach.
        ii. The dissolution rate of one or more such products is slow.
        iii. The particle size and/or surface area of the drug is critical to bioavailability.
        iv. Physical structural characteristics of the drug (e.g., polymorphic forms, conforms, solvates, complexes, and crystal modifications) dissolve poorly, and such poor dissolution may affect absorption.

   v. Drug product has a high ratio of excipients to active ingredients.
   vi. Presence of specific inactive ingredients (e.g., hydrophobic or hydrophilic excipients and lubricants) are required for drug absorption or conversely interfere with it.

f. Pharmacokinetic evidence that:

   i. The drug or its precursor is absorbed in large part in a particular segment of the gastrointestinal tract or from a localized site.
   ii. The degree of absorption (compared to an intravenous dose) is poor.
   iii. Presence of first pass metabolism.
   iv. Rapid drug metabolism or excretion.
   v. The drug is unstable in specific portions of the gastrointestinal tract and requires special coatings or formulations.
   vi. The drug product is subject to dose dependent kinetics in or near the therapeutic range.

3. Criteria met by previous manufacturers.

With rare exception, the FDA has not required bioequivalence data on products when it has been determined that the first product was marketed prior to 1938. For those drug products evaluated in the Drug Efficacy Study Implementation (DESI), first marketed between 1938 and 1962 on the basis of safety data, and later determined as being both safe and efficacious, the biopharmaceutic basis of generic drug product approval is listed below:

1. An in-vivo test in humans.
2. An in-vivo test in animsls other than humans that has been correlated with human in-vivo data.
3. An in-vivo test in animals other than humans that has not been correlated with human in-vivo data.
4. An in-vitro bioequivalence standard, i.e., an in-vitro test that has been correlated with human in-vivo bioavailability data.
5 A currently available in-vitro test (usually a dissolution rate test) that has not been correlated with human in-vivo bioavailability data.

Within the meaning of the regulation, the following in-vivo approaches, in descending order of accuracy and sensitivity, are acceptable where such testing employed the most accurate, sensitive, and reproducible approach available.

1. In-vivo testing in humans in which the concentration of the therapeutic moiety and/or its metabolites in whole blood, plasma, serum, or other appropriate biological fluid is measured as a function of time, or in which the urinary excretion of the therapeutic moiety and/or its metabolites is measured as a function of time. This approach is particularly applicable to dosage forms intended to deliver the therapeutic moiety to the blood stream for systemic distribution within the body, such as injectable drugs, most oral dosage forms, most suppositories, certain drugs administered by inhalation, and some drugs administered by local application to mucous membranes.
2. In-vivo testing in humans in which an acute pharmacological effect of the therapeutic moiety is measured as a function of time, where such effect can be measured with sufficient sensitivity and is reproducible. This approach has been successfully employed when analytical methods are not available for measuring the concentration of the therapeutic moiety or its metabolites in biological fluids, but a method is available for measuring an acute pharmacological effect.
3. Well-controlled clinical trials in humans that establish the effectiveness of the drug product. This approach is almost always the least sensitive of the general approaches for demonstrating in-vivo bioavailability in humans. The authors do not recommend this approach, not only because it is insensitive, but also because it is much more expensive.
4. Any other in-vivo approach approved by the FDA. This provision is intended for special situations and includes those in which the in-vivo bioavailability of the drug product might be determined in a suitable animal model rather than in humans, or by using a radioactive or nonradioactive isotopically labeled drug product.

Since the regulations state that bioavailability/bioequivalence testing will be conducted using the most accurate and sensitive approach available, it would be wise to prepare the reviewer by explaining why a particular analytical procedure was employed. When the procedure is nonspecific, the authors recommend that applicants, prior to the presentation of their data, explain why a nonspecific assay was employed. Since the FDA pharmacokineticist cannot be aware of the state-of-the-art for each of the many drugs under review prior to initiating his evaluation, such an explanation will bring him quickly up to speed, and will prevent him from needlessly (where justification exists) searching for a better procedure.

The in-vivo bioavailability/bioequivalence of a drug product is demonstrated if the product's rate and extent of absorption, as determined by comparison of measured parameters (e.g., concentration of the active drug ingredient in the blood, urinary excretion rates, or pharmacological effects), do not indicate a *significant difference* from the reference material's rate and extent of absorption. The usually accepted reference product for a bioequivalence study is a marketed product (pharmaceutical equivalent) that is the subject of a New Drug Application. Recently, because of bioavailability problems associated with some of the approved marketed products, the FDA has been recommending two reference products: the use of a solution as well as the marketed approved brand.

A drug product that differs from the reference material in its rate, but not its extent, of absorption, is considered to be bioavailable if (*1*) the difference in the rate of absorption is intentional and appropriately reflected in the labeling, and/or (*2*) the difference in the rate of absorption is not detrimental to the safety and effectiveness of the drug product.

The FDA, of course, requires that the statistical techniques used be of sufficient sensitivity to detect differences in the rate and extent of absorption that are not attributable to subject variability.

1.2.3 *Dose Proportionality Studies*

One purpose of dose proportionality studies is to demonstrate the linearity (or lack of it) within the dosage range. This is best accomplished by using the most bioavailable dosage form for a particular route of administration, for example, a solution in the case of oral administration. A second purpose is to demonstrate adequate bioavailability of some, if not all, strengths of a particular dosage form. Although appropriate dissolution data may be acceptable for generic versions of many drugs where the drug content and excipients maintain the same ratio and where bioavailability data has been supplied on one strength, in-vivo data will usually be required for new chemical entities or where the drug-excipient content ratio varies. In either case, the applicant should clearly establish the basis for the studies performed, so as to enable the reviewer to make a quick determination about the adequacy of the study design.

1.2.4 *Statistical Consideration*

Statistical designs usually reviewed by the FDA include:

1. *Two-way crossover study*. In general this design can be used to compare a test product with a reference product.

2. *Three-way crossover study*. This general design can be used to compare a test product, reference product, and a readily available dosage form (e.g., oral solution). This design is especially useful when there is doubt about the acceptability of a reference product, and when inter-subject variation is expected to be large.
3. *Four-way and larger crossover studies*. These designs are generally useful for comparing multiple test products to readily available dosage forms. These designs offer direct comparisons of many test products, but require a very stable and dependable subject population for the successful completion of a study.
4. *Parallel studies*. Parallel studies are recommended when long periods of time would be required between test periods, if a crossover design was employed, and when changes in the subject's pharmacokinetic and/or physiologic parameters could be anticipated.
5. *Balanced incomplete block designs*. These designs are useful in some cases instead of resorting to parallel designs, or for very large crossover studies (e.g., those used to access the bioequivalency of five or more dosage forms).

When studying drugs whose bioavailability has not been previously reported in the literature, it is strongly recommended that a pilot study be initiated to determine the number of subjects necessary to provide sufficient power for evaluation.

The statistical analysis for a typical crossover design should include the following:

ANOVA with partitioning of effects, for example,

Typical Crossover Design

Source of Variation	Degrees of Freedom
Total	$KN-1$
Subjects	$N-1$
Treatments	$K-1$
Periods	$K-1$
Error	$(K-1)(N-2)$

where K = the number of treatments (equal to the number of phases) and N = the number of subjects in the study.

The use of Paired T test comparisons is *not* adequate to evaluate data when a crossover design is used, because it fails to consider period effects. In addition, the FDA would prefer a general linear model that includes treatments, subject, and period as the main effects, as well as any interaction effects where appropriate.

The FDA reviewer first determines whether the study is able to detect a significant difference of 20% at an alpha=0.05 and beta=0.2. This rule (Power Test) is suitable for most drugs. However, some drugs (among them the Beta Blockers) present problems in this regard because of large intersubject variabilities. Studies of more than 100 subjects would be required to meet the "power rule" for these drugs. The rule also has a shortcoming associated with the determination of the proper number of subjects to be used. When too many subjects are used, the test may indicate a statistically significant difference between a test and reference product, even though the two drug products are bioequivalent.

The use of a 95% symmetrical confidence interval of the test formulation around the reference standard has been suggested. Under this procedure, the test product would be required to fall within an interval of 0.80–1.2 of the reference product. One advantage of this method is that increasing the number of subjects makes determinations of bioequivalence easier, provided there is indeed no difference between the products tested. Although this has not found favor with FDA reviewers, evaluation of the data by this procedure is recommended by the authors as an ancillary technique where study coefficients of variation become rather large, since it provides the reviewer with additional important information useful in making a final decision.

When more than 24 subjects are used in a two-period crossover study, and a 20% difference cannot be obtained with an alpha of 0.05 and beta of 0.2, consideration should be given to employing FDA's 75/75 rule. According to this rule, at least 75% of the subjects administered the test drug will have a bioavailability of at least 75% and no greater than 125%, relative to that of the administered reference material, utilizing each subject as their own control. The analytical and statistical techniques used will be of sufficient sensitivity to detect differences in rate and extent of absorption that are not attributable to subject variability. Although the use of this test by the FDA has recently been criticized, a retrospective study, using data files generated under the Division of Biopharmaceutics Contract Program, demonstrated that the rule holds for coefficients of variation less than 40%. For those rare cases where coefficients of variation are larger than 40%, the FDA reviewer will consider all the blood and urine data and each of the above statistical evaluations.

The use of this rule will not eliminate the comparison of a test product to a readily bioavailable dosage form, when the reference product is found to be unacceptable as a reference. Consideration should also be given to the use of stable isotopes for highly variable drugs. The Agency has determined through its own studies that as few as four subjects would be required to perform a bioavailability study using the relative area and/or relative peak concentration by the stable isotope approach employing concomitant nonlabel drug and label drug administration, when in excess of 24 subjects using conventional assays failed to do so.

1.2.5 *Pharmacokinetic Modeling*

Pharmacokinetics, which is usually defined as the study of the time course of drug and metabolite(s) levels in different fluids, tissues, and excreta of the body, also includes the mathematical relationships required to develop models that permit data interpretation.

For most pharmacokinetic/bioavailability/bioequivalance studies, consideration should be given to using normal healthy adult (preferrably male) subjects unless the drug is designed specifically for female, pediatric, or geriatric patients. In these cases, consideration should be given to gearing the study population toward the specified patient population. Since the number of subjects to be included in the study depends on the variability of the drug, it may be necessary to conduct some pilot studies. The degree of confidence in estimating the pharmacokinetic parameters is the important consideration in pharmacokinetic studies, rather than the number of subjects, since the pharmacokinetic parameter derived from the study will be used to predict drug concentrations in-vivo.

After administration of the drug, blood samples should be collected from the subjects to characterize the blood profiles of the parent drug and its therapeutically active metabolites over a period of 3–4 half-lives, as determined by the drug/active metabolite species having the longest half-life. Consideration should be given to collecting urine and saliva samples that could provide important collaborative information on drug elimination, metabolism, and distribution.

From the blood profiles of the parent drug and its active metabolites, experimental values of $C_{\max}$, $T_{\max}$, and AUC (by trapezoidal rule) from each of the drug species should be compared among treatments to determine drug bioavailability. Careful consideration should be given to the method of estimating the theoretical pharmacokinetic parameters. Compartmental model fittings, using computer programs such as AUTOAN, NONLIN, SAAM, and prophet are well-known and easily interpreted. Basic mathematical equations and pharmacokinetic parameters associated with each linear model should be presented for the reviewers consideration. If a time lag exists, then all t's presented in equations should be replaced by '$t-t_0$'s before the fitting is processed.

Computer programs AUTOAN, NONLIN, and SAAM are written in Fortan IV and are used for pharmacokinetic model fitting and data analysis. AUTOAN–NONLIN is designed specifically for choosing the best fitted model and the corresponding pharmacokinetic parameters. SAAM is not capable of model selection, but is able to fit and simulate more sophisticated pharmacokinetic models than those in the AUTOAN library.

AUTOAN–NONLIN. This package provides adequate pharmacokinetic analysis of blood profiles after inputting blood data and route of drug administration. AUTOAN executes all operations normally performed during manual pharmacokinetic analysis including:

1. Evaluating the type of elimination kinetics (whether drug elimination is best described by nonlinear or linear mechanisms or by first order kinetics, etc.).
2. Estimating the number of exponential terms by sequential stripping or peeling of the blood profile beginning at the terminal phase.
3. Selecting pharmacokinetic models based on the number of exponential terms that best describe the blood profiles.
4. Estimating the initial values of the various kinetic parameters.

Based on the information obtained from AUTOAN, the subsequent NONLIN program is able to use the Gauss-Newton iterative method to find the least-square estimate of the various parameters associated with the model.

At present, the AUTOAN library has 10 sets of linear one- and two-compartment models described by no more than three exponential terms, and four sets of nonlinear one-compartment models where the Michaelis–Menten kinetic is operative only in the process of drug elimination.

SAAM. Because SAAM contains no program to handle model selection and initial parameter estimation, these two steps are done manually or by AUTOAN, prior to using SAAM. The advantage of SAAM is its ability to simulate and fit kinetic models under various situations, provided that a solution exists. Consequently, models involving any number of compartments, nonlinear and/or linear kinetics, time delay, forcing functions, and a deconvolution function can all be processed through SAAM. If SAAM is not available, the fittings can still be done by incorporating suitable model equations in Fortran statements into the NONLIN program.

2. GENERAL APPROACH FOR DETERMINING IN-VIVO BIOEQUIVALENCE/BIOAVAILABILITY

FDA pharmacokineticists routinely approach their review according to the categories listed below. Although dissolution data is listed separately, it is a fundamental part of all solid oral dosage form bioavailability and bioequivalence evaluations.

2.1 Bioavailability Studies

Bioavailability studies are required by the FDA when the drug product meets one or more of the following conditions:

1. The drug product is a subject of the bioavailability requirement.
2. The sponsor wishes to market a new drug product that is not the subject of an approved new drug application.
3. The sponsor makes a change in the manufacturing process, or manufacturing site for a dosage form, or in dosage strength different from the drug product that is the subject of an approved new drug application.
4. The sponsor makes a change in the labeling to provide for a new dosage regimen or for an additional dosage regimen for a special patient population (e.g., infants, children, etc.) if clinical studies are required to support the new or additional dosage regimen.

Bioavailability may be determined by several direct or indirect in-vivo methods, generally involving testing in humans. The selection of the method depends upon the purpose of the study, the analytical method available, and the nature of the drug product. These limitations affect the degree to which precise pharmacokinetic studies can be applied, and in some cases necessitate the use of other methods. As with bioequivalence, the regulations require that bioavailability testing be conducted using the most accurate, sensitive, and reproducible approach available.

2.2 Dose Proportionality Studies

Dose proportionality or linearity in pharmacokinetic systems can be defined by a direct proportionality of transfer rates between compartments to concentrations within those compartments. This proportionality is a characteristic of first order kinetics. Several features indicate the presence of linearity or first order kinetics in a pharmacokinetic model: (*1*) the area under the concentration versus time curve is proportional to the administered dose; (*2*) the amount of drug eliminated is proportional to the dose; and (*3*) the time required to remove half the remaining drug from the body is constant. Other parameters remain constant in linear or first order systems, including the fraction of drug reaching the general circulation, the percent of drug bound to plasma proteins, renal and total body clearances, and the ratio of amount of drug in tissue, saliva, or other body fluids to the amount of drug in the blood.

Since any or all of the characteristics mentioned above may be influenced by enzyme or carrier-mediated systems, the processes have a finite capacity or maximum velocity, and can therefore be referred to as saturable or capacity limited. When the maximum capacity of one or more of these processes is approached, the linearity of the system is altered and transfer rates are no longer proportional to the dose. A pharmacokinetic model in which one or more of the transfer processes can be saturated is a nonlinear model.

It is also possible that enzyme-mediated processes governing the transfer of drug into or out of compartments may be enhanced or induced. The process of enzyme-induction, which is primarily a time dependent function, is influenced by previous drug administration and causes deviation from proportionality between doses.

The one area reviewed most critically by FDA pharmacokineticists involves possible evidence of lack of dose proportionality in the therapeutic dosing range. The authors suggest that where such data exist, close attention to the data be paid by the applicant in the discussion.

The dose proportionality study report should contain: (*1*) a brief summary description of the drug, its intended clinical use, and its potential clinical advantages; any background information about its pharmacokinetics or metabolism should introduce the protocol (a brief summary of previous meetings with FDA where the general design of the study was outlined and any pertinent regulatory history should be included; and (*2*) the purpose of conducting an in-vivo dose proportionality study (generally to determine the pharmacokinetics of the drug at a minimum of three dosage levels).

3. GUIDELINES FOR IN-VIVO STUDIES IN HUMANS

The objective of the study should be stated explicity and the purpose of conducting the study should be clearly established lest the reviewer try to make more of your data than you intended.

1. *Principal investigator*. The person responsible for the conduct of the

study, and the safety and welfare of the subjects participating in the study, should be identified. Any coinvestigators should also be listed in the protocol.

2. *Clinical/analytical facilities.* The suitability for the proposed study of clinics, hospitals, private offices, or other facilities, or location from one in which subjects may be secured and/or followed in the course of the study, should be set forth. Because most of the study data rejected by the FDA has been rejected on the basis of deficiencies in the area of analytical chemistry, the qualification requirements of laboratories to be performing tests should be determined prior to initiation of the study. It is advisable that provision be made for determining the accuracy and precision of any routine baseline or entry tests done for the study through established voluntary programs (e.g., National Accrediting Agency for Clinical Laboratory Sciences). In addition "unknowns," replications, and so forth, should be conducted throughout the study to establish daily consistency or lack of column breakdown done in conjunction with the study.

3. *Institutional Review Boards (IRB's).* There should be a discussion of the specific requirements of the study for institutional review, periodic review, and evidence of the patient's informed consent. The procedures of study should be explained to the volunteers, together with the potential hazards involving drug allergies and adverse reactions. Informed consent should be obtained in writing. Each volunteer should be assured that they are entirely free to withdraw from participation in the study at any time.

4. *Experimental plans.*

   a. Subject selection. Although normal healthy subjects are ordinarily selected, patients may also be used. The source of the volunteers (i.e., healthy subjects or patients) should be specified (e.g., in-house personnel, convicts, students, in-patients, out-patients, etc.). Where studies may last for some time, the authors recommend that the potential volunteers be screened for their availability for the duration of the study.

   In the case of healthy volunteers, nonobese, adult volunteers with no history of gastrointestinal, hepatic, renal, and/or hematological disease should be eligible for participation in the study. Subjects with a history of chronic alcohol consumption should not be eligible. In the ideal situation, subjects should be 21–50 years of age and should not greatly deviate from their ideal weight as described in the Metropolitan Insurance Company's Height and Weight Tables, 1983. Subjects should have normal vital signs and present normal values for certain clinical tests. These tests should include, but not be limited to hematocrit, hemoglobin, WBC, differential, BUN, creatinine, alkaline phosphase, SGOT, total bilirubin, and urinalysis (plus microscopic). Particular emphasis should be placed on normal renal and hepatic functions. Subjects with test values outside of the normal range, which are confirmed on reexamination, should generally not be eligible to participate in the study. For certain drugs, additional tests could include creatinine clearance, EKG, and so forth.

When other than healthy volunteers are utilized, their use should be characterized and the criteria for selecting them described. A medical history should be submitted for all patients indicating current or recent medications. Where patients may be used, there should be consideration of concurrent diseases that should be excluded because they may mask or confuse the conditions required to assess the drug, or because the medications taken will prevent assessment of the drug.

When the drug is primarily designed to be used in women, the study should be performed in females. In certain instances (e.g., pediatrics), studies must be performed in children to support pediatric labeling.

Except for the drug under study, normal subjects should not have received any other medication including OTC for a period of 7 days prior to testing. They should not have received any similar drug to the drug under study for 15 days or more, depending on the biological half-life of the drug.

In the case of patients, if any concurrent drugs are permitted, the conditions under which they may be used should be carefully defined. If concurrent medication is permitted, the patient should be in approximately steady state condition and should not deviate from his usual therapy during the entire study. Patients receiving drugs that potentially may cause drug interaction should be avoided, unless the purpose is specifically to study the possibility of drug–drug interaction.

b. Study design. A randomized crossover design offers many advantages in that each subject is his own control. They are generally used, unless a parallel design or other design is more appropriate for valid scientific reasons. The drug elimination period should be either at least 3 times the half-life of the active drug ingredient or therapeutic moiety or its metabolites measured in the blood or urine, or at least 3 times the half-life of decay of the acute pharmacological effect if crossover design is employed;

no less than 7 half-lives washout period should be allowed between the treatments.

c. Products tested. The formulation and the planned batch or lot size of the test product(s), and whether it will be a pilot lot or production lot, should be identified. If the reference product is another manufacturer's product or a different batch of the sponsor's product, the lot(s) should be identified. In addition, to rule out the unanticipated problem that occurs when the test product shows much greater bioavailability than the reference product, the use of a solution is strongly encouraged.

d. Proper physiochemical tests. The protocol should specify what in-vitro tests the sponsor plans to do for the test drug products and the reference standards products. Content uniformity and, where applicable, disintegration tests and dissolution tests for drug products are required in the final reports.

e. Drug administration. Ordinarily, for an orally administered dosage form, the drug should be given under fasting conditions. The subject should be fasted overnight (at least 10 hours) prior to and for 4 hours after dosing, unless it is scientifically or medically necessary to give the drug on a postprandial state. Beverages such as coffee, milk, and diet drinks, are generally not permitted during the first period.

f. Observations. Chemical measurement of drug and/or metabolites: where blood and/or urine assays are to be the only measurements, the biological samples should ordinarily be assayed employing a crossover design to safeguard against malfunctioning or period interaction. Although not always possible, and in a number of situations not recommended, the test samples submitted for laboratory analysis are blinded as to the drug being tested. It would be very helpful to the reviewer to know the procedure employed as well as the reason behind it.

When analytical methodology is either totally lacking, chemically nonspecific, or less precise than pharmacological or physiological endpoints (e.g., heart rate, blood pressure, pupillometry changes, etc.), these parameters may be used provided the drug response can be quantified with adequate accuracy and precision. Generally, a dose response should be established for the drug, and it should be possible to measure the onset and duration of activity of the test drug compared to the reference drug. The protocol should document the adequacy of the pharmacological endpoint to detect clinically significant differences in bioavailability.

When applicable, data elements should be considered in two categories:

i. Those observations recorded as entry requirements and not intended to be used in the actual analysis.
ii. Those observations recorded as critical basic measurements and intended to be used in the final analysis.

If blood and/or urine samples of drug and/or metabolites are collected, the time schedule of these collections in relationship to the time(s) of drug administration(s), as well as to meals, fluid intake, and activities should be outlined. If applicable, the nature, timing, and amounts of food and fluid intake and exercise should be specified.

Whenever possible, active metabolites should be identified and quantitated in blood and/or urine.

The protocol and/or study report should discuss the plans for the collection of blood and urine samples, including when and how samples will be processed and stored.

Blood samples should be drawn from each subject receiving the test and reference drug product just before dosing and again at specified time intervals, which will adequately describe the absorption and elimination phases of the drug. The exact times for sample collection will depend on the nature of the drug and its dosage form; usually 8–10 samples need to be taken over a period of 3–4 biological half-lives of the drug. Three or four collections should be made during the rising phase of the blood levels profile. Provisions should be made to record and report the actual clock times when samples are drawn, as well as the elapsed time related to drug administration.

Generally, plasma or serum, depending on the specific need of the analytical procedure, should be separated from each blood sample as soon as possible after collection and, if not assayed immediately, be quickly frozen and stored at deep freeze temperature (−20°C). Specimens requiring shipment over long distances from clinic to laboratory should be packed in sufficient dry ice to insure keeping them frozen in transit. In dealing with drugs that are relatively unstable, plasma samples can be cooled immediately in an ice bath prior to centrifugation. In certain instances, whole blood may be required (e.g., for drugs bound to red blood cells), and in specific cases preservatives may be required to insure drug stability.

Urine should be collected prior to drug administration and

during specified time intervals thereafter over three to four biological half-lives of the drug so as to enable elimination rate determination, and to adequately compute (by kinetics) the asymptotic value or demonstrate that the cumulative excretion curve has reached an asymptotic value. Urine volume, creatinine levels, and, if pertinent, pH should generally be measured for each collection period and the data reported together with the drug and/or metabolite assay results. Storage precautions for urine samples should be as carefully thought out as those for blood samples. Whenever feasible, urinary creatinine results should be used to verify completeness of collections and to eliminate data on samples from outside the ranges established in the protocol.

Generally, each subject should be questioned at least once following each medication about whether he experienced any side effects or adverse reactions attributable to the medication. The occurrence or the absence of any such effects should be part of the final report.

Definitive criteria establishing a priori, the conditions under which a subject or patient would be removed from a study (i.e., in the event of an adverse reaction that warrants removal), should be clearly explained. This does not include drop-outs, but provisions should be made to contact lost volunteers to ascertain why they did not return and their subsequent course. Records of the follow-up efforts should be part of the sponsor's records. Any treatment required by a volunteer owing to an adverse reaction should also be part of the record. The circumstances that would require following the course of any or all volunteers after they have been in the study should be considered.

The procedure for replacing a volunteer should also be discussed, in terms of how the data from both the original subject (or patient) and the replacement will be treated, to minimize biasing the results. The protocol should contain a justification of the decision to use or not to use incomplete or partial data, from the standpoint of the bias that such a decision may introduce.

Where subjects have been dropped or added, reference to the protocol procedures should be cited to facilitate quick review. Otherwise, the reviewer will look up the appropriate IND to assure himself that preferred procedures have been followed. Such reviews take additional time, given that the particular volume could be quickly located in the Bureau. When it cannot be readily located, additional delays occur.

The circumstances surrounding an early termination or an extension of the study should be discussed (i.e., if p value is established before the projected number of patients is used, or if p will not be established with the particular experimental design or projected number of patients). The guiding principles should be to maximize productive and minimize unproductive or unnecessary human experimentation. It should be outlined with particular attention in the latter case as to how the study data will be analyzed.

The analytical method used in an in-vivo bioequivalence study to measure the concentration of the active drug ingredient, therapeutic moiety, or its metabolites in body fluid or excretory products, or the method used to measure an acute pharmacological effect, should be demonstrated to be accurate and of sufficient sensitivity to measure, with appropriate precision, the actual concentration of the active drug ingredient, therapeutic moiety, or its metabolites achieved in the body.

Although a published method may be referenced, the specific details of the analytical procedure for estimating the concentration of drug and/or its metabolites in the biological specimens should be furnished if they are not clearly and completely discussed in the reference. Because of different laboratory capabilities, the FDA reviewers will insist that the laboratory assigned to assay the biological samples demonstrate that the analytical method has the required specificity, sensitivity, and linearity at the concentration of drug and/or metabolite anticipated in the test specimens. In dealing with active metabolites of approximate equal activity, the use of combined assays may be justified if methodology for the parent drug is totally lacking.

All data that supports the assay method regarding recovery, standard assay curves, and so forth, should be included in the NDA. Whenever possible, recovery samples should be included with the test samples to assure drug assay reliability.

In dealing with drugs that are susceptible to assay interference from dietary intake or commonly used drugs, the investigator should take precautions to rule out such interfering agents by adequately monitoring the volunteers and assaying the predrug samples.

The authors recommend that the following pharmacokinetic parameters be computed from each individual's data when blood samples are collected: AUC, $C_{\max}$, $T_{\max}$, relative bioavailability, and urinary excretion (if applicable).

When feasible, the use of pharmacokinetic models and equations is encouraged. The pharmacokinetic models and equations should be described and referenced. The pharmacokinetic parameters, such as absorption rate constant (k_a), elimination rate constant (K), elimination half-lifes ($T_{1/2}$), volume of distribution (Vd), lag time ($T_{\log}$), and AUC should be determined.

5. *Results.* The study report should contain:

i. Each subject's raw data and computed pharmacokinetic parameters.

ii. Summary data (i.e., mean and standard deviation) for the plasma and/or urine level profile or any other appropriate observations and pertinent pharmacokinetic parameters for each treatment.

iii. A statistical report.

6. *Conclusion.* A brief paragraph summarizing the pertinent conclusion from the study. With multiple dose studies, whenever comparison of the test product and the reference material is based on blood concentration–time curves at steady state, sufficient samples of blood should be taken to define adequately the minimum ($C_{\min}$) blood concentrations on three or more consecutive days, using each individual subject as his control, to establish that steady state conditions are achieved. The individual subject during a dosing interval must be at steady state.

Whenever comparison of the test product and the reference material is to be based on cumulative urinary excretion–time curves at steady state, sufficient samples of urine should be taken to define the rate and extent of urinary excretion on three or more consecutive days, to establish that steady state conditions are achieved.

CHAPTER 7

Computer Resolution of Bioavailability and Pharmacokinetic Data from Recorded Physiological Signals Exemplified for Organic Nitrates

VICTOR F. SMOLEN
DANIEL B. TUEY

PharmaControl Corporation
Englewood Cliffs, New Jersey

CONTENTS

Measures of the activity of hypotensives, hypoglycemics, antiglaucoma agents, mydriatics, miotics, adrenergics, and anticoagulants can be obtained directly from blood pressure, blood glucose, intraocular pressure, pupil size, heart rate, and clotting times, respectively. That such measures can be used for quantitative pharmacokinetic analysis and the computation of absolute bioavailabilities has been demonstrated. The growing sophistication of biomedical recording instrumentation and methods of computerized analysis of biologic signals is providing a concomitantly increasing capability for quantitating drug effects when such direct measures do not apply. This is accomplished through the computerized resolution of drug-induced time variations in the characteristics of the signals. The final results of the analysis of drug-affected biosignals are presented as pharmacokinetic response profiles that resemble blood level versus time curves. Often, several response variables versus time profiles can be resolved from the recording of a single signal, such as evoked and spontaneous electroencephalography (EEG), electrocardiography (ECG), plethysmography, electroenterogastrography (EEnG), electromyography (EMG), displacement cardiography (DCG), and phonocardiography (PCG).

A Drug Effectiveness Study Implementation (DESI) of organic nitrates, by the FDA (3, 36) resulted in a classification of oral and controlled release formulations as only possibly effective. This classification was a consequence of clinical studies that produced conflicting and inconclusive results because of the large variability in response seen with the patients tested, and the relative insensitivity of clinical endpoints. A Federal Register notice issued by the FDA approved and recommended the pharmacological response monitoring procedures described herein, which quantitate drug-induced physiologic changes underlying the clinical effectiveness of organic nitrate antianginal drug products by recording noninvasive biologic signals as a valid method for assessing their bioavailability and pharmacological effectiveness (3).

1. DEVELOPMENT OF THE METHOD

This investigation was initiated with the intent that, if success were achieved with sublingual nitroglycerin, the methodology could also be employed to evaluate the controversial bioavailability and effectiveness of drugs such as isosorbide dinitrate and pentaerythritol tetranitrate; the pharmacological effectiveness and bioavailability of sustained action or "long-acting" dosage forms are of special interest, since these particular products are most susceptible to bioavailability problems (1). When more than one simultaneously occurring drug effect is monitored for such purposes, the use of pharmacological data, relative to direct assay data, has the added advantage that bioavailability differences suspected on the basis of a single response can be further corroborated by the other, simultaneously monitored, responses. Comparisons of time profiles for different drug effects can also provide insights into the mechanisms operative in reducing systemic drug bioavailability from oral drug products (20).

Sublingual nitroglycerin (NG) was chosen as an exemplary drug product for developing a physiological response methodology, suitable for assessing the bioavailability and pharmacological effectiveness of organic nitrate products, because sublingual nitroglycerin provokes pronounced hemodynamic changes and is generally effective in the treatment of angina pectoris. Moreover, in sublingual nitroglycerin dosing, the quantity of administered nitroglycerin is small (0.3–1.2 mg); the resulting nitroglycerin blood levels are low, and because of the rapid elimination of the drug (2), it is difficult to sample the blood with a frequency that is compatible with the construction of accurate pharmacokinetic profiles.

1.1 Experimental Design

All of the dosage forms used in the study were provided by the FDA and each dosage form was certified to conform to compendial or other appropriate standards (Table 1). The experimental design consistently employed was a duplicated balanced 6×6 Latin square. Prior to beginning the Latin square experiments, each subject was given a preliminary sublingual 0.3 mg nitroglycerin screening dose to detect any hypersensitivity to nitroglycerin. These preliminary screening experiments also acclimated the subjects to the test routine. In some of the Latin squares, sublingual nitroglycerin was tested in conjunction with oral dosage forms of nitroglycerin and other organic nitrate drugs. A placebo dose was always included in each Latin square, along with a 0.6 mg nitroglycerin reference dose. Each dose treatment was separated from the subsequent dose treatment by a one-week washout period.

1.2 Subject Selection

All candidates for participation in the study were interviewed by a psychiatrist to exclude subjects with potential psychological or drug abuse problems. All subjects were male volunteers, 21–35 years old, and each was required to read and execute an informed consent statement approved by the FDA Committee on Human Experimentation. A staff nurse took a family and personal medical history from each volunteer; any history of serious or chronic illness or allergy immediately disqualified him from further consider-

Table 1. Listing of Organic Nitrate Drug Products Received from the FDA and Studied in Human Subjects

Drug[a]	Dosage Form	Trade Name	Manufacturer	Lot Number	Date Received
NG	0.3 mg sublingual tablets	Nitrostat	Parke-Davis	RJ131	1/5/75
NG	0.4 mg sublingual tablets	NitroPRN	Warner/Chilcott	4911094A	3/15/76
NG	2.6 mg sustained action tablets[b]	Nitroglyn	Key Pharmaceuticals, Inc.	56221	12/19/75
NG	6.5 mg sustained action tablets[b]	Nitroglyn	Key Pharmaceuticals, Inc.	56201	12/19/75
ISDN	2.5 mg sublingual tablets	Isordil Sublingual	Ives Laboratories	1750321	4/30/75
ISDN	5.0 mg sublingual tablets	Isordil Sublingual	Ives Laboratories	1742248	4/30/75
ISDN	10.0 mg oral tablets	Isordil Oral	Ives Laboratories	1750162	4/30/75
ISDN	40.0 mg sustained action tablets	Isordil Tembids	Ives Laboratories	1750337	4/30/75
ISDN[b]	5.0 mg chewable tablets	Chewable Sorbitrate	ICI United States, Inc.	188DB	5/13/75
ISDN[b]	5.0 mg sublingual tablets	Sublingual Sorbitrate	ICI United States, Inc.	174DB	5/13/75
PETN	10.0 mg tablets	Peritrate	Warner/Chilcott	006P065C	10/8/75
PETN	20.0 mg tablets	Peritrate	Warner/Chilcott	0053P065C	10/8/75
PETN	80.0 mg sustained action tablets	Peritrate SA	Warner/Chilcott	2032V065A	10/8/75

[a]NG—Nitroglycerine; ISDN—isosorbide dinitrate; PETN—pentaerythritol tetranitrate.
[b]Received from ICI United States.

ation. The candidate then received a complete physical examination, which included a fasting blood chemistry, electrocardiogram, hematology, and urinalysis. The experiments were conducted double blind as far as possible Subjects refrained from taking any medication during the study, and excessive use of alcohol was also forbidden. Subjects were given an equitable payment for each test in which they participated.

1.3 Experimental Procedures

In each Latin square, six subjects were tested per week, usually two per day for six consecutive weeks. To minimize effects attributable to circadian biorhythms, subjects were always tested on the same day of the week beginning at the same time of day. On each test day, subjects arrived 15 minutes prior to testing, and their general state of health, including respiration, body temperature, and pulse rate was checked. They then reported to a specially equipped room where they were dressed in hospital attire, weighed, and placed in bed with the upper part of their body slightly elevated at about 30° from horizontal. Electrocardiography (ECG) leads were attached to their upper arms and left leg in the #1 ECG lead configuration. A stethyscope funnel connected by tubing to a pressure transducer was placed over the carotid artery; this carotid plethysmography (CPG) monitoring device was held in place with an elastic bandage. A microphone was placed on the chest over the heart to record phonocardiography (PCG) data. In early experiments, a circular 5-cm-diameter electromagnetic field coil sensor for monitoring displacement cardiography (DCG) signals (4) was also placed on the chest over the heart. A piezoelectric pressure pulse transducer (Harvard Apparatus, Waltham, MA) for recording digital plethysmography (DPG) data was attached to the index finger of the left hand of each subject. For the purposes of this study, the piezoelectric sensor was judged to be superior to the photoelectric, pneumatic, and impedance type plethysmographic devices, as was determined from preliminary experiments. The placement of the DCG and CPG sensors occasionally required lengthy adjustment before satisfactory electronic signals were obtained; this was especially the case for the DCG coil, which often functioned erratically. Attempts to determine the effect of NG on peripheral circulation by recording big toe temperature using a thermistor sensor attached to different toe locations proved unsuccessful. Room temperature was maintained at 24 ± 2°C.

The sensors were connected to a 4- or 8-channel physiological recorder (Beckman Dynograph Model 411 or 511). Data were recorded on rectilinear strip chart paper and on magnetic tape using FM 4-channel analog tape recorders (Hewlett-Packard Model 3960) equipped for voice recording. Examples of typical predrug and postdrug data waveforms obtained during monitoring of NG pharmacological activity are shown in Figure 1. The waveforms were traced from a strip chart recording taken with the recorder operating at a chart speed of 100 mm per second. The acquisition and processing of the experimental data are summarized by the flow chart in Figure 2.

The procedural sequence shown in Table 2 was utilized to obtain the biosignal data at predrug and postdrug monitoring periods. This sequence of each recording time before and after administering the drug consisted of a baseline nonrecording interval in which a test subject remained quiet but breathed normally, followed by a 10-second data acquisition interval in which the subject held his breath following partial expiration. This interval was succeeded by another normal breathing interval, which was in turn

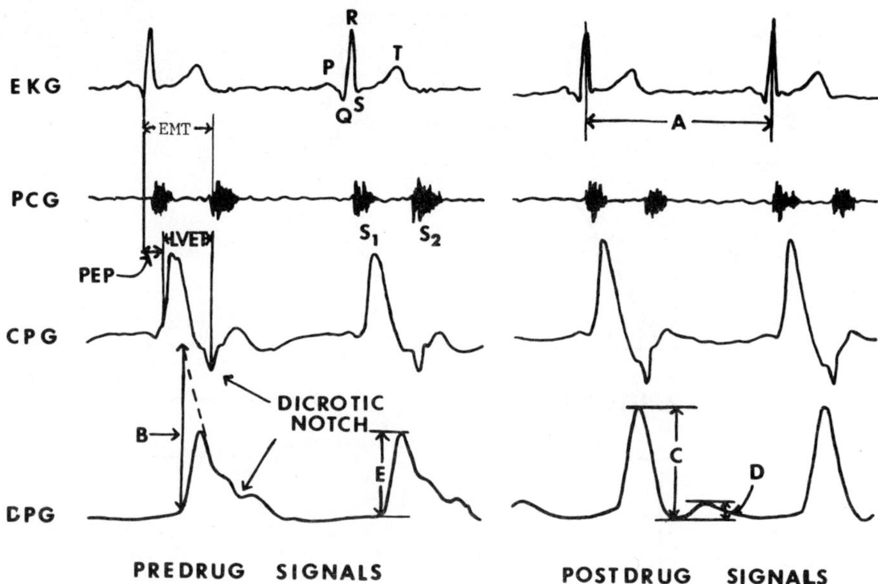

Figure 1. Comparison of typical predrug and peak response postdrug physiological signals monitored to gauge the effect of organic nitrate drugs on cardiovascular functions: ECG—electrocardiogram [heartrate = 60/A]; PCG—phonocardiogram (S_1, first heart sound; S_2 second heart sound); CPG—carotid plethysmogram; DPG—digital plethysmography [(B) pulse volume; (C) systolic amplitude; (D) diastolic amplitude]; EMT—electromechanical systole; PEP—pre-ejection period; LVET—left ventricular ejection time.

followed by another 10-second breath-holding interval. The electromagnetic field from the DCG monitoring distorted the other electronic signals; therefore, DCG was not recorded during the first breath-holding interval. DCG monitoring was halted after the first several experiments, and the second breath-holding interval was discontinued. Six to ten predrug testing sequences and 16–20 postdrug sequences were utilized for sublingual NG. The subjects were directed to alter their respiration from normal breathing to breath-holding to nonbreath-holding on command of the test supervisor, who timed each breathing interval in each testing sequence with a stopwatch.

The drug was administered immediately after the last predrug testing sequence was completed, and the first postdrug sequence was initiated immediately after dosing. Each subject was asked to signal the time at which the sublingual tablets dissolved under his tongue, the onset of any drug-induced sensations, and the stopping of drug sensations, by raising his right hand slowly and carefully, but not during a breath-holding interval. These times of onset and duration were noted on an information sheet. Other pertinent information for the experimental run, which included dosing

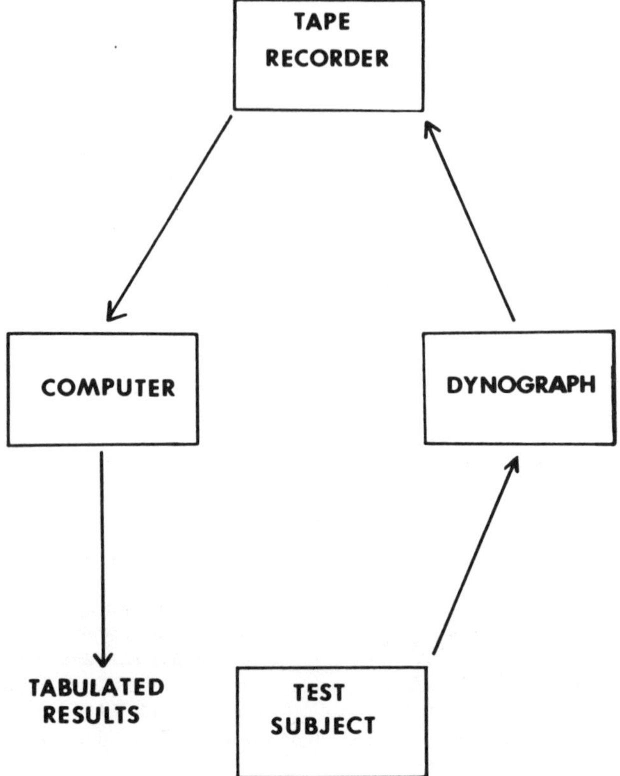

Figure 2. The flow of experimental data collection and processing.

times and physiological recorder and tape recorder settings, were also written on a subject information sheet.

1.4 Computerized Analysis of Organic Nitrate Affected Biological Signals

Time variations of drug induced changes in the form of physiological signals were resolved from the recorded biological signals by manual or computerized processing to obtain pharmacokinetic response profiles characterizing the pharmacological effectiveness of the drugs and the bioavailability of their dosage forms. The biological signals were recorded in analog form on magnetic tape and on strip charts. The electrocardiogram (ECG) and digital plethysmogram (DPG) were routinely recorded in all experiments. The carotid (pulse pressure) plethysmogram (CPG) and phonocardiogram (PCG) were deleted for the later experiments.

Table 2. Testing Sequence for Monitoring the Pharmacological Activity of Organic Nitrate Drugs in Humans

Dynograph and Tape Recorder Channel	Data Collection on Magnetic Tape and Chart Paper (2 minutes)			
	Resting Interval	First 10 second Breathing Interval	Resting Interval	Second 10 second Breath-Holding Interval
Electrocardiogram (EKG)[a]	ND[b]	D[c]	ND	D
Phonocardiogram (PCG)	ND	D	ND	D
Carotid plethysmogram (CPG)	ND	DND[d]	ND	NDD[e]
Digital plethysmogram (DPG) and displacement cardiogram (DCG)	ND	DND	ND	NDD

[a]Equipment operator's voice was placed on the tape on this channel during the resting interval to identify particular sequences (i.e., "Predrug Number 1"). Dynograph recorder settings for each signal were also recorded on the voice channel.
[b]No data.
[c]Data recorded.
[d]CPG and DPG data recorded; DCG data not recorded.
[e]DCG data recorded; CPG and DPG data not recorded.

1.4.1 *Computer Equipment*

The equipment used by the authors to analyze the data included a Hewlett-Packard 5451B Fourier Analyzer system comprised of an H-P 2100S minicomputer with 32K 16-bit words of central memory, a teletype, a high speed paper tape reader, a digital plotter, a display oscilloscope, the Fourier keyboard, a 4-channel 12-bit analog to digital converter, a 5-megabyte disc, a 4010 Tektronix terminal, and a Centronics printer. Also used in the processing is a Rockland analog filter, a Tektronix storage oscilloscope, and a Hewlett-Packard (Model 3960) FM analog data tape recorder. The computational procedures described below can also be accomplished by other systems. A program for an IBM 370 computer was also developed by the authors for use on the FDA (Parklawn Building) computer system in Rockville, Maryland.

1.4.2 *Response Variables*

The electrocardiogram and the digital plethysmogram were routinely computer processed. The response variables were computed in a single operation. The electrocardiogram was analyzed for heart rate and the location of the *R* peaks was used for subsequent delimitation of individual digital plethysmographic waveforms contained in 10 second epochs of data.

As defined in Figures 1 and 3, the response variables obtained from the digital plethysmogram are: (*1*) the slope before (S_1) and after (S_2) peak systole (reflective of the net arterial blood inflow and the rate of run-off, respectively); (*2*) the apparent LVET (i.e., the time interval between the beginning of systole and the dicrotic notch); (*3*) systolic pulse volume (the amplitude between the DPG wave baseline and S_2 through the DPG wave after peak systole; S_2 is extrapolated to the beginning of the upsweeps of the peak systole); (*4*) min–max amplitude between the peak systole and the dicrotic notch; (*5*) min–max amplitude between the peak systole and the beginning of the systolic upsweep; (*6*) relative cardiac output (product of pulse volume and heart rate); (*7*) slope before (D_1) and after (D_2) the diastolic pulse wave (reflective of net venous inflow and venous run-off, respec-

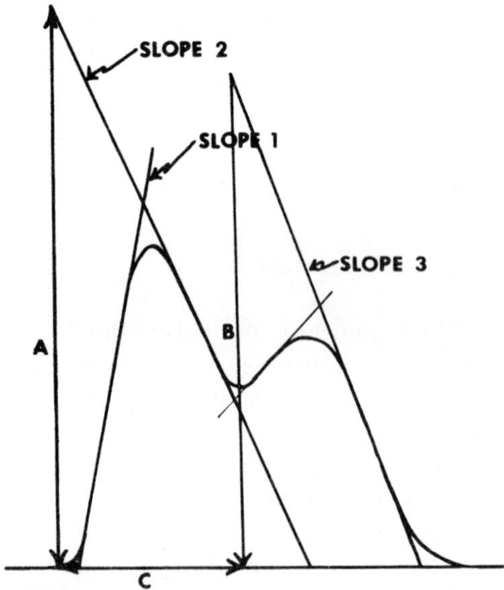

Figure 3. Digital pulse pressure responses: (*A*) systolic pulse volume; (*B*) diastolic pulse volume; (*C*) duration of systole; slope 1, arterial inflow rate; slope 2, arterial outflow rate; slope 3, venous outflow rate; slope 4, venous inflow rate.

tively, and therefore an indication of total peripheral resistance); (*8*) diastolic pulse volume (analog to *3*); and (*9*) minimum-maximum diastolic amplitude.

1.4.3. *Digital Plethysmogram*

The response variables obtained from the DPG waveform were computed in the following manner. First, each 10 second interval of data was filtered at 40 Hz and digitized at 204.8 Hz into the computer. The data were checked by the operator for acceptability, scaled according to amplification changes on the dynagraph recorder at the time the signal was recorded, and stored.

The heart rate was determined from the electrocardiogram as well as the location of the *R* peaks. The *R* peaks were used to pass individual DPG waveforms to the waveform analysis subroutine. Each waveform was then analyzed according to the following algorithm:

1. Find the largest point in the waveform—label it as peak systole.
2. Differentiate the data blocks stored in computer memory.
3. Find the maximum first derivative prior to peak systole—this is the inflection point of the leading slope.
4. Find the point where the slope drops below .03 volts before the inflection point. Mark it as the beginning of the upsweep of the peak systole.
5. Find the longest positive slope following the peak systole for 520 milliseconds. The beginning of this range is the dicrotic notch. If this point is not found by the computer, provision is made to display the waveform on an oscilloscope, from which the operator can determine the dicrotic notch manually and return this information to the computer. Alternatively for batch operation, the computer outputs a plot of the waveform to the line printer and goes on to process the next epoch of data. The operator later determines the location of the dicrotic notches of all such waveforms and inputs them; the computer then completes the data processing.
6. Find the maximum negative point in the first derivative between the peak systole and the dicrotic notch. This is the inflection point of the slope trailing the peak systole.
7. Find the points before and after the inflection point of the leading edge of the peak systole that are $\frac{1}{2}$ the amplitude of the inflection point. This is the range for the linear portion of the leading slope.
8. Find the points before and after the inflection point of the trailing slope that are $\frac{1}{2}$ the amplitude after the inflection point. This is the range of the linear portion of the trailing edge.

9. Integrate the data blocks.
10. Obtain the value of the peak systole, the dicrotic notch, and the beginning of the upsweep of the peak systole. The difference between the amplitude at the peak systole and at the dicrotic notch is the systolic amplitude. The difference between the amplitude at the peak systole and at the beginning of the systolic upsweep for the last five predrug intervals is stored for later use (see step *18*).
11. Generate the least-squares line through the already defined (in step *7*) range for the leading slope. The slope of this is the arterial blood flow.
12. Generate the least-squares line through the already defined (step 8) range for the trailing slope. The slope of this line is the net arterial outflow.
13. Calculate the value of the line from step *12* at the time of the beginning of the upsweep of the peak systole. Subtract the value of the DPG at the time of the upsweep. This is the pulse volume.
14. Label the dicrotic notch as the beginning of the waveform and return to step *1* for the calculation of the relevant diastolic parameters.
15. Multiply heart rate by systolic pulse volume to obtain cardiac output.
16. Average all the parameters for all the waveforms in the interval, except the first, then average all the parameters for the second, third, fourth, and fifth waveforms in the interval.
17. Compute the response intensity for both averages of all parameters for each postdrug interval, by subtracting the average of the last five predrug interval values from the postdrug interval average values computed in step *16* and dividing by the average value of the last five predrug intervals. Thus, for a particular response,

$$\text{Intensity} = \frac{(\text{postdrug interval average}) - (\text{average of last five predrug interval average values})}{(\text{average of last five predrug interval average values})}$$

    This procedure normalizes postdrug response values with respect to predrug values.
18. Compute the ratio of the difference between the post drug interval average for the diastolic amplitude and the average of the last five predrug interval averages for the diastolic amplitude over the average of the last five predrug interval averages for systolic amplitude, as measured from the beginning of the systolic upsweep.

Each of the computed response intensity variables are stored on magnetic disk and later printed in tables form with individual subject values, averages over all subjects, standard deviations, and standard errors of the mean.

1.4.4 *Displacement Cardiogram, Phonocardiogram, and Carotid Plethysmogram*

The displacement cardiogram (DCG) signals were recorded with a device supplied by Dr. Ron Vas (Carnegie Mellon University, Pittsburgh, PA) on magnetic tape, as well as being output to a strip chart recorder. The procedure to extract the systolic time intervals and process the DPG signal involved the ECG, PCG, and DCG signals being digitized together. The ECG's were cross-correlated and the displacement cardiogram was rotated to properly align the waveform with the first ECG and PCG. The DCG wave was smoothed by taking the Fourier Transform, blanking out all frequency components above 15 Hz to zero, and taking the inverse Fourier Transform. The computer program then extracted the location of the *Q* peaks from the ECG. It does this by finding the *R* peaks as the maximum point of the ECG. The program then looks back from the *R* peak to find the slope change at the *Q* peak. Since the onset of the *Q* is approximately 20 milliseconds before the *Q* peak, the *Q* onset is moved back 20 milliseconds from the *Q* peak. The maximum of the *T* wave is then found by looking forward in the ECG from the *R* peaks. This is located because the second heart sound always follows the *T* wave. The onset of the second heart sound is detected following the *T* wave by picking the first value greater than a number determined by the operator. The time between the onset of the *Q* and the second heart sound is the total electromechanical time (EMT) of the heart. The EMT was corrected for the effects of variable heart rate by adding a factor of 2.1 times the heart rate, in milliseconds, to the computed value. The left ventricular ejection time (LVET) was extracted from the carotid pulse pressure wave (CPG) as the time between the beginning of the upsweep of the pressure wave to the dicrotic notch. The LVET was obtained by finding the peak systole and looking backward to find the point where the slope changes from positive to negative, so as to find the beginning of the upsweep of the wave. The entire wave is then differentiated, and the first positive slope following the peak systole is defined as the dicrotic notch. The time between the upsweep of the wave and the dicrotic notch is corrected for heart rate by adding 1.7 times the heart rate (milliseconds). The pre-ejection period (PEP) was calculated as EMT−LVET. The relative apparent myocardial energy expended during PEP, LVET, and EMT was calculated from the following formula, where DCG indicates the displacement cardiographic signal.

$$\int_{\text{Onset of } Q}^{\text{Onset of } Q+\text{PEP}} \frac{d^2(\text{DCG})}{dt^2} \times [\text{DCG}] \ dt = \begin{array}{l}\text{Apparent, relative myocardial} \\ \text{energy expended during PEP}\end{array}$$

$$\int_{\text{Onset of } Q \text{ and PEP}}^{\text{2nd heart sound}} \frac{d^2(\text{DCG})}{dt^2} \times [\text{DCG}] \ dt = \begin{array}{l}\text{Apparent, relative myocardial} \\ \text{energy expended during LVET}\end{array}$$

$$\int_{\text{Onset of } Q}^{\text{2nd heart sound}} \frac{d^2(\text{DCG})}{dt^2} \times [\text{DCG}] \ dt = \begin{array}{l}\text{Apparent, relative myocardial} \\ \text{energy expended during EMT}\end{array}$$

Predrug and postdrug intensities of change in the amplitude of the DCG waveform were determined in a manner similar to DPG amplitude changes, except that this was done manually from the strip chart recordings with the aid of calipers. The intensity of the DCG amplitude response variable was computed (as described above for DPG) as the ratio of the postdrug–predrug difference to the predrug average.

The apparent, relative myocardial energy expenditure response variables provided response intensity versus time profiles similar to the DPG amplitude response variables, except that the data were more scattered. Such results served no additional purpose, and the computation of the apparent, relative myocardial energy expenditure response variables was discontinued at an early stage of the experimentation.

The use of computerized methods of analysis of the recorded physiological data can save considerable time and effort. However, the same results are obtainable by direct estimation of parameters from chart paper recordings. For example, systolic and diastolic DPG amplitudes can be read from the charts using a pair of calipers; heart rate is obtainable from ECG recordings by counting the R peaks occurring in an interval of time (e.g., 10 seconds, then multiplying by 6 to obtain beats/minute) or by estimating the times between R peaks in seconds and dividing into 60.

Comparisons of DPG amplitude response intensities obtained by computer processing with manually computed values show that they are not statistically different, although the manually computed results are more variable. For example, DPG systolic amplitude 60-minute area under the curve values had a coefficient of variation of 0.79 when obtained by manual computation and 0.40 when the data were computer processed. The manual estimation of pharmacological response variables that involve determining slopes and/or intercepts (e.g., systolic pulse volume, which when multiplied by heart rate gives values proportional to cardiac output) is difficult, and the results are even more variable and dependent upon the specific individual making the estimates. Although manual estimates can be obtained, computer programs employing consistent algorithms to perform such computations are obviously preferred, and should be used whenever the required equipment is available. Program listings and detailed descriptions of the approaches used in the author's laboratory for the computerized analysis of ECG, DPG, PCG, CPG, and DCG signals are available in reports submitted to the FDA.* Detailed procedures for manually estimating response variables from strip chart recordings are also provided. Reference should be made to a document entitled "Recommended Guidelines and Methodology for the Evaluation of Pharmacological Effectiveness and Comparative Bioavailability of Organic Nitrate Antianginal Drug Products," contained in a report submitted to the FDA on March 22, 1977.

2. RESPONSE VARIABLES AND THEIR PROPERTIES

In developing and applying physiological recording methodology to the evaluation of the pharmacological effectiveness and bioavailability of organic nirate drug and drug products, an enormous quantity of data was generated. Typical results, which are exemplary of the methods employed and the behavior of the drugs studied, are described below. In preliminary experiments, a variety of transducers, biological signals, and methods of analysis were screened and discarded. For example, impedance plethysmography measured on limbs and the thorax offered no advantage for our purposes over digital plethysmography, which is far more simply recorded; power spectral density analysis of the phonocardiogram (PCG), electrocardiogram (ECG), and electroencephalogram (EEG) revealed these signals to be only negligibly affected by the actions of sublingual nitroglycerin and was discontinued; skin temperature recorded on the big toe and other locations on the body was not useful. As seen from the plots in Figure 4 of the time course of change in the displacement cardiogram (DCG) amplitude response intensity induced by 0.3 and 0.4 mg sublingual doses of nitroglycerin, this measure is both time and dose sensitive. The small amount of data obtained on only two and three subjects suggests that this measure could be potentially useful. The results in Figure 4 indicate that a NG-induced increase in myocardial contractility has occurred, as reported by other investigators (5). However, due to experimental difficulties with the apparatus (4) and its interference with other measurements, DCG was not included in the routine experimentation.

*Bureau of Drugs, 5600 Fishers Lane, Rockville, Md. 20852. The project title is "Bioavailability as Related to Physiological Response," V. F. Smolen, Principal Investigator (FDA Contract No. 223-73-3023).

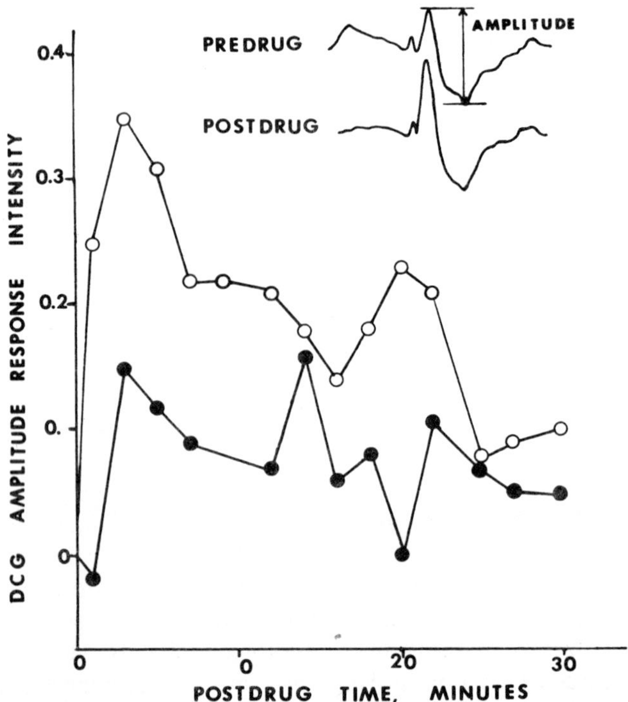

Figure 4. Temporal variation of the mean displacement cardiogram amplitude response intensity in healthy volunteers dosed sublingually with nitroglycerin (NG). ●, 0.3 Mg NG (2 subjects); ○, 0.9 Mg NG (3 subjects).

Figure 5 exemplifies the influence of 0.9 mg sublingual NG and placebo on heart rate corrected changes in systolic time intervals (STI) averaged for 12 subjects. Drug-induced changes in STI parameters (6) such as EMT, LVET, and PEP, which were calculated from ECG, CPG, and PCG data as defined in Figure 1, were small and quite variable. Because LVET increased as PEP decreased following the administration of NG, the (PEP/LVET) ratio is more sensitive to the drug than LVET or PEP considered separately. Nevertheless, the effect of NG on this ratio is small (Figure 5). Inhalation of amylnitrite by normal human subjects decreases PEP/LVET, but the ratio is unchanged for patients with ischemic heart disease (7). The failure of the ratio to decrease is attributed to failure of the drug to increase the cardiac stroke volume of the patient (the PEP/LVET ratio is inversely proportional to stroke volume). Sawayama and coworkers (8) reported that NG does increase cardiac stroke volume. The monitoring and analysis of the PEP/LVET response is complex, since it involves syn-

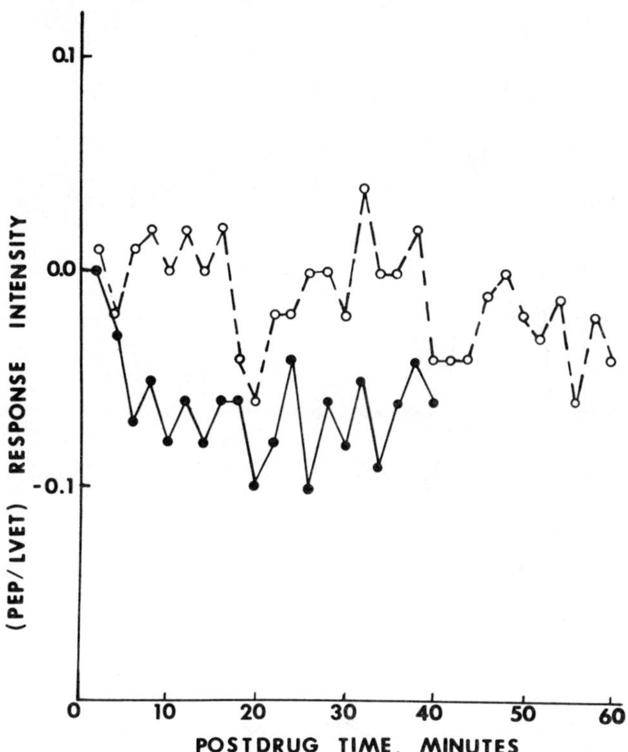

Figure 5. Temporal variation of the mean heart rate-corrected systolic time interval response variable (PEP/LVET), intensity for 12 healthy volunteers dosed sublingually with nitroglycerin (NG). ○, Placebo; ●, 0.9 Mg NG.

chronized monitoring and analysis of PCG, ECG, and CPG data (Figure 1). The PEP/LVET response placebo baseline is also much more variable than other response variable placebo baselines, which was an additional reason for concluding that this ratio is of limited value as a suitable pharmacological response for NG and other organic nitrate drugs.

Digital plethysmography (DPG) and electrocardiography (ECG) can be easily and conveniently monitored and either manually or computer processed to provide at least ten different, physiologically relevent, pharmacological response variables. All of the DPG response variables, as defined in Figures 1 and 2, were both time and dose sensitive and were routinely computed. However, as can be seen for the heart rate, systolic amplitude, and diastolic amplitude response variables shown in Figure 6 as the averages for 19 subjects, the time patterns of change are somewhat redundant for each of the variables, although they differ in the relative magnitudes of the drug-

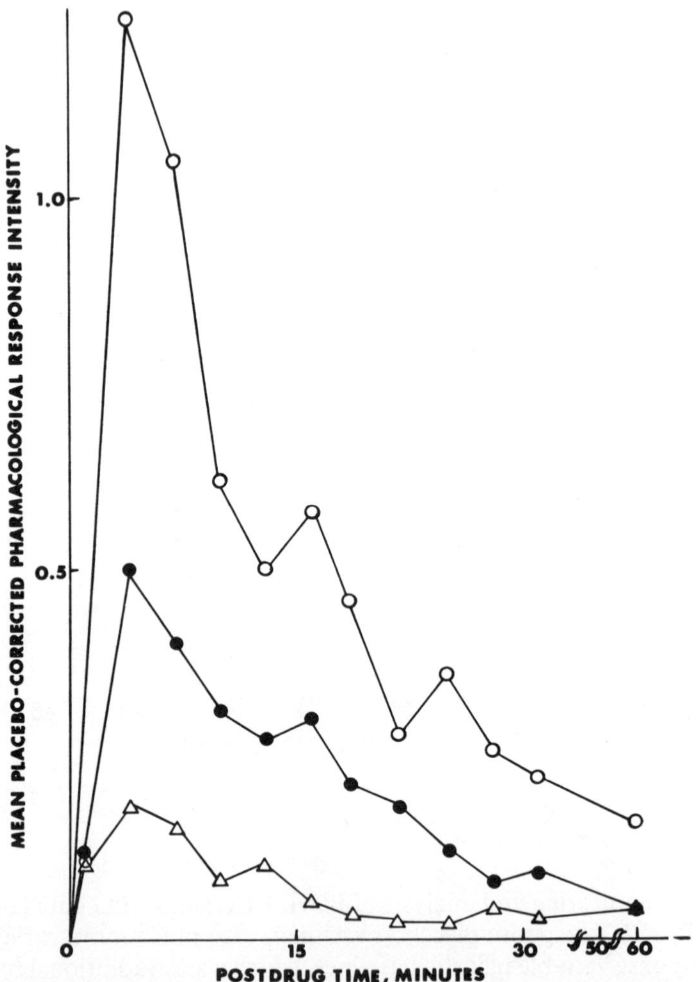

Figure 6. Temporal variation of the pharmacological response intensity of 19 healthy male volunteers dosed sublingually with 0.6 mg of nitroglycerin: △, heart rate response; ○, DPG systolic amplitude response; ●, DPG diastolic amplitude response.

induced changes. The results plotted in Figure 6 represent drug-induced changes relative to the magnitude of placebo baseline effects occurring at the same time after dosing. Each subject's data were individually placebo corrected before averaging. Figure 7 presents semilog plots of the DPG amplitude response variables as a function of time. Recently reported (9) average NG plasma levels for six subjects are also shown in Figure 7, with their standard errors of the mean. The plasma levels were obtained from healthy

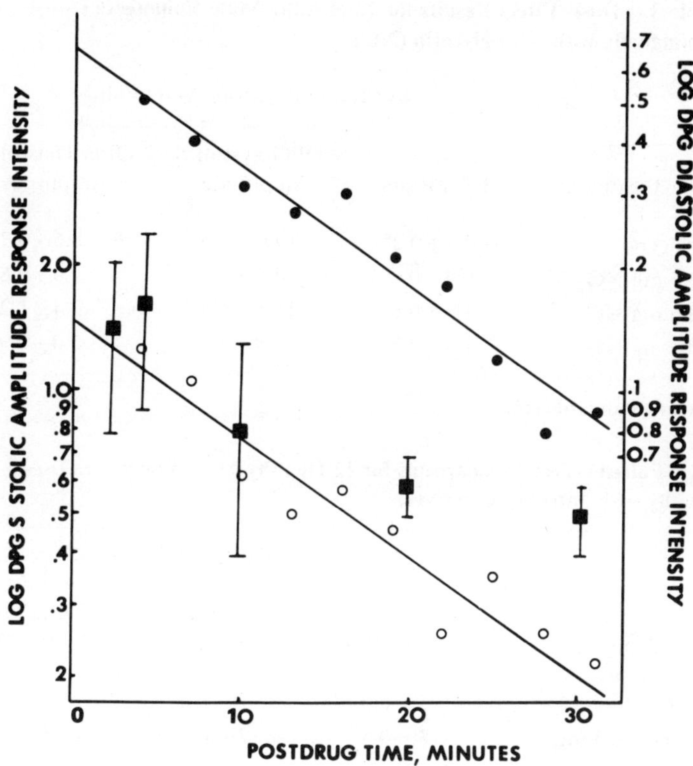

Figure 7. Linear regression plots of mean, placebo-corrected DPG systolic and diastolic amplitude response intensity data from Figure 6: ○, systolic amplitude; ●, diastolic amplitude. Equations of the lines and their correlation coefficients are: systolic amplitude, log $1=0.140-0.265t$; $R=0.96$; diastolic amplitude, log $1=0.172-0.029t$; $R=0.97$. Average six subject NG plasma levels (■) are also plotted with their standard errors of the mean as reported in reference 9.

human subjects following dosing with 0.6 mg sublingual NG. The half-lives of the DPG amplitude response intensities are approximately 10 minutes. Except for DPG determined LVET, which is more similar to the results shown in Figure 5, the heart rate and other DPG response variables exhibit patterns of change following sublingual NG dosing similar to those seen in Figures 6 and 7.

The dose dependency of the heart rate and DPG amplitude response intensities are demonstrated by the 40 minute areas under the curve (AUC) values listed in Table 3 for placebo, 0.3, 0.6, and 0.9 mg sublingual NG doses, along with the paired t-test statistical comparisons of these values contained in Table 4. The dose dependency is graphically shown for the DPG systolic

Table 3. Dose–Effect Results for 12 Healthy Male Volunteers Dosed Sublingually with Nitroglycerin (NG)

	40-Minute Postdrug AUC Values		
Dose Treatment	Heart Rate	DPG Systolic Amplitude	DPG Diastolic Amplitude
Placebo	-0.6 ± 0.2[a]	-7.4 ± 3.9	-0.6 ± 0.2
0.3 mg NG	0.4 ± 0.6	4.2 ± 2.8	3.6 ± 0.8
0.6 mg NG	1.6 ± 0.6	15.5 ± 4.9	5.4 ± 1.2
0.9 mg NG	1.4 ± 0.5	14.8 ± 5.7	6.0 ± 0.9

[a]Mean ± standard error.

Table 4. Paired *t*-Test Comparisons for 12 Healthy Male Volunteers Dosed Sublingually with Nitroglycerin (NG)

	t-Test Probabilities[a]		
Dose Comparison	Heart Rate	DPG Systolic Amplitude	DPG Diastolic Amplitude
0.3 mg NG versus placebo	$P<0.05$	$P<0.01$	$P<0.005$
0.6 mg versus 0.3 mg	$P=0.5$	$P<0.005$	$P<0.025$
0.9 mg versus 0.6 mg	NS[b]	NS	NS
0.9 mg versus 0.3 mg	$P=0.5$	$P<0.05$	$P<0.05$

[a]Based on 40-minute postdrug AUC values.
[b]Not significant, $P>0.10$.

amplitude variable by the response curves in Figure 8 and the dose–effect curve in Figure 9. In general, the response intensities approach a maximum plateau level at 0.6 mg NG; very little, if any, additional response intensity is achieved with a 0.9 mg dose.

An indication of the intersubject variability of the heart rate and DPG amplitude responses is provided in Table 5, with 0.3 mg NG dosing data obtained from 24 subjects composing 4 separate groups. The intrasubject variability of these response variables can be judged from the results of successive doses of 0.3 mg NG administered to 12 subjects, as listed in Table 6. Judging from the AUC's in Table 6, no tolerances in the responses to the drug develop as a consequence of the previous doses; the effects of each previous 0.3 mg NG dose were completely dissipated prior to the administra-

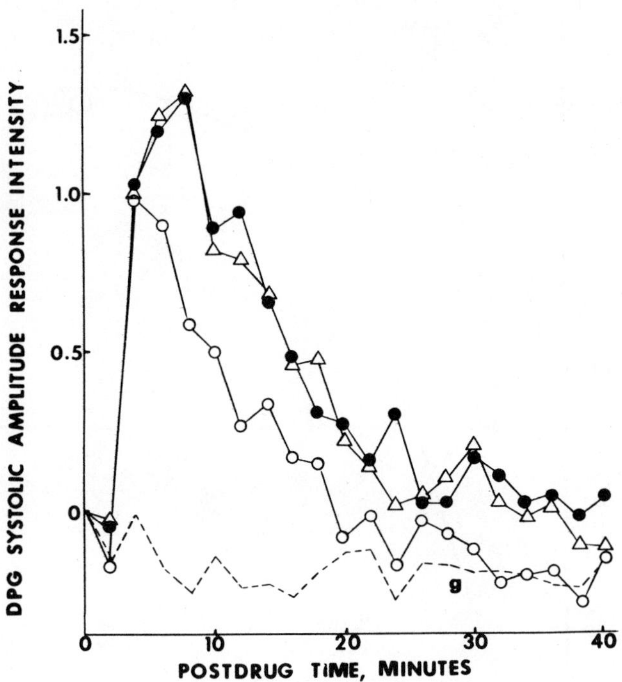

Figure 8. Temporal variation of the mean DPG systolic amplitude response intensity for 12 healthy male volunteers dosed sublingually with nitroglycerin: ---, placebo; ○, 0.3 mg; ●, 0.6 mg; △, 0.9 mg.

Table 5. Mean Placebo-Corrected Pharmacological Response AUC Data for Four Groups of Healthy Male Volunteers Following Dosing with 0.3 mg Sublingual Nitroglycerin[a]

Pharmacological Response	AUC Data (Dimensionless Units) Group 1	Group 2	Group 3	Group 4	Total Mean[b]	CV[c]
Heart rate	1.1	1.1	0.9	1.1	1.0	0.10
DPG Systolic amplitude	8.5	15.3	17.4	9.3	12.6	0.35
DPG Diastolic amplitude	4.9	3.1	6.0	4.1	4.5	0.27

[a]Data obtained 0–31 minute postdrug; six volunteers per group.
[b]Of all four groups.
[c]Coefficient of variation = standard deviation/mean.

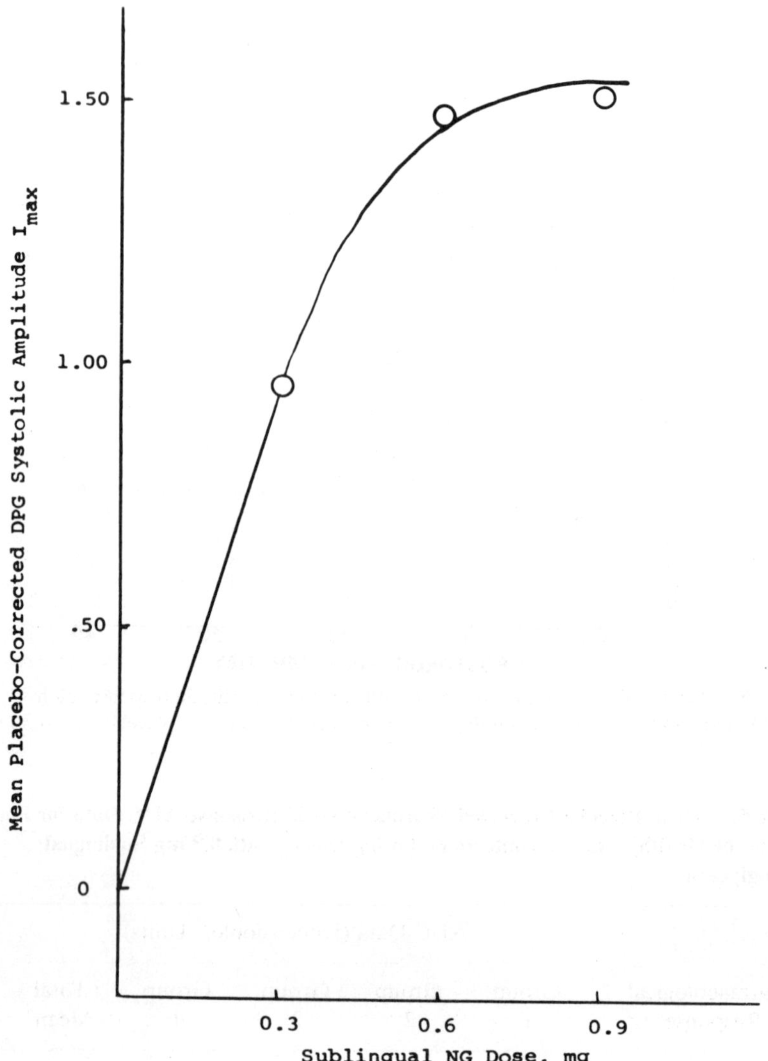

Figure 9. Dose–effect curve for sublingual nitroglycerin induced average increase in the DPG systolic amplitude in healthy male volunteers (12), constructed as a plot of the maximum response intensity versus dose.

tion of the succeeding doses. A comparison of the average DPG systolic amplitude response intensity versus time profiles obtained for 10 subjects, with the same result obtained when 0.6 mg NG was administered 1 hour later, is shown in Figure 10; the two response profiles do not differ significantly.

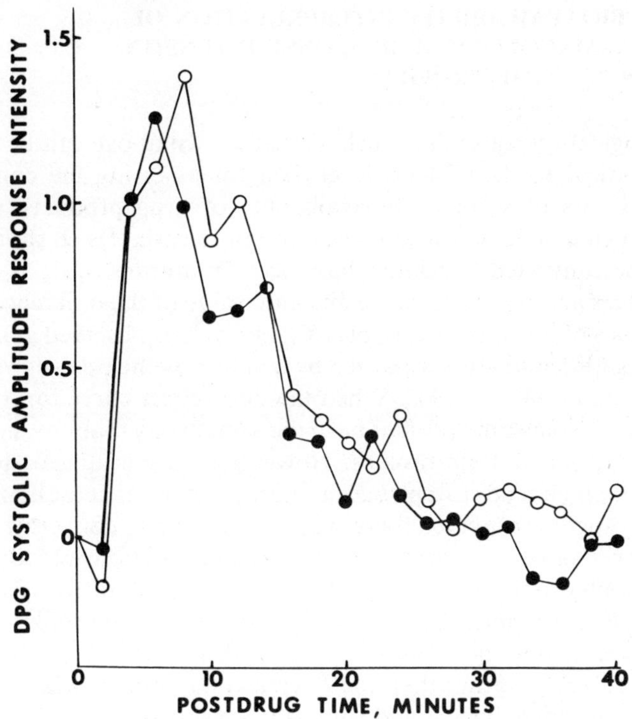

Figure 10. Temporal variation of the mean DPG systolic amplitude response intensity for 10 volunteers dosed sublingually and repetitively with 0.6 mg of nitroglycerin: ○, first dosing; ●, second dosing (1 hour after first dosing).

Table 6. Mean Placebo-Corrected Pharmacological Response AUC Data for Twelve Healthy Male Volunteers Dosed Successively with Single 0.3 mg Nitroglycerin Sublingual Tablets[a]

	AUC Data (Arbitrary Units ± SE)[b]		
Postdrug Interval (min)	Heart Rate	DPG Systolic Amplitude	DPG Diastolic Amplitude
0–31	0.9 ± 0.7 (1.1)[d]	13.4 ± 3.3 (11.9)[d]	5.0 ± 0.7 (4.0)[d]
210–240[c]	1.3 ± 1.0	14.0 ± 3.3	4.6 ± 1.1
390–420	1.3 ± 0.9	16.2 ± 4.5	4.8 ± 1.2

[a]Study included three dosings.
[b]SE—standard error.
[c]Lunch break interval was 150–210 minutes postdrug.
[d]Mean value for 12 different subjects in another study.

3. BIOAVAILABILITY INTERPRETATION OF PHARMACOLOGICAL RESPONSE INTENSITY VERSUS TIME PROFILES

Pharmacological response data such as that shown above can be used in a manner identical to drug blood level data for assessing the comparative rates and extents of systemic bioavailability of drug products. Observed intensities of change in pharmacological response variables (I) should, when necessary, be converted to relative biophasic drug levels (Q_B); as discussed above, I values are expressed as the absolute value of the difference between predrug values of a response variable (X_0) and values observed at some time t after dosing (X_t), and are normalized by dividing by the predrug value. This is expressed as $I = |X_t - X_0/X_0|$. When the dose–effect curve for a drug is a straight line, I versus time profiles have the same bioavailability significance as blood level versus time profiles. However, if a curvilinear dose–effect relationship (which tends to a plateau at the highest doses at the extreme of its therapeutic range) is observed for a drug, it is correct to convert the I values observed for a particular dosage form under evaluation into their corresponding biophasic drug levels (Q_B) to assess its comparative systemic bioavailability. For example, the areas under Q_B versus time profiles are in this case directly related to the quantities of active drug entities absorbed into the systemic circulation, rather than the I versus time profiles which, however, are of more pharmacological and clinical interest. For the rigorous evaluation of the comparative bioavailability of different drug formulations, the observed I values can be converted to Q_B values using parenteral, sublingual, or oral dose–effect curves in the manner of calibration curves. This is analogous to the use of a nonlinear Beer's law type plot to convert observed absorbances into corresponding plasma drug concentrations when using a spectrophotometric assay to analyze blood samples. Bioavailability parameters computed from Q_B values are then directly proportional to bioavailability. For example, a 25% difference between AUC's, computed from I values of a generic brand dosage form and the innovating drug company's brand chosen as a standard, would in all cases indicate that at least a 25% difference exists in the amount of active drug systemically bioavailable from the two brands of drug products. If the dose–effect curve (constructed from the results of studying various doses of the standard product) is linear or the I values of interest lie on the lower, linear segment of the dose–effect curve, then it is not necessary to convert I values into Q_B values, since AUC's computed from Q_B values are directly proportional to those computed from I values; the proportionality constant is the slope of the dose–effect curve. However, if the I values lie on a curvilinear dose–effect curve, only the AUC's computed from Q_B values are directly proportional to amounts of drug absorbed and indicate larger differences than those computed from I values. For example, a 25% difference in AUC's obtained from I values may actually transform to indicate that a much larger difference exists in the amounts of active drug systemically bioavailable from the two products. This is exemplified by the DPG systolic amplitude response intensities curves shown in Figure 11 for two brands of sublingual nitroglycerin, as compared to the corresponding dose normalized Q_B versus time curves plotted in Figure 12; the curves in Figure 12 were obtained by converting the I values plotted in Figure 11 into Q_B values, using the dose–effect curve DPG systolic response intensity contained in Figure 9 and dividing the resulting Q_B values by dose.

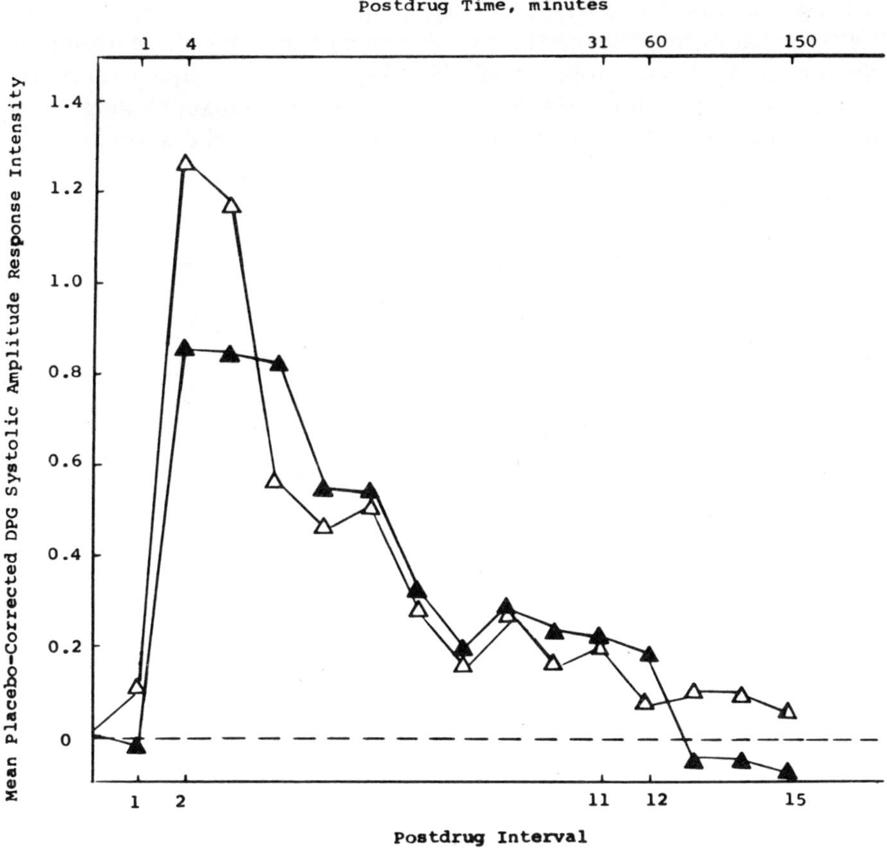

Figure 11. Comparison of mean placebo-corrected DPG systolic amplitude response intensity data for 12 healthy male volunteers dosed sublingually with: △, 0.6 Mg NG; ▲, 0.8 Mg NG (Warner-Lambert).

In effect, the conversion of I values to Q_B values, when appropriate, and their subsequent use to compute bioavailability parameters such as AUC's, increases the sensitivity of the measures and renders them directly proportional to the amounts of active drug systemically absorbed into the body from the drug products. Details of the theoretical basis and verification of this approach to the quantitative pharmacokinetic treatment of pharmacological data have been well-described (10–16). However, for bioequivalency comparisons of allegedly identical drug products, it is generally sufficient to compare I versus time profiles directly. This is especially the case if the majority of the I values lie on the lower, approximately linear, segment of the dose–effect curve, as is often the case. For example, the greater response obtainable with two 0.3 mg sublingual Parke-Davis tablets, relative to two 0.4 mg Warner-Lambert tablets is apparent from mere inspection of the DPG cardiac output response profiles shown in Figure 13, which corroborate the results for DPG systolic amplitude in Figure 11. Whenever I values are converted into Q_B values to more precisely make bioavailability judgments, it is important to note that dose–effect curves are used as calibration curves to

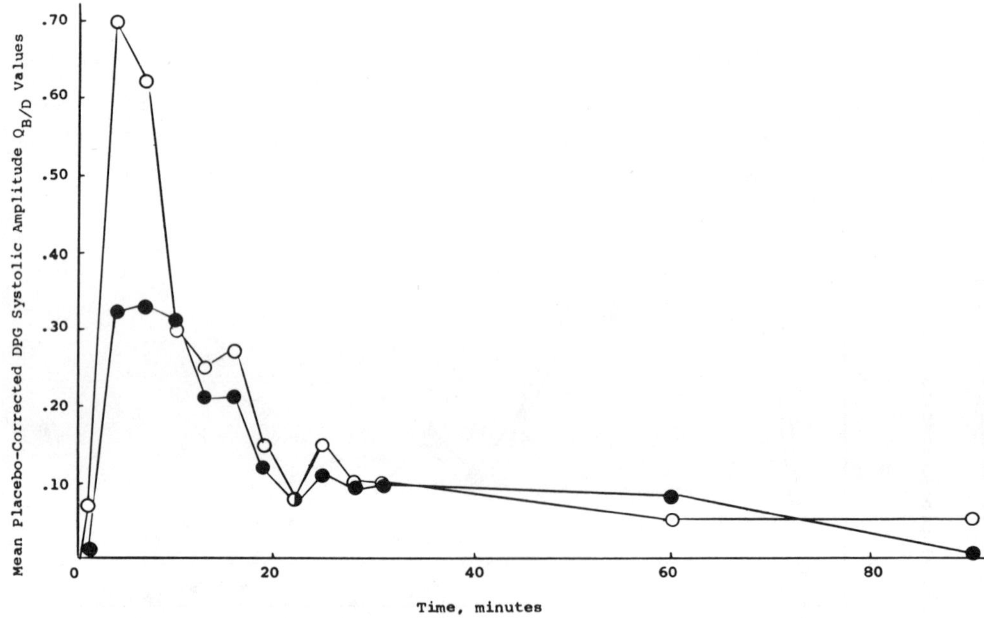

Figure 12. DPG systolic amplitude response intensities transduced to Q_B values (relative biophasic drug levels) using the sublingual nitroglycerin dose–effect curve as a calibration curve normalized by dividing by the corresponding dose: ○, two 0.3 mg molded nitroglycerin tablets; ●, two 0.4 mg compressed nitroglycerin tablets. The areas under the two curves represent the systemic bioavailabilities.

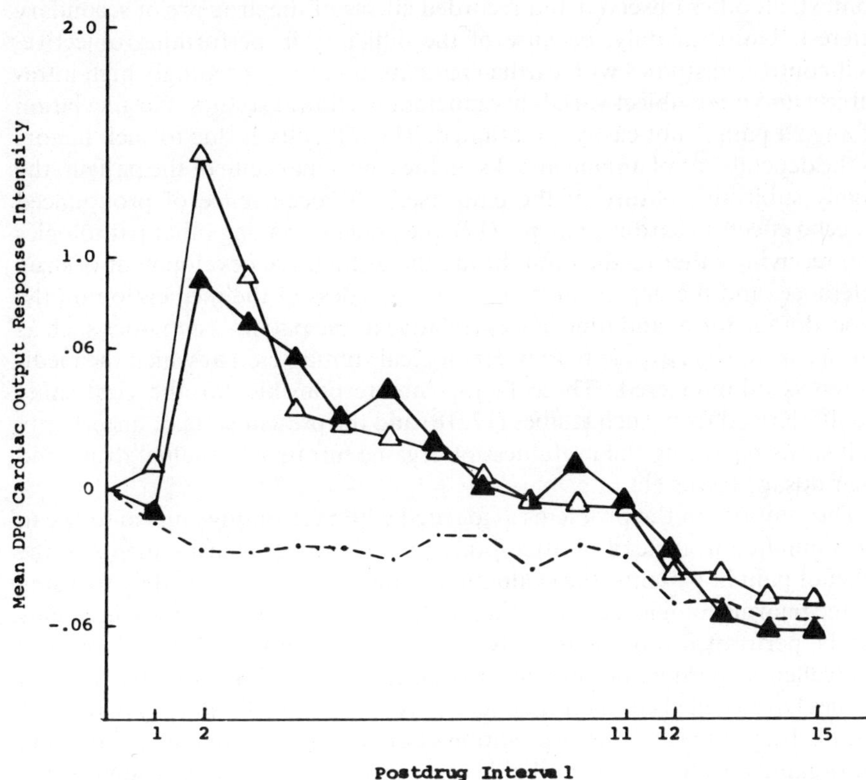

Figure 13. Temporal variation of the mean DPG cardiac output response intensity for 12 healthy male volunteers dosed with: ---, placebo tablet; △, 0.6 mg sublingual nitroglycerin; and ▲, 0.8 mg sublingual nitroglycerin (Warner-Lambert).

convert I into Q_B, not log(dose)–effect curves. The former are generally hyperbolic in shape and approximate straight lines at lower doses; the latter are usually sigmoidal and often give the impression that a threshold dose must be exceeded to elicit any response.

4. DISCUSSION

The utility of the methodology described here for determining the pharmacological effectiveness of sublingual NG and other organic nitrates may primarily be judged for each pharmacological response on the basis of its relevance to clinical activity. The principal, desired clinical action of organic nitrates is the prophylaxis and alleviation of the pain of angina pectoris. In this context, all other observed and recorded effects of the drug are of secondary interest. Unfortunately, because of the difficulty in performing objective, well-controlled studies with cardiac patients, and the exceedingly high intra-subject and intersubject variability inherent in clinical studies, the alleviation of angina pain is not easily quantitated. The difficulty is due to such factors as the dependence of angina attacks on the emotional state of the patient, the highly subjective nature of the pain itself, the occurrence of pronounced placebo effects in cardiac patients (17), the patient's having other pathologies and receiving other medication during the testing, the development of drug tolerance, and the dependence of the effectiveness of the medication on the dose, dosage form, and time of day (relative to the patient's activities such as eating, exercising, exposure to psychological stimuli, etc.) at which the medication is administered. These factors are responsible for the conflicting results derived from such studies (17, 18) and the present state of uncertainty that exists regarding the usefulness of organic nitrate antianginal drugs and their dosage forms (1).

The majority of the problems associated with performing clinical tests can be eliminated if, instead of attempting to make direct measurements of the relief of pain in patients, the evaluation of the drug is performed by focusing on the pharmacological activity that underlies the relief. Such measurements can be performed most sensitively with normal subjects using a rigorously controlled experimental design. Considering that (*1*) extensive clinical studies have yielded conflicting conclusions concerning the efficacy of organic nitrate drugs and (*2*) the interpretation of direct sampling and assay of blood for organic nitrates, when a reliable assay is available, is complicated by the activity of the metabolites, the use of pharmacological response variables as criteria to assess the effectiveness of these drugs constitutes a practical approach to the problem. Although there is presently a sufficient understanding of the mechanisms operative in relieving the pain of angina (17, 19) to validate the contention that pharmacological measurements of the actions of these drugs on the heart and peripheral circulation of normal subjects are clinically relevant, such measurements should ultimately be corroborated with the results of direct clinical studies of the prophylaxis and relief of pain in angina patients, as far as this is practical to achieve.

In reviewing the literature, it appears that all the organic nitrates, at least qualitatively, act by the same physiological mechanisms. The relief of angina pain is most commonly attributed to a drug-induced decrease in myocardial energy expenditure with a concomitant diminuition in oxygen consumption requirements. This reduced need for oxygen consumption derives both from a reduction in left ventricular end diastolic pressure (LVEDP) preload and systolic work load, which is manifested by a decrease in left ventricular distension. The decrease in LVEDP also leads to an increased blood flow to deep (endocardial) layers of the ventricular wall. These central (heart) changes occur as a consequence of drug-induced peripheral arteriodilation and venodilation, which results in decreased peripheral vascular resistance and venous return. However, there also appears to be some evidence that an increased oxygen supply to the myocardium, owing to a drug-induced coronary vasodilation as opposed to a decreased oxygen demand, also contributes to the antianginal activity of nitrates (17, 19).

As secondary indicators of the pharmacological actions that mechanistically underlie the antianginal activity of organic nitrates, central measurements of drug effects [such as DCG and systolic time interval (STI) measurements] and peripheral measurements (i.e., the vascular response variables derived from DPG) are interrelated by homeostatic control mechanisms. Although differing in certain response characteristics, such as dose sensitivity, time of onset, and duration of action, each of these measurements is a clinically relevant secondary indicator of nitroglycerin's clinical effects. The DPG response variables, however, are more reflective of the drug's direct effect in relaxing vascular smooth muscle, whereas the other measurements result less directly from this primary action.

Requisite features of acceptable pharmacological response variables used for routine testing of drugs in human subjects are: (*1*) simplicity of the monitoring equipment and test procedures; (*2*) capability of the measurement to provide accurate time and dose-dependent data; (*3*) a satisfactorily low degree of intrasubject and intersubject variability; (*4*) ease of processing the recorded data; and (*5*) correlation of the pharmacological response variable to physiological effects known to be relevant to the clinically sought effects of the drug. Heart rate and DPG amplitude measurements, in particular, meet these requirements, as demonstrated for sublingual nitroglycerin. Heart rate can be obtained easily from the ECG or DPG signals recorded on magnetic tape and either computer processed by reading the signals into a cardiotachometer, or manually processed from chart paper recordings.

Figure 3 and Tables 3 and 4 demonstrate that the heart rate response is both time- and dose-dependent; it is widely recognized that NG induces transient tachycardia in healthy humans and angina patients alike (17, 21–24). DPG amplitude measurements also possess these desired requisites. Attachment of a piezoelectric detector to the finger is uncomplicated, and Figure 4 and Tables 3 and 4 demonstrate that the DPG systolic and diastolic amplitude responses are also time- and dose-dependent. DPG data on magnetic tape can be computer analyzed or data on the chart paper can be analyzed manually; either method of analysis is uncomplicated. Furthermore, there is little question that NG induces peripheral vasodilation, which can be detected plethysmographically (25–28). In a digital plethysmographic investigation of sublingual and oral controlled-release NG and isosorbide dinitrate tablets, using angina patients and healthy subjects, Winsor (25, 36) also detected a drug-induced DPG response that was time-dependent. The other eight pharmacological response variables computed from DPG signals are largely redundant of the systolic and diastolic amplitude responses. Although such responses as systolic and diastolic pulse volumes, arterial inflow and outflow rates, and the duration of systole (6, 29) are of physiological interest, these other DPG variables are more variable than the two amplitude responses; the processing of the data is also more complex. Therefore, the principal emphasis in subsequent experiments with NG and other organic nitrates was primarily focused on heart rate and the two DPG amplitude response variables. The DCG and STI response variables cannot be recommended, as they lack the requisite features described above. From the temporal variation of heart rate, DPG systolic amplitude, and DPG diastolic amplitude following dosing with 0.6 mg sublingual NG shown in Figure 3, it can be observed that all three pharmacological response variables peaked at 4 minutes following administration of drug. This observation is in accord with the reported rapid onset and decay of sublingual NG antianginal activity (17). In sublingual NG therapy, it is recommended that the tablets be taken 2–4 minutes prior to an expected exertion to obtain maximum prophylactic benefits. Reichek (8) stated that a clinically effective organic nitrate dose is usually associated with an increase in heart rate of at least 10 beats per minute. This corresponds to a response intensity value of approximately 0.14 and establishes a direct connection between clinical activity and pharmacological activity. Since an increase in heart rate signifies an undesirable increase in myocardial energy expenditure, the heart rate response is not a direct measure of the therapeutic activity, as are the DPG amplitude responses. In some of the individuals who do not benefit from sublingual NG, an exaggerated drug-induced increase in heart rate may counteract the therapeutic hemodynamic effects of the drug.

The DPG systolic amplitude response appears to be most sensitive to NG, with heart rate being least sensitive. Although the effect of NG on the DPG diastolic amplitude is smaller than its effect on the DPG systolic amplitude, the diastolic amplitude is less variable (Table 5). The greater variability of the systolic amplitude response is related to a more pronounced variation in intersubject responsiveness to the drug, which may be a consequence of the variability of the condition of the vascular system of the test subjects. Whereas the systolic amplitude response is a manifestation of a drug-induced decrease in the resistance to ventricular ejection, which decreases myocardial oxygen demand, the diastolic amplitude response primarily represents a drug-induced decrease in venous return from venous pooling; this also decreases the oxygen demand. It is generally acknowledged that

NG and similar drugs are clinically effective because of their peripheral vasodilatory activity, although there is evidence that they also dilate non-sclerotic coronary arteries. An increase in DPG systolic and diastolic amplitude response intensity signifies peripheral vasodilation.

All three of the pharmacological responses depicted in Figure 3 are reproducible with relatively small intrasubject variation. Hirshliefer (27) reported that the DPG response for successive dosings of human patients with sublingual nitroglycerin was very reproducible and showed no indication that the patients had developed a sensitivity or tolerance to nitroglycerin. This observation coincides with the results of the present study. All three responses are dose-sensitive, as demonstrated by the statistical comparisons of AUC's in Table 4. The leveling off of the DPG amplitude responses at sublingual doses approximating 0.6 mg is in accord with observations that the therapeutic benefit from sublingual nitroglycerin tends to saturate at moderate nitroglycerin doses. The elimination half-life value for nitroglycerin estimated from Figure 7 is approximately 10 minutes, which corresponds to the short duration of sublingual nitroglycerin clinical activity. The maximum duration of the three responses, as judged from detectable differences compared to placebo baselines, is approximately 60 minutes for a 0.6 mg nitroglycerin sublingual dose. It is generally acknowledged that the duration of the therapeutic benefit from sublingual nitroglycerin rarely exceeds 1 hour (17).

5. ISOSORBIDE DINITRATE

Isosorbide dinitrate (ISDN) is an effective antianginal drug (30). Nevertheless, there is uncertainty that the duration of action of a sublingual isosorbide dinitrate dose is appreciably greater than that of a comparable sublingual nitroglycerin dose, (17, 30) and this is not universally accepted (30). Isosorbide dinitrate is more expensive than nitroglycerin and induces severe headaches in certain individuals, hence some physicians have questioned its usefulness. Since the experiments described and discussed in this section were performed in conjunction with the testing of sublingual nitroglycerin tablets, some direct comparisons can be made. The NG results were presented above. Blood levels of ISDN were measured in humans following the administration of various ISDN dosage forms, including sublingual and chewable tablets (31–33). The availability of blood level data permits a comparison and correlation of this data with the pharmacological response data obtained in the present investigation.

5.1 Experimental Methods

Isosorbide dinitrate was tested with nitroglycerin and a placebo in a duplicated, balanced 6 × 6 Latin square design. The isosorbide dinitrate dose treatments consisted of a single 2.5 mg and a single 5 mg sublingual tablet. A placebo and three sublingual nitroglycerin tablet doses constituted the remaining four dose treatments in each of the two identical Latin squares. After completion of each set of Latin square experiments, the test subjects were given a seventh dose treatment; those who participated in the first square received another brand of a 5 mg sublingual isosorbide dinitrate tablet, whereas those in the second square received a 5 mg chewable isosorbide dinitrate tablet. A 0.3 mg nitroglycerin sublingual screening dose was administered to each subject prior to his acceptance into the study. Details of the protocol for selecting the 12 healthy male volunteers who participated in the study were described in Section 1.2. All of the same procedures described in that section, including data collection and data analysis methodology, were also used to obtain the results reported with isosorbide dinitrate.

5.2 Results

Sublingual dosing with nitroglycerin and isosorbide dinitrate is advantageous because the systemic absorption of these drugs from sublingual tablets is rapid, and their hepatic metabolism to less active and inactive derivatives is not as pronounced as following oral dosing (34). However, the rapid elimination of nitroglycerin is a particular disadvantage for patients subject to frequently recurring angina attacks, since these patients must carefully anticipate situations that might provoke an attack and must often resort to habitual repetitive dosing. It has been claimed that the duration of the therapeutic effect of sublingual isosorbide dinitrate is longer than that of sublingual nitroglycerin—although just how much longer is questionable (17, 35)—and that isosorbide dinitrate is, therefore, preferable to NG in chronic dosing situations.

Figure 14 shows that the three pharmacological response intensities selected for routine use, that is, heart rate, digital plethysmographic (DPG) systolic amplitude, and DPG diastolic amplitude, peak 7–11 minutes after administration of sublingual 5 mg isosorbide dinitrate tablets; evidence of pharmacological activity remains for approximately 60 minutes postdrug. The maximum intensities (I_{max}) of the responses, with the exception of the heart rate response, are generally smaller in magnitude for sublingual 5 mg isosorbide dinitrate, as compared to sublingual nitroglycerin. This is exemplified in Figure 15, where the DPG diastolic amplitude response to 5 mg isosorbide dinitrate and 0.9 mg nitroglycerin in the same 12 subjects is

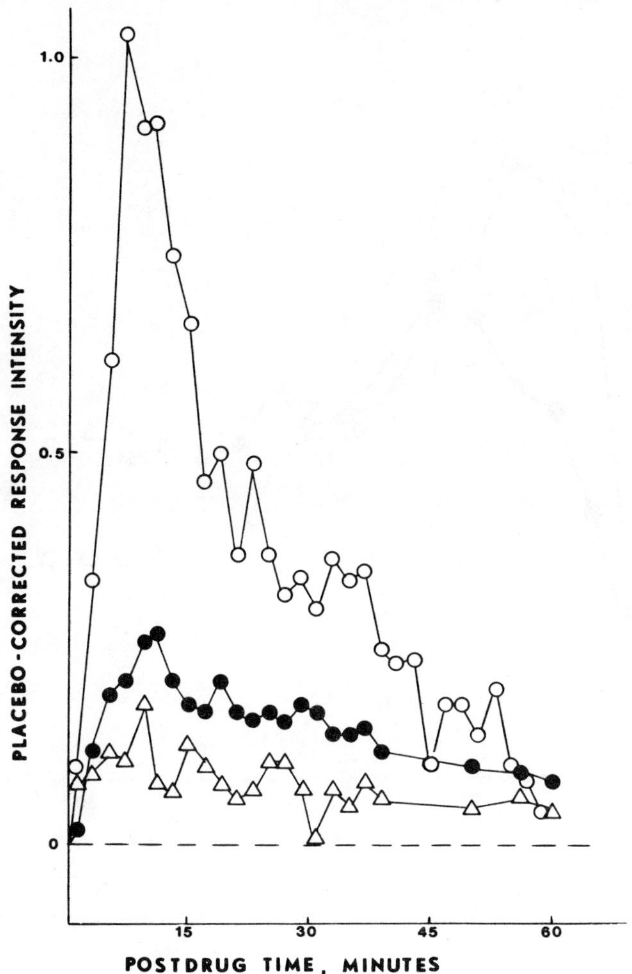

Figure 14. Temporal variation of the pharmacological response intensity of 12 healthy male volunteers dosed sublingually with a 5 mg isosorbide dinitrate tablet: △, heart rate response; ○, DPG systolic amplitude response; ●, DPG diastolic response.

compared. Referring to Figure 14, the heart rate response appears less sensitive to isosorbide dinitrate, as compared to the DPG amplitude responses. This same pattern was also observed for sublingual nitroglycerin and in general for all organic nitrate drugs and dosage forms (36).

Table 7 and Figures 16–18 indicate that all three pharmacological responses are dose dependent. Table 7 also shows that the dose differences are statistically significant. The AUC values in Table 7 do not level off with

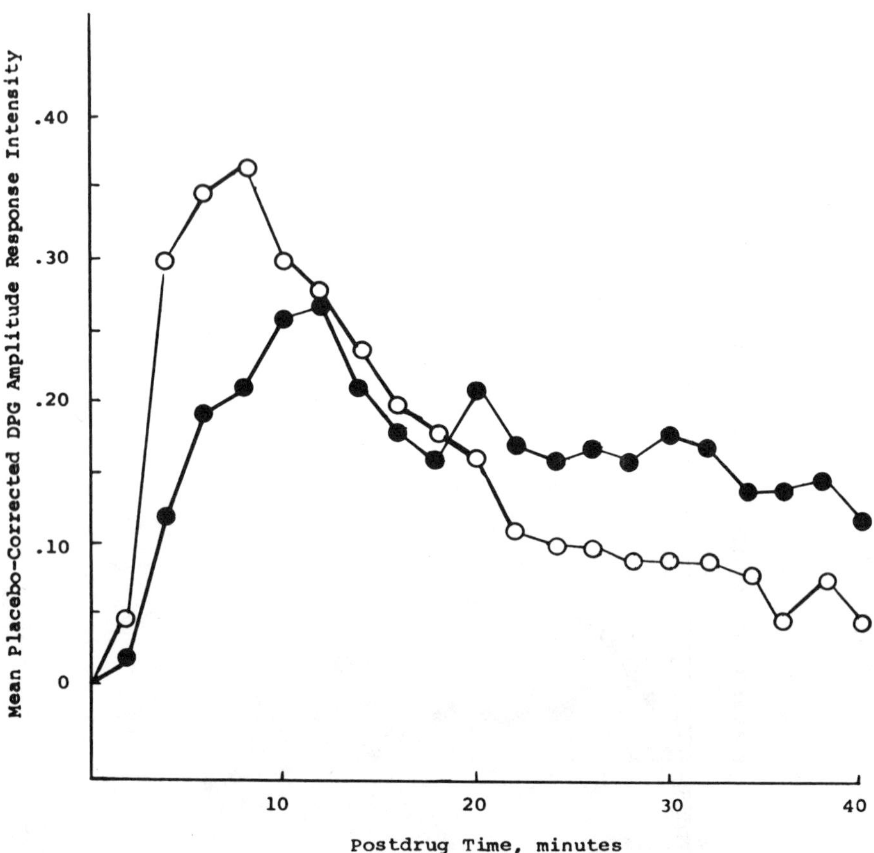

Figure 15. Temporal variation of the mean placebo-corrected digital plethysmographic diastolic amplitude response intensity for 12 volunteers dosed sublingually with: ○, 0.9 Mg NG, ●, 5 mg Isordil®.

increasing drug dose as abruptly with isosorbide dinitrate as previously reported for sublingual nitroglycerin. This is presumed to be a consequence of the longer duration of the drug effect obtained with isosorbide dinitrate relative to nitroglycerin, since only a small increase in the maximum intensity of isosorbide dinitrate effects occur with increased dosage. Extension of the AUC time from 40 to 60 minutes or longer would preferentially increase the AUC estimates for isosorbide dinitrate even more. A 0.5 mg nitroglycerin sublingual dose is as effective clinically as a 5 mg isosorbide dinitrate sublingual dose (37). The results in Table 8 appear to support this observation.

The delayed peaking of the three isosorbide dinitrate pharmacological responses, relative to sublingual nitroglycerin, can be attributed to a slower

Table 7. 40-Minute AUC Dose–Effect Data for 12 Volunteers Dosed Sublingually with Nitroglycerin (NG) and Isosorbide Dinitrate (ISDN)

	Physiological Responses		
Dose Treatment	Heart Rate	DPG Systolic Amplitude	DPG Diastolic Amplitude
(I) Placebo	-0.6 ± 0.3[a]	-7.4 ± 3.8	0.6 ± 0.2
(II) 0.6 mg NG	1.6 ± 0.6	15.5 ± 4.9	5.4 ± 1.1
(III) 2.5 mg ISDN	0.6 ± 0.6	5.9 ± 4.0	4.9 ± 1.0
(IV) 5 mg ISDN	3.0 ± 0.7	11.9 ± 3.7	6.0 ± 1.0
AUC Comparison	**Paired *t*-Test Significance Levels**		
III versus I	$p < 0.05$	$p < 0.025$	$p < 0.005$
IV versus I	$p < 0.005$	$p < 0.01$	$p < 0.005$
IV versus III	$p < 0.005$	$p < 0.05$	$p < 0.05$

[a]Mean 40-minute postdrug AUC values ± standard error.

Table 8. Subjective Data for the Sublingual Dosing of 12 Healthy Male Volunteers with Nitroglycerin (NG) and Isosorbide Dinitrate (ISDN) Tablets

Drug Dose	Tablet Disappearance Time (min)	Drug Effect Onset Time (min)	Drug Effect Disappearance Time (min)
0.3 mg NG (one NG tablet and two placebo tablets)	$1.2 + 0.2$[a]	2.8 ± 0.3	12.2 ± 1.2
0.6 mg NG (two 0.3 mg NG tablets and one placebo tablet)	0.9 ± 0.1	2.3 ± 0.2	13.5 ± 1.7
0.9 mg NG (three 0.3 mg NG tablets)	1.9 ± 0.1	2.0 ± 0.2	14.3 ± 2.6
2.5 mg ISDN (one tablet)	1.8 ± 0.4	4.4 ± 0.3	15.1 ± 3.8
5.0 mg ISDN (one tablet)	1.8 ± 0.5	4.3 ± 0.7	15.9 ± 1.9
Placebo (three tablets)	1.0 ± 0.2	—	—

[a]Mean ± standard error.

disintegration–dissolution of the isosorbide dinitrate tablets, as seen from the results in Table 8. The data in Table 8 were obtained by having the volunteers in the study signal the time of disappearance of the sublingual tablets placed beneath their tongues, and times of appearance and cessation of

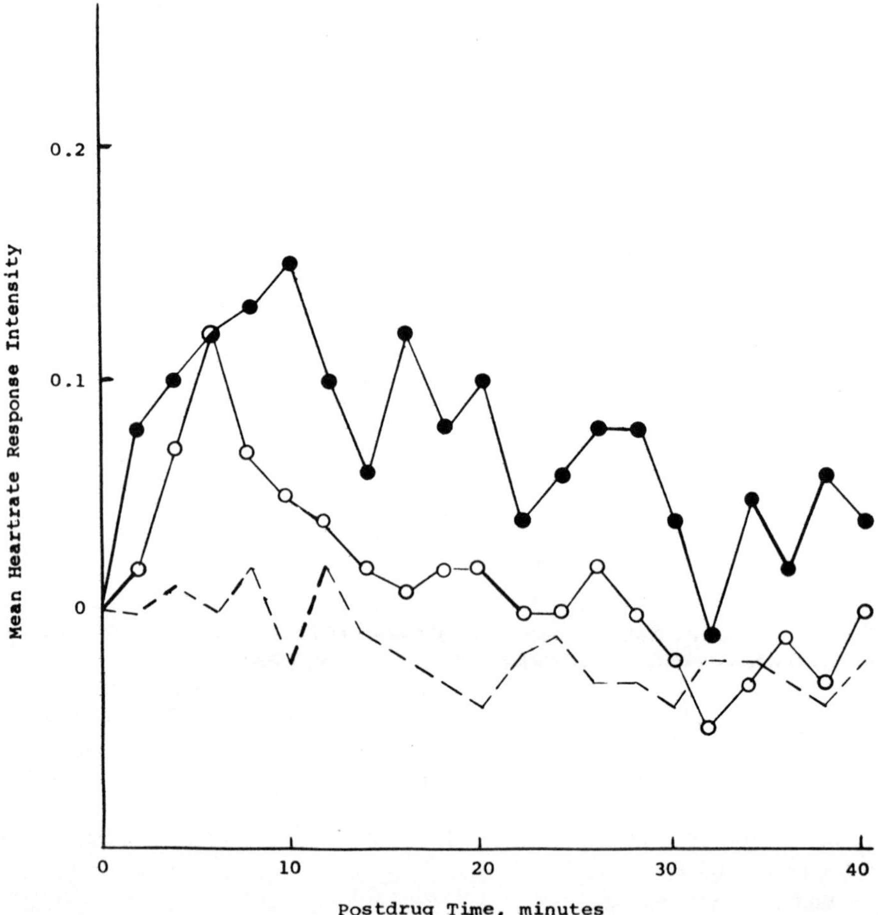

Figure 16. Temporal variation of the mean heart rate response intensity for 12 volunteers dosed sublingually: ---, placebo; ○, 2.5 mg Isordil®; ●, 5 mg Isordil®.

subjective sensations of the drug's effects (feelings of "expansion"); the values in Table 8 are averages obtained from 12 subjects listed with their standard deviations.

The estimated tablet disappearance times, which are directly related to their in-vivo disintegration–dissolution characteristics, are almost twice as long for the isosorbide dinitrate tablets as compared to nitroglycerin. In all cases, before administering the tablets, the subjects were directed to generate some saliva in their mouths so that the tablets would be introduced into a more consistent disintegration–dissolution environment. Since the isosorbide

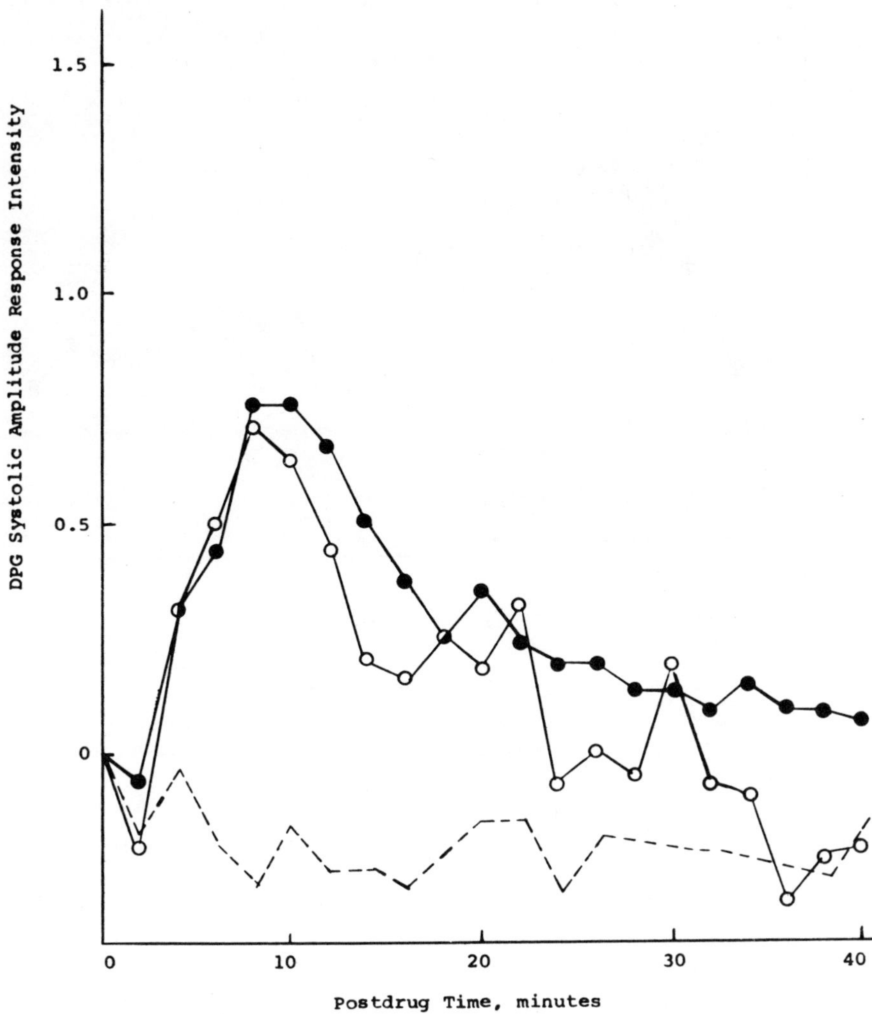

Figure 17. Temporal variation of the mean digital plethysmographic systolic amplitude response intensity for 12 volunteers dosed sublingually with isosorbide dinitrate: ---, placebo; ○, 2.5 mg Isordil®; ●, 5 mg Isordil®.

dinitrate tablets are larger than the nitroglycerin tablets, the differences in Table 8 are not surprising. The difference in the estimated drug effect onset times are consistent with the differences in the times of maximum pharmacological response for the isosorbide dinitrate and nitroglycerin tablets. The drug effect cessation times are shorter than either the durations of the pharmacological responses or the reported durations of the therapeutic benefits

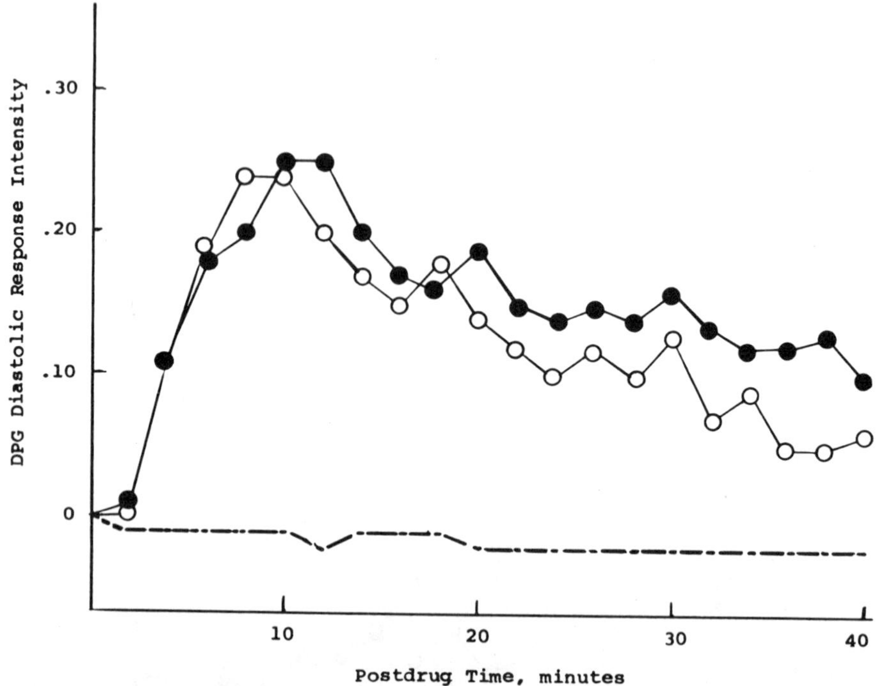

Figure 18. Temporal variation of the mean digital plethysmographic diastolic amplitude response intensity for 12 volunteers dosed sublingually with: ---, placebo; ○, 2.5 mg Isordil®; ●, 5 mg Isordil®.

for sublingual isosorbide dinitrate (17), which indicates that antianginal drug effects cannot be evaluated solely on the basis of subjective questioning.

A purpose for developing a pharmacological response methodology for monitoring the influence of sublingual nitroglycerin and isosorbide dinitrate on cardiovascular functions was to apply this methodology to the bioavailability assessment of a variety of organic nitrate antianginal drugs and drug products. In the investigation, two bioavailability comparisons were made. Figure 19 presents a comparison of Stuart's Sorbitrate® and Ives' Isordil® brands of sublingual 5 mg ISDN tablets based upon the DPG diastolic response intensity. The difference between the 60 minute AUC values for the two tablets, using a paired *t*-test comparison, is significant at the 0.05 probability level, despite the data having been derived from only six subjects. The same statistical significance also holds for the results shown in Figure 20, where a 5 mg sublingual Sorbitrate® ISDN tablet is compared with a 5 mg chewable ISDN tablet of the same brand. There is little difference in the times to reach peak effects for these two ISDN dosage forms. Definitive

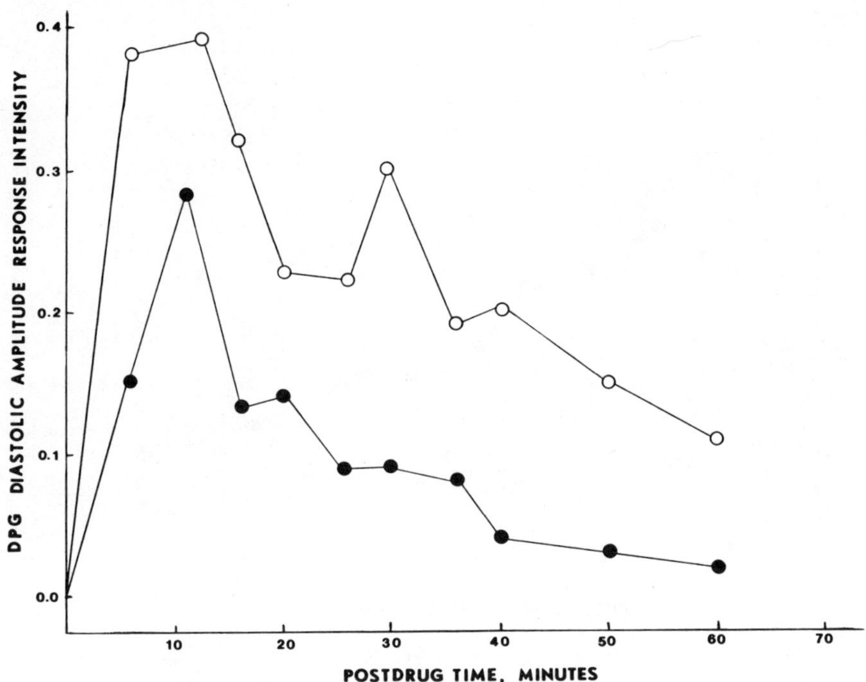

Figure 19. Temporal variation of the mean DPG diastolic response intensity of six healthy male volunteers dosed sublingually with a 5 mg isosorbide dinitrate tablet: ○, Sorbitrate®; ●, Isordil®.

conclusions concerning the duration of clinical antiangina activity cannot be made from the present data, although it is likely that the ISDN dose treatments with the smaller 60 minute AUC's will also have shorter durations. Results obtained for the ISDN tablets using other pharmacological response variables, such as the DPG systolic amplitude response intensity, corroborate the conclusions obtained on the DPG diastolic amplitude response versus time profiles shown in Figures 19 and 20. However, these other responses are not as satisfactory as the diastolic amplitude response for bioequivalency comparisons because they are somewhat more variable.

Reported (31, 33) blood-level data for sublingual and chewable ISDN tablets, although limited, permit comparisons to be made with pharmacological response data such as that shown in Figures 21–24. It is quite apparent in these figures that there is a definite correlation between ISDN plasma levels and the pharmacological responses, even though the subject populations were different and the sublingual data were obtained with two different brands of ISDN tablets. The agreement for peak times between the blood

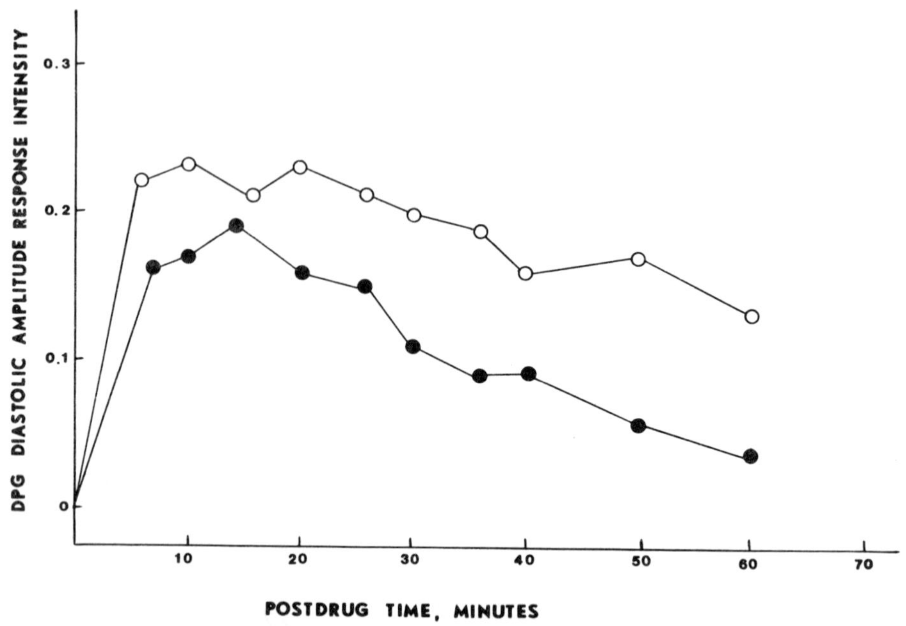

Figure 20. Temporal variation of the mean DPG diastolic response intensity of six healthy male volunteers dosed with 5 mg isosorbide dinitrate (Sorbitrate®) tablets: ○, sublingual tablet; ●, chewable tablet.

levels and pharmacological response variables is very close in every case. Although only pharmacological response intensities corresponding to the blood sampling times were plotted in Figures 21–23, a far greater frequency of pharmacological response data points can be obtained in a 60 minute postdrug interval than with blood samples, since the pharmacological measurements can be made every minute, or almost continuously if desired. The pharmacological response recording approach is also noninvasive and sensitive; the computation of drug response variables is nearly automatic and relatively simple. It should be apparent that this approach can provide a more satisfactory method for performing bioavailability studies of sublingual and chewable NG and ISDN tablets than the chemical assay of blood samples. Another advantage of using the pharmacological response approach is the more direct relationship between pharmacological effects and clinical activity. The use of pharmacological response intensity data for bioavailability evaluations of organic nitrate drug products has been recommended by the Food and Drug Administration (3).

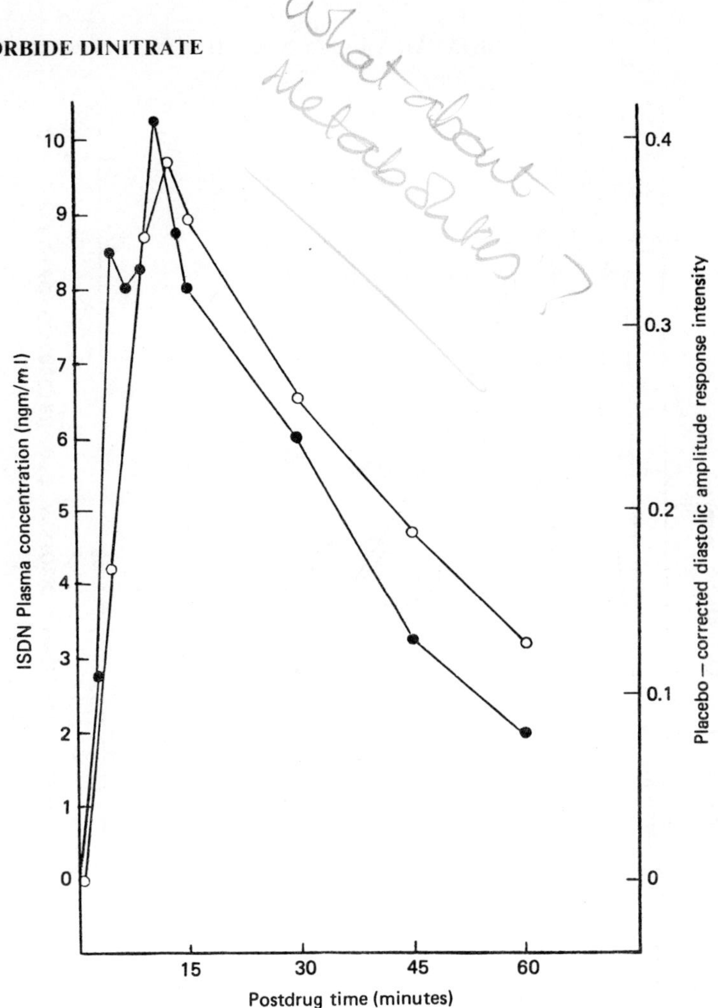

Figure 21. Temporal variation of the mean isosorbide dinitrate plasma concentration and the mean placebo-corrected DPG diastolic amplitude response intensity following sublingual dosing of six healthy male volunteers with 5 mg isosorbide dinitrate tablet; ○, plasma concentration; ●, diastolic response intensity.

5.3 Absorption and Elimination Half-Lives

Monitoring the absorptive phase of a pharmacokinetic profile of ISDN following sublingual and chewable tablet dosing, using blood level data, is difficult because of the extremely rapid drug absorption. However, using pharmacological response data allows a more complete representation of the time curve to be achieved.

Table 9 lists and compares values for the apparent half-lives of absorption

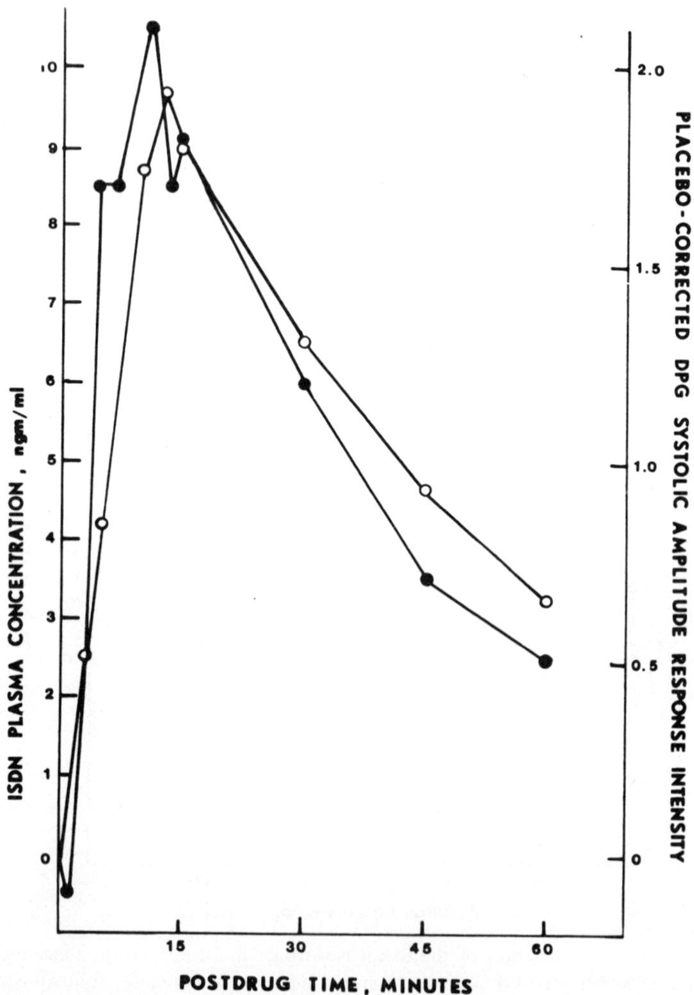

Figure 22. Temporal variation of the mean isosorbide dinitrate plasma concentration and the mean placebo-corrected DPG systolic response intensity following sublingual dosing of six healthy male volunteers with a 5 mg isosorbide dinitrate tablet: ○, plasma concentration; ●, systolic response intensity.

and elimination of ISDN obtained from plasma level, diastolic amplitude, and systolic amplitude response variables for sublingual and chewable tablets. The absorption half-life estimates listed in Table 9 are remarkably similar, as expected from the observation that the blood levels and pharmacological response data with plasma levels is satisfactory, although not as

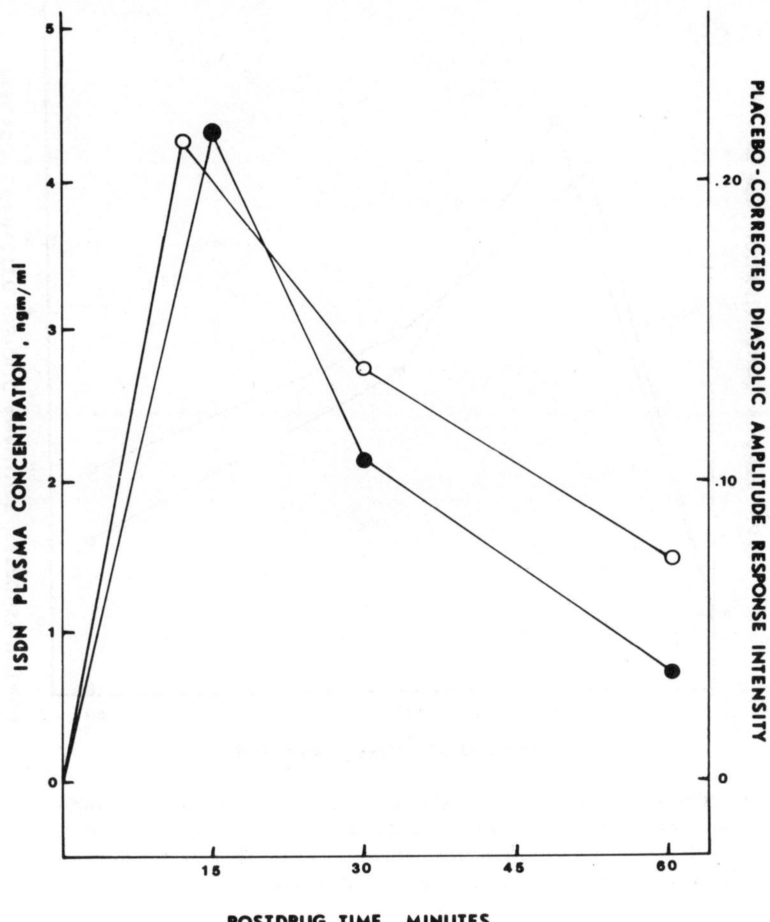

Figure 23. Temporal variation of the mean isosorbide dinitrate plasma concentration and the mean placebo-corrected DPG diastolic response intensity following dosing of healthy male volunteers with a 5 mg chewable isosorbide dinitrate tablet; ●, plasma concentration, 4 volunteers; ○, diastolic amplitude response intensity, 6 volunteers.

good as the absorption results. Differences between plasma level elimination half-life values for the two types of tablets, and between plasma level values and pharmacological response values, can largely be attributed to the data having been derived from different subject populations in each case. Considering that the absorption of the drug across the oral mucosa is very rapid and the rate limiting step is likely the release of the ISDN from the tablet, the use of different subject groups would be expected to have little or

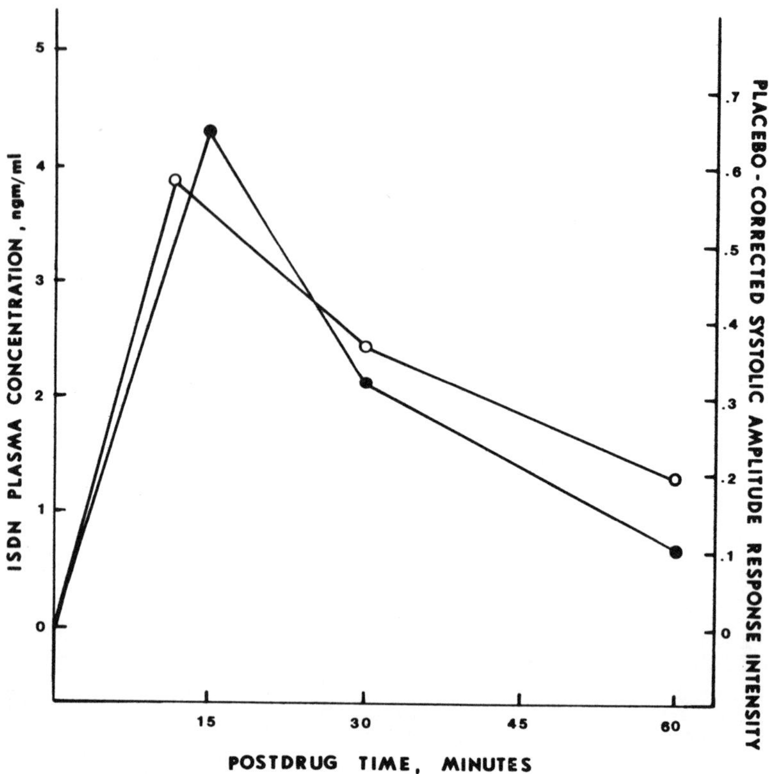

Figure 24. Temporal variation of the mean isosorbide dinitrate plasma concentration and the mean placebo-corrected DPG systolic response intensity following dosing of healthy male volunteers with a 5 mg chewable isosorbide dinitrate tablet: ●, plasma concentration, 4 volunteers; ○, systolic amplitude response intensity, 6 volunteers.

no influence on the absorption half-lives obtained from the three different measures. The shortest elimination half-life listed in Table 9, 18 minutes, was observed in a study involving only four subjects. The elimination half-life values for sublingual ISDN are approximately three times as long as elimination half-life values determined for sublingual NG, which accounts for the longer duration of sublingual ISDN. The enhanced duration of ISDN has been ascribed to slower metabolic degradation of the drug (34). The results in Table 9 indicate that DPG pharmacological response monitoring is capable of providing useful pharmacokinetic information, which corroborates similar information derived from blood level measurements.

Table 9. Drug Absorption and Elimination Half-Life Values for the Dosing of Healthy Male Volunteers with 5 mg Sublingual and Chewable Isosorbide Dinitrate (ISDN) Tablets

	Half-Life (min)			
	Absorption		Elimination	
Source of Data	(Sublingual tablet)	(Chewable tablet)	(Sublingual tablet)	(Chewable tablet)
ISDN Plasma concentration	2.4[a]	—	30.3[a]	18[c]
DPG Systolic amplitude response	3[b]	3[b]	25[b]	34[b]
DPG Diastolic amplitude response	3[b]	3[b]	22[b]	32[b]

[a]Isordil®, 6 healthy volunteers.
[b]Sorbitrate®, 6 healthy volunteers (not the same as for *a*).
[c]Sorbitrate®, 4 healthy volunteers (not the same as for *a* and *b*).

6. ORAL SUSTAINED ACTION DOSAGE FORMS OF NITROGLYCERIN, ISOSORBIDE DINITRATE, AND PENTAERYTHRITOL TETRANITRATE

The effectiveness of oral sustained action organic nitrate antianginal drug products in the treatment of ischemic heart pain and their bioavailability has been controversial (38–40). Although studies have been conducted to prove that these widely used products are effective for prolonged periods of time (26, 40), the experimental design and execution of many of the studies has been criticized (17). In some studies a placebo comparison is lacking; in others insensitive or imprecise drug activity assessment procedures were used; in still others the lack of statistical evaluations of the data were a deficiency. The problem has been compounded, at least until relatively recently (31–33) by the lack of suitable assays for determining concentrations of organic nitrate drugs and their metabolites in biological fluids. The metabolites are worthy of consideration, since most are pharmacologically active. Although less active than the parent drugs, relatively high concentrations of metabolites are present, and often predominate, in the systemic circulation soon after organic nitrate drugs have been administered orally because of a pronounced hepatic "first pass" effect (34, 41, 42).

In the preceding sections of this chapter it was demonstrated that a pharmacological response methodology is capable of sensitively and reliably assessing the bioavailability and hemodynamic effectiveness of sublingual nitroglycerin (NG) and sublingual isosorbide (ISDN) tablets. The methodology, which has been recommended by the Food and Drug Administration (3), is noninvasive, sensitive, and relatively uncomplicated to implement. The present section presents the results of applying this method to the investigation of oral sustained action nitroglycerin (NG), isosorbide dinitrate (ISDN), and pentaerythritol tetranitrate (PETN) dosage forms. In 1971 a NRC, DESI review classified the oral sustained action dosage forms of organic nitrates as only possibly effective, but they were allowed to remain on the market through a judicial ruling in 1972 (3). Relatively little definitive information concerning these products has been reported since that time.

6.1 Experimental Methods

Of the drug products listed in Table 1, the duplicated 6×6 Latin square experiments constituting the present study included: (*1*) oral placebo tablets; (*2*) 0.6 mg sublingual NG (two tablets of 0.3 mg Nitrostat®); (*3*) 40 mg oral ISDN administered as 10 mg conventional tablets (Isordil®) at 0, 2, 4, and 6 hours; (*4*) 40 mg oral ISDN sustained action (Isordil® Tembids); (*5*) 80 mg oral PETN administered as 20 mg conventional tablets at 0, 2, 4, and 6 hours; and (*6*) 80 mg oral PETN sustained action tablets (Peritrate®).

The daily testing procedure was as previously described, each experimental run beginning at the same time of day and repeating each subject's run on the same day of the week after a 7-day washout period. The time of dosing was considered zero postdrug time. Following dosing, biosignal recordings were made over a 10 second breath-holding period at intervals, for 0.6 mg sublingual nitroglycerin, of every 3 minutes for the first 30 minutes postdrug and every 6 minutes for the next 30 minutes. The same recording schedule was maintained for the placebo, except that after the first hour recordings were made at intervals of every 30 minutes for up to 8 hours postdrug. The recordings were similarly made every 30 minutes following oral doses of the drug. The recorded data were computer processed as previously described to resolve the time course of drug-induced changes in the DPG signals.

6.2 Bioavailability Comparison of Oral Dosage Forms

The hemodynamic efficacy of sustained action oral NG and ISDN tablets has been demonstrated by several investigators. Digital plethysmographic (DPG) measurements were used by Winsor and coworkers (26) to show that, relative to a placebo control, a 2.6 mg NG tablet and a 40 mg ISDN tablet each increased peripheral vasodilation for several hours. Unfortunately, statistical assessment of the hemodynamic effects were not made, nor were any pharmacokinetic bioavailability parameters calculated. In a well-controlled, rigorous clinical study using angina patients, Winsor and Berger (40) observed that 2.6 mg NG tablets elicited statistically significant effects, relative to placebo, by increasing the duration of exercise and decreasing the pathological depression of the ST segment of the electrocardiograms for several hours. However, since the patients in the study were maintained on a 2.6 mg NG tablet t.i.d. dosage regimen for a lengthy period of time, the results are representative of a "steady-rate" dosing situation and not of a single dose or chronic dosing situation. The measured drug effects are, therefore, due to residual NG and pharmacologically active metabolites, as well as to NG from a single specific dose. Nevertheless, the results of this study do conclusively demonstrate the inherent effectiveness of orally administered NG given on a repetitive dosing regimen. A well-controlled study performed by Danahey and coworkers (30) on a conventional oral ISDN tablet indicated that orally administered ISDN also is an effective antianginal agent. Of the three drugs considered in this report, PETN is the one most in doubt. Its major drawback is low aqueous solutility (34). The majority of an oral PETN dose reaching the systemic circulation is absorbed as metabolites that are much less active (34, 45, 46) than PETN itself.

The results of the present study comparing the AUC responses of the sustained action dosage forms to each other, and to the 0.6 mg sublingual reference dose treatment included in the complete crossover study with 12 subjects, are summarized in Tables 10 and 11. Table 10 reveals that the vasodilation induced by the sustained action PETN tablets is least when compared to the other sustained action tablets, even though the PETN tablets contain the largest quantity (by weight) of antianginal drug. The heart rate response to PETN is exceptionally large, which may result from certain PETN metabolites being unusually active inducers of tachycardia. These results for PETN demonstrate that it is useful to measure more than one pharmacological response, since some may be sensitive to the parent drug and others may reflect the presence and activity of its metabolites (47).

Table 10 also shows that the oral 6.5 mg NG tablet is more active pharmacologically than the 2.6 mg NG tablet, as expected. This observation has been confirmed in a subsequent study of different brands of 2.6 mg and 6.5 mg NG tablets (44, 47). It was noted that increasing the oral dose of sustained action NG above 6.5 mg does not increase the response, either in magnitude of individual response intensity time points or in total AUC, and may actually diminish it. Although the mechanism of this phenomenon is not known, it can be speculated that relatively inactive metabolite(s) are being formed, which antagonize the active drug species by competing for their receptor

Table 10. Results for Oral and Sublingual Organic Nitrate Antianginal Drug Dosing Experiments Using Human Subjects[a]

	Heart Rate				DPG Systolic Amplitude				DPG Diastolic Amplitude			
Statistical Calculations	($\bar{x}$)	(σ)	(SE)	(CV)	($\bar{x}$)	(σ)	(SE)	(CV)	($\bar{x}$)	(σ)	(SE)	(CV)
0.6 mg sublingual nitroglycerin (NG); 19 subjects, 60 minute postdrug AUC	3.3	3.2	0.73	1.0	24.6	23.1	5.2	0.9	9.7	4.2	0.95	0.4
2.6 mg oral sustained action NG; 11 subjects, 7.5 hour postdrug AUC	4.6	35.0	10.6	7.1	76.8	140.7	42.4	1.8	21.9	24.6	7.4	1.1
6.5 mg oral sustained action NG; 11 subjects, 7.5 hour postdrug AUC	8.6	40.1	12.1	4.7	177.0	142.4	42.9	0.8	48.1	49.5	14.9	1.0
40 mg oral sustained action Isosorbide Dinitrate; 11 subjects, 7.5 hour postdrug AUC	−38.2	47.6	14.3	0.8	164.2	167.6	50.5	1.0	92.5	118.1	35.6	1.3
80 mg oral sustained action Pentaerythritol Tetranitrate; 12 subjects, 7.5 hour postdrug AUC	24.5	26.7	7.7	1.1	−29.2	121.4	35.0	4.2	7.2	37.0	10.7	5.2

[a] $\bar{x}$, Mean; σ, standard deviation; SE, standard error; CV, coefficient of variation.

Table 11. Paired *t*-Test Comparisons of 7.5 hour AUC for Oral Sustained Action Antianginal Organic Nitrate Tablets to Placebo Doses

Placebo-Sustained Action Tablet Comparison	Heart Rate Response	DPG Systolic Amplitude Response	DPG Diastolic Amplitude Response
2.6 mg nitroglycerin tablet[a]	NS[b]	$p \simeq 0.05$	$p < 0.01$
6.5 mg nitroglycerin tablet[a]	NS	$p < 0.005$	$p < 0.005$
40 mg isosorbide dinitrate[a]	NS	$p < 0.005$	$p < 0.025$
80 mg pentaerythritol tetranitrate[c]	$p < 0.005$	NS	NS

[a]For 11 test subjects.
[b]Not significant at 0.05 probability level.
[c]For 12 test subjects.

site(s). In any event, the maximum response intensity elicited by an oral dose of NG is always less than that obtained for a sublingual dose; this is demonstrated in Figure 25 for the DPG diastolic amplitude response and is also the case for heart rate and DPG systolic amplitude responses. However, a 5 mg buccal NG tablet dosage form slightly exceeded the maximum DPG diastolic response intensity elicited by 0.6 mg sublingual NG and maintained at least 50% of this maximum response intensity for nearly 4 hours (44). This is presumably a consequence of the drug being largely absorbed through the oral mucosa directly into the systemic circulation, and thereby circumventing first pass hepatic metabolism in the same manner as occurs with sublingual dosing.

An informative approach to evaluating the bioavailability of controlled-release oral dosage forms is to compare their response profiles to those obtained from repeated dosing with conventional immediate release tablets (48). This approach was used in testing oral sustained action 40 mg ISDN and 80 mg PETN tablets. The results of these comparisons are presented in Figures 26–29 and Table 11. Figure 29 is similar to Figure 28 in summarily presenting the results of the present study for all the dose treatments by plots of the partial AUC's for each dose treatment versus the midpoint of the time period over which the AUC was calculated. Partial AUC's that are significantly different by paired *t*-tests from the placebo baseline, to which all the plotted values should be referred, are indicated in the figure. It is apparent from inspection of the results in Figures 26–29 and Table 12, that the performance of the 80 mg sustained action PETN tablet, when compared to

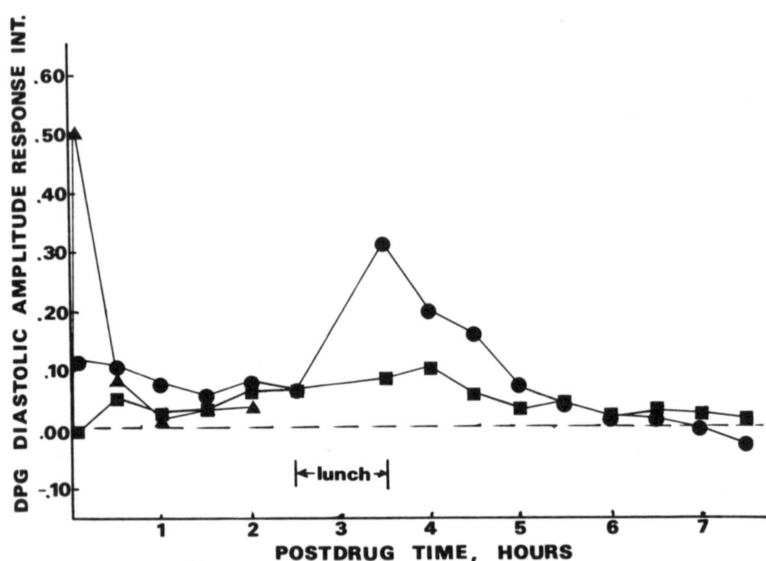

Figure 25. Temporal variation of mean, placebo-corrected DPG diastolic amplitude response intensities for 11–12 healthy male volunteers dosed with; ▲, 0.6 mg sublingual nitroglycerin (two 0.3 mg tablets); ■, an oral 2.6 mg sustained action nitroglycerin tablet; ●, an oral 6.5 mg sustained action nitroglycerin tablet.

Table 12. Paired *t*-Test Statistical Comparisons of 7.5 Hour AUC's for Oral Sustained Organic Nitrate Dosage Forms to Repeated Dosing with Conventional Tablets

Oral Tablet Dose Treatment Comparison	Heart Rate Response	DPG Systolic Amplitude Response	DPG Diastolic Amplitude Response
Susained action 40 mg isosorbide dinitrate versus 4 × 10 mg isosorbide dinitrate[a]	$p<0.1$ (multiple dosing better)	NS[b]	NS
Sustained action 80 mg pentaerythritol tetranitrate versus 4 × 20 mg pentaerythritol tetranitrate[c]	NS	$p<0.05$ (multiple dosing better)	$p<0.005$ (multiple dosing better)

[a]For 11 test subjects.
[b]Not significant at 0.05 probability level.
[c]For 12 test subjects.

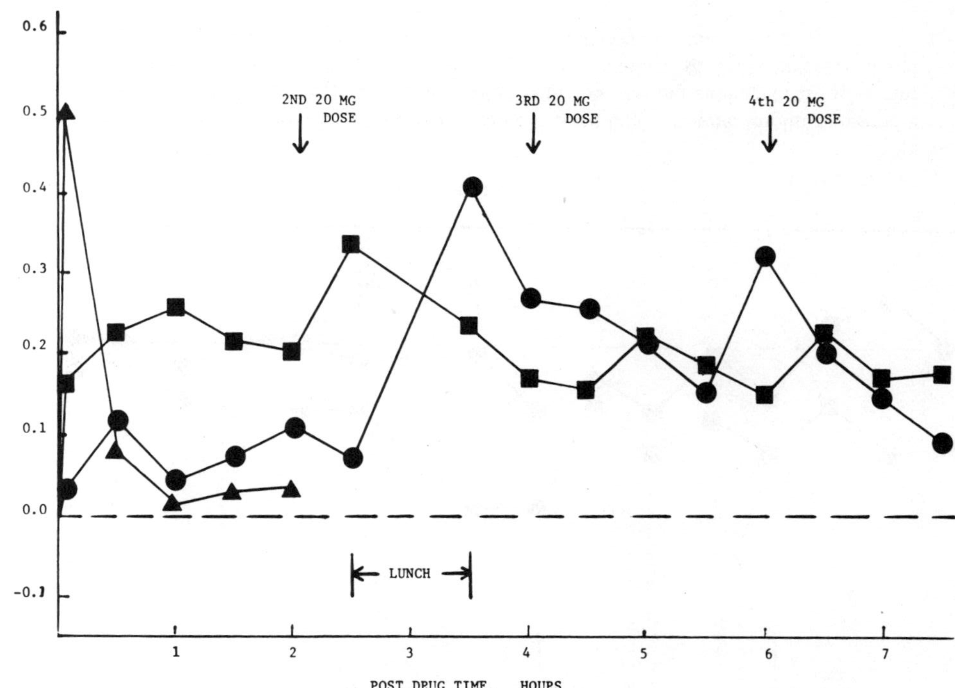

Figure 26. Temporal variation of mean, placebo-corrected DPG diastolic amplitude response intensities for 11–12 healthy male volunteers dosed with: ▲, 0.6 mg sublingual nitroglycerin; ●, an oral 40 mg isosorbide dinitrate sustained action tablet; ■, four conventional oral 10 mg isosorbide dinitrate tablets, one administered every 2 hours.

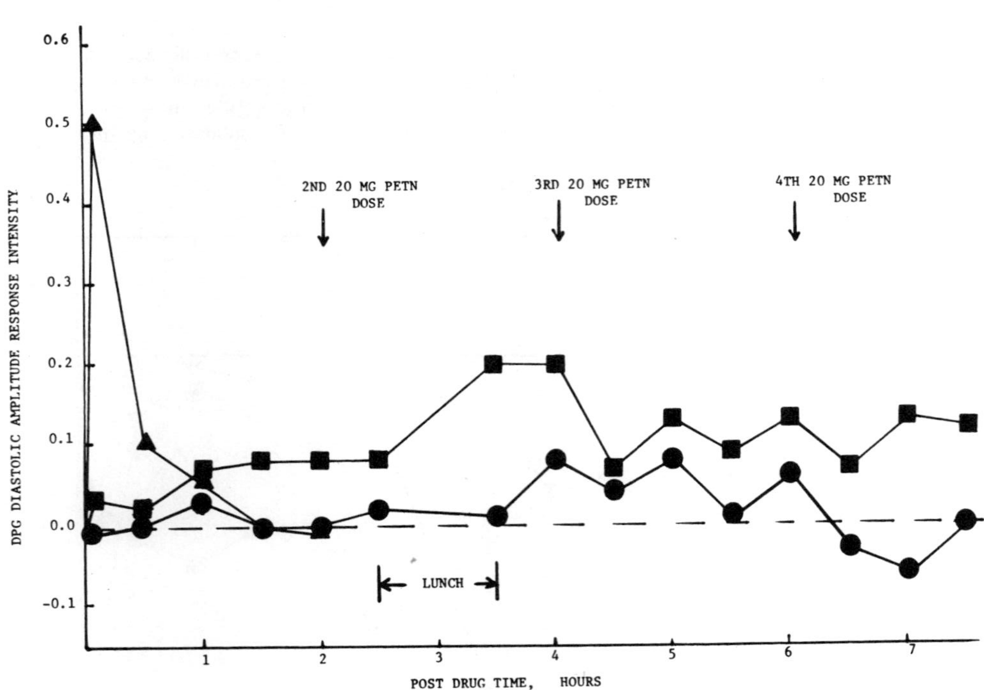

Figure 27. Temporal variation of mean, placebo-corrected DPG diastolic amplitude response intensities for 12 healthy male volunteers dosed with: ▲. 0.6 mg sublingual nitroglycerin; ●, an oral 80 mg pentaerythritol tetranitrate sustained action tablet; ■, four conventional oral 20 mg pentaerythritol tetranitrate tablets, one administered every 2 hours.

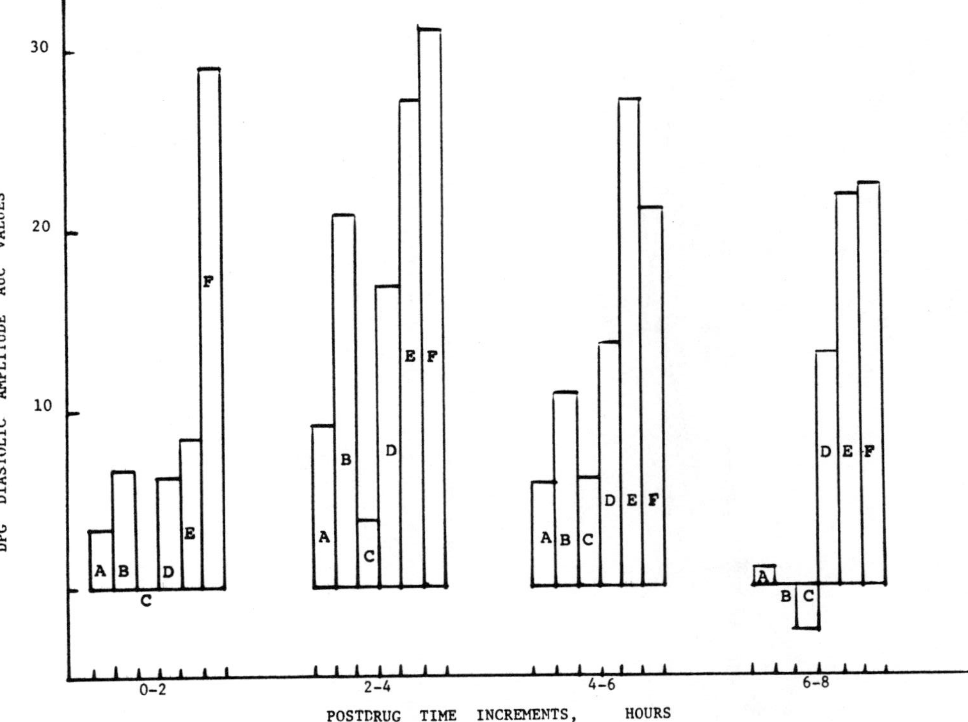

Figure 28. Bar graphs of incremental 2 hour AUC data for oral antianginal organic nitrate tablets. AUC values are mean, placebo-corrected values for 11–12 healthy male volunteers: (*A*) 2.6 mg sustained action nitroglycerin tablet; (*B*) 6.5 mg sustained action nitroglycerin tablet; (*C*) 80 mg sustained action pentaerythritol tetranitrate tablet; (*D*) 4×20 mg pentaerythritol tetranitrate tablets (one tablet administered every 2 hours); (*E*) 40 mg sustained action isosorbide dinitrate tablet; (*F*) 4×10 isosorbide dinitrate tablets (one tablet administered every 2 hours).

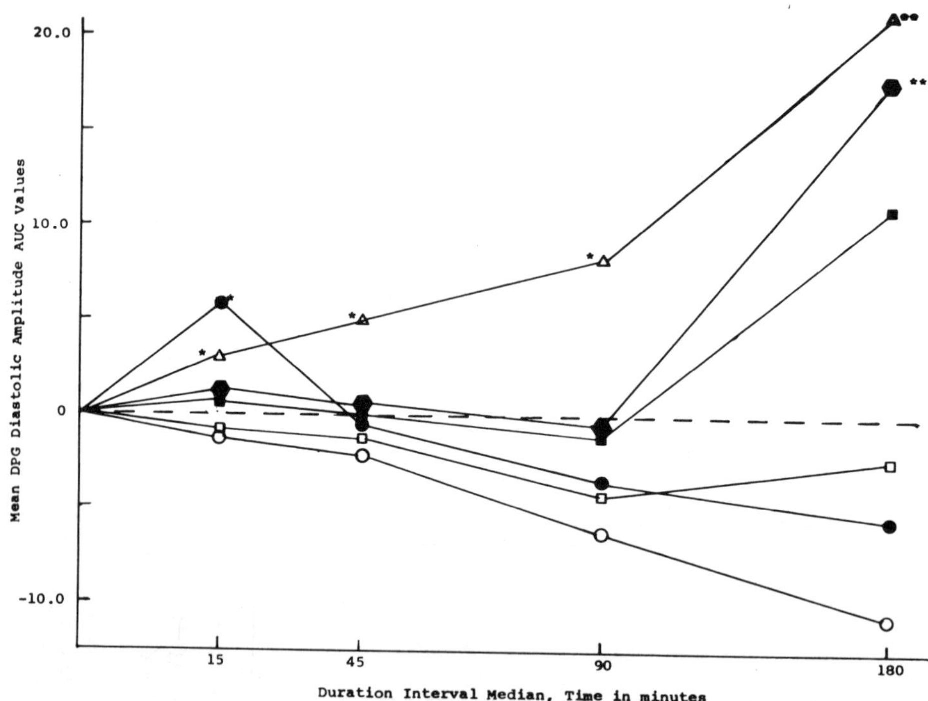

Figure 29. Mean DPG diastolic amplitude response AUC values for the 0–30, 31–60, 61–120, and 121–240 minute duration intervals plotted versus the midpoint time of the four sequential area duration intervals observed for 12 healthy male volunteers dosed with organic nitrate antianginal drugs: ○, placebo; ●, 0.6 mg nitroglycerin (NG) sublingual (two 0.3 mg tablets); □, 2.6 mg NG oral sustained action tablet; ■, 6.5 mg NG oral sustained action tablet; △, repeat dosing 10 mg isosorbide dinitrate (ISDN) oral tablets (one tablet administered at 0, 0+120, 0+240, and 0+360 minutes); ⬢, 40 mg ISDN oral sustained action tablet. (*) Statistically different from placebo at 5% level at this particular duration interval. (**) Statistically different from placebo at 1% level.

conventional 20 mg PETN tablets given every 2 hours, is quite poor, relative to that of the sustained action 40 mg ISDN tablet results. As shown in Figures 28 and 29, both the controlled release 6.5 mg NG and the 40 mg ISDN elicited an appreciable vasodilatory activity over the 8-hour monitoring period.

Referring to Table 10, it is quite apparent that the intersubject variability observed with the oral controlled release dosage forms was much greater than with sublingual nitroglycerin. This can in part be attributed to a large irregularity in the ability of individual subjects to hepatically metabolize the drug after oral dosing. Table 10 also illustrates that the least bioavailable 80 mg sustained PETN tablets have the greatest variability in DPG responses.

Based on 60-minute placebo-corrected AUC results, all the test subjects responded to the sublingual NG dose treatment. Based on 7.5-hour AUC results, 9 out of 11 subjects responded to the 40 mg ISDN and 6.5 mg NG sustained action tablet dose treatments, whereas only 7 out of 12 subjects responded to the 80 mg PETN sustained action dose treatment. The unusually small response to the sustained action PETN tablet during the first 2-hour postdrug interval indicates that PETN is not readily absorbed from this dosage form.

In as much as measured body fluid levels or pharmacological response variables reflect clinical antiangina activity of the drugs, the bioavailability evaluations of organic nitrate drug products based on these measures will also have direct clinical relevance. It is well-known that following oral dosing organic nitrate drugs are extensively metabolized (45, 46, 49–51) to lesser active metabolites that contribute significantly to the drugs' actions. For example, following oral dosing of ISDN, the levels of 2-ISDN in the plasma were reported to be 2–5 times higher than the parent drug, and the 5-ISDN metabolite of ISDN 12–24 times higher than the parent drug (42). These ISDN metabolites are active (34, 51, 52); in such cases, plasma level determinations of the parent drug alone are an inadequate and misleading basis for the bioavailability assessment of such drugs. An extreme example is that of PETN, which following oral dosing is not detectable in the blood as the parent drug (45). However, oral PETN exhibits pharmacological activity through the actions of its metabolites. If plasma level data are used, they must include determinations of the metabolites as well as the parent drug, and the results must weigh on considerations of the bioactivity of each species detected. It is considerable less complex to directly employ pharmacological measures to achieve the same result.

In a recent, well-controlled clinical investigation of oral ISDN and sublingual NG, Danahy and coworkers (30) concurrently obtained exercise tolerance and hemodynamic information on angina patients. The reported results of their study with ISDN has been converted to response intensities, placebo-corrected, and replotted in Figure 30. The 8-hour data points were obtained by extrapolation of the linear, semilogarithmic plots of the data in Figure 30 that are shown in Figure 31. Estimates of the half-lives of the exercise tolerance, exercise heart rate, and resting heart rate responses can be derived from the plots in Figures 30 and 31. Since the half-life of ISDN is approximately 30 minutes, these half-life estimates of 3–5 hours suggest that a major part of the response elicited by oral ISDN tablets is due to the 2-moninitrate and 5-mononitrate metabolites. Plasma level measurements following ISDN dosing of rats and dogs indicate that the elimination half-life of the two metabolites range from 2 to 2.5 hours, whereas the half-life of ISDN is very short (34). Plasma level (32, 33) and exercise tolerance (34)

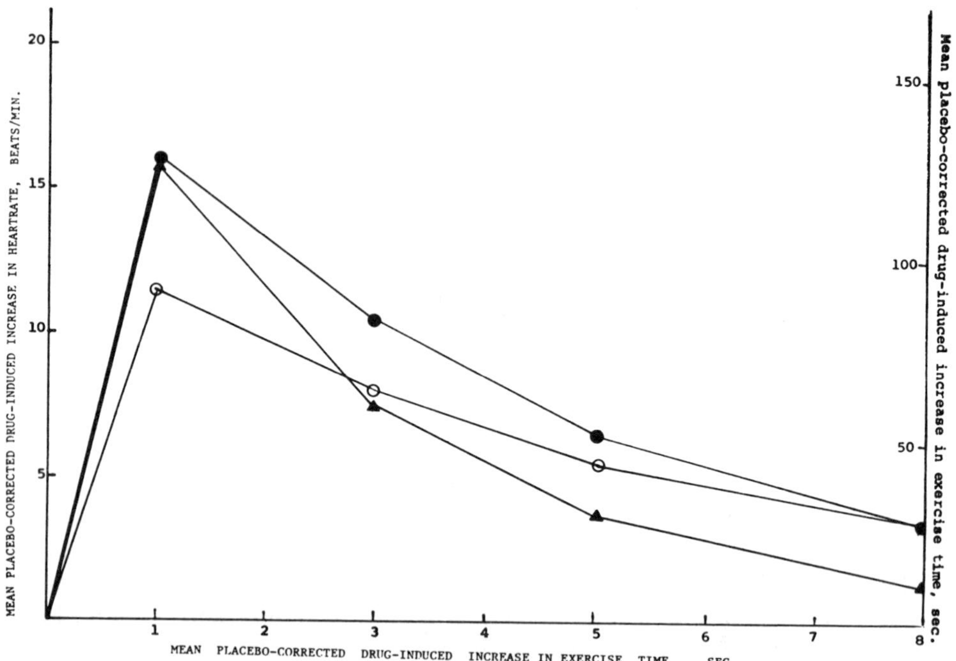

Figure 30. Time dependence of drug-induced increases in exercise time, ▲, exercise heart rate, ○, and resting heart rate, ● following dosing of 21 angina patients with oral isosorbide dinitrate (ISDN) tablets (20–50 mg ISDN; average dose = 29 mg). Data taken from reference 30.

data obtained in humans indicate that the elimination half-life of ISDN is 20–40 minutes, the half-life of the 2-mononitrate metabolite is 2.5 hours, and the half-life of the 5-monometabolite is 4.5 hours (32). Even though the 5-mononitrate compound is more abundant, the 2-mononitrate compound is much more active pharmacologically (34). A similar situation is probably true for NG, since there is evidence that the elimination half-life of NG is shorter than that of ISDN, and the half-lives of the 1,2- and 1,3-dinitro NG metabolites are analogous to the half-lives of the ISDN metabolites in being longer than the parent drug (34). Although the pharmacological activities of the ISDN and NG metabolites are small compared to unchanged NG and ISDN, moderate conventional oral doses of these drugs conceivably supply sufficient active material to the systemic circulation to exert significant pharmacological effects. The observed prominent activity of submilligram sublingual NG doses attests to the potency of this class of drugs.

The two active ISDN metabolites may have qualitatively different pharmacological activities, and alteration of the relative abundance of the two

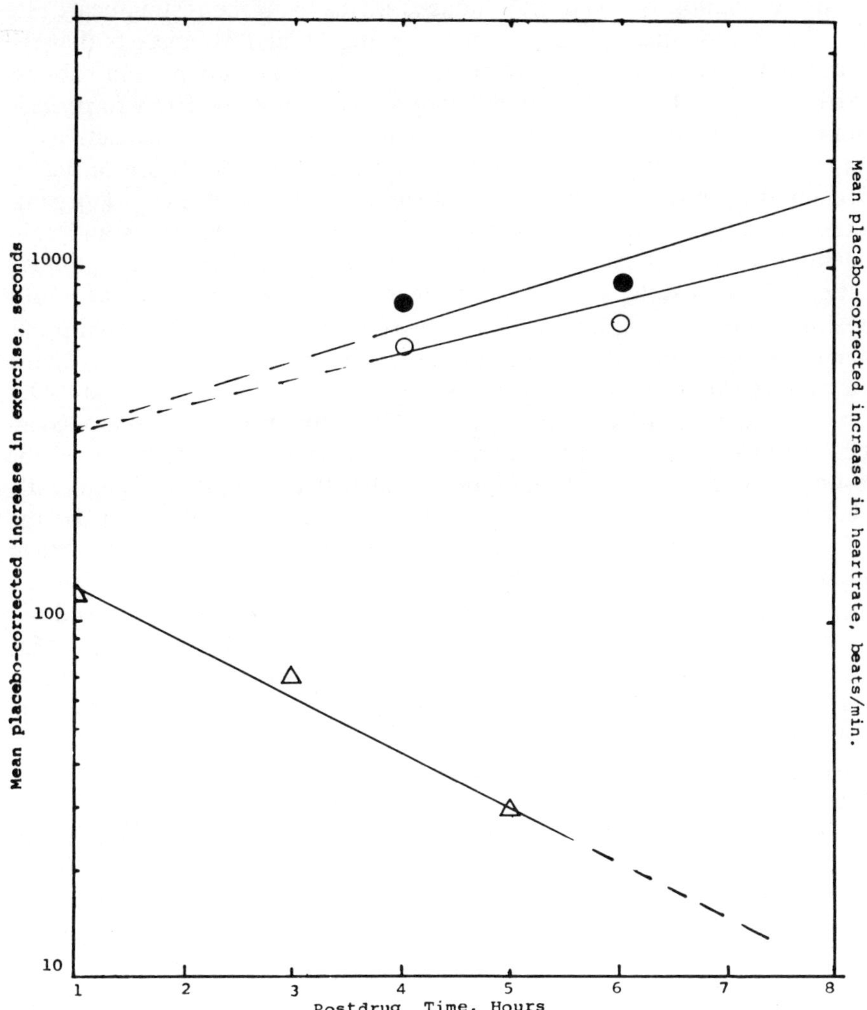

Figure 31. Semi-log plots of data from Figure 30. Exercise tolerance data linear correlation coefficient = 0.98; exercise heart rate data linear correlation coefficient = 0.95; resting heart rate data linear correlation coefficient = 0.93.

metabolites due to intersubject differences in metabolism could explain the need to titrate patients to their proper dosage (30), why some individuals experience severe headaches (42) during ISDN treatment, and the reason certain people benefit from sublingual NG therapy but not from oral ISDN therapy (54).

The correlation between drug-induced increases in the resting heart rate and the exercise duration apparent in Figures 30 and 31 suggests that the pharmacological response measurements made on healthy human subjects participating in the bioavailability studies required by the FDA to precede clinical studies, can also be used to predictively assess the clinical activity of ISDN (and other organic nitrates) in angina patients. Such use of hemodynamic response variables to assess the clinical effectiveness of organic nitrate drug products depends upon the following assumptions and considerations: (*1*) that the effect of ISDN on the resting heart rate of angina patients does not differ significantly from its effect on the resting heart rate of healthy volunteers (except for extreme conditions, this is a valid assumption) and (*2*) the need and acceptance of a clinical criterion, or a clinical standard, for comparison purposes. For example, 5 hours after dosing with oral ISDN tablets, 48% of the angina patients studied by Danahy et al. still exhibited an increase in exercise duration compared to placebo (30). At this time, the resting heart rate was 6.5 beats/minute higher than the placebo heart rate. Therefore, accepting that the drug is clinically effective at this time, on the basis that nearly 50% of the patients are deriving therapeutic benefits, then it could be surmised that an increase in resting heart rate of approximately 10% is an alternate indication of clinical effectiveness. Three hours postdrug, approximately 70% of the patients in the Danahy et al. study had an increased exercise duration, and the corresponding increase in resting heart rate is 10.5 beats/minute; this is an increase of approximately 15% over the placebo control rate.

Although approximately half of the patients still demonstrated clinical drug effects 5 hours after the ISDN tablet dosing, there was no statistically significant difference between the drug treatment and placebo. This is due to the quite large variability inherent in the exercise tolerance data. The digital plethysmography (DPG) diastolic amplitude response—the primary pharmacological response on which to base conclusions in bioavailability studies (43)—is approximately $\frac{1}{3}$ as variable as the exercise tolerance response and $\frac{1}{2}$ as variable as the resting heart rate response. The DPG diastolic amplitude response, which is related to the therapeutic effect of organic nitrate drugs since it reflects a decrease in myocardial energy expenditure resulting from peripheral vasodilation (53), could therefore provide a less variable secondary measure of clinical activity than resting heart rate since fewer subjects are required to demonstrate a statistically significant difference in the clinical activity of oral ISDN 5–6 hours postdrug. Three hours postdrug, the difference between the drug treatment and placebo, based on the exercise tolerance results, is statistically significant ($p<0.01$). A significant difference in the Danahy exercise tolerance data probably also exists 4 hours postdrug, when the increase in resting heart rate is 8.5 beats/minute (12% increase).

If so, it could be concluded that ISDN administered in oral tablets is clinically effective as long as the increase in resting heart rate resulting from the drug exceeds 12% of the placebo resting heart rate.

7. SUMMARY

Hemodynamic response variables provide a sensitive and reliable means for evaluating the comparative bioavailability of organic nitrate dosage forms (3). The use of these pharmacological response variables for bioavailability determinations is analogous to using a nonspecific chemical assay that does not discriminate between the drug and its metabolites, except that the assay sensitivity for each chemical species, and therefore each species' contribution to the assayed body fluid drug levels, is equal to its potency for inducing the measured pharmacological response intensity. Hence, the use of pharmacological data is a measure of the presence of all bioactive chemical entities present at the site(s) of action and contribute to the observed intensity of the measured response. In this way, the use of pharmacological response data for bioavailability studies exactly fulfills the official definition of bioavailability stated in the Federal regulations (3, 48).

The accepted use of secondary measures of hemodynamic response variables, which underlie the clinical activity of organic nitrates, to assess the clinical effectiveness of drug products would allow efficacy judgments to be made from the results of mandatory bioavailability studies on these products (3) at a tremendous saving of expense and effort; the ethical concern in clinical studies of placing patients in need of medication on drug products of unproved effectiveness would also be obviated. In any event, the best that can usually be accomplished in clinical studies is to maintain a record of the frequency of angina attacks and periodically make a few exercise tolerance measurements following dosing. For example, even in the excellent study done by Danahy and coworkers (30), only three sets of exercise tolerance measurements were made in a 5-hour postdrug testing period. Pharmacological data recording permits the measurements to be made nearly continuously and noninvasively, without disturbing the subjects.

REFERENCES

1. Coronary Vasodilator Efficacy. *FDA Drug Bull.*, February, 1972.
2. P. Needleman. Biotransformation of Organic Nitrates. In P. Needleman (ed.), *Organic Nitrates*, Springer-Verlag, New York 1975, p. 57.

3. Department of Health, Education, and Welfare, FDA. Single-entity coronary vasodilators: Drugs for human use; drug efficacy study implementation; permission for drugs to remain on the market; amendment. *Fed. Regist.* **42**:43127 (1977).

4. J. B. McGuinness, T. Semple, M. Van Lith, and R. Vas. Displacement Cardiographic Studies in Ischemic Heart Disease. In R. M. Kenedi (ed.), *Biomedical Engineering*, Macmillan, New York 1972, p. 250.

5. G. C. Gensini, A. E. Kelly, B. C. B. DaCosta, and P. B. Huntington. Quantitative angiography: The measurement of coronary vasomobility in the intact animal and man. *Chest* **60**:522 (1971).

6. A. M. Weissler, R. P. Lewis, and R. F. Leighton. In P. N. Yu and J. F. Goodwin (eds.), *Progress in Cardiology*, Lea and Febiger, Philadelphia, 1972, p. 155.

6. A. M. Weissler, R. P. Lewis, and R. F. Leighton. In P. N. Yu and J. F. Goodwin (eds.), *Progress in Cardiology*, Lea and Febiger, Philadelphia, 1972, p. 155.

7. N. Reichek. Long-acting nitrates in the treatment of angina pectoris. *J.A.M.A.* **236**:1399 (1976).

8. T. J. Sawayama, M. Ochiai, S. Marumoto, T. Matsuura, and I. Niki. Influence of amylnitrite inhalation on the systolic time intervals in normal subjects and in patients with ischemic heart disease. *Cirulation* **40**:327 (1969).

9. J. Y. Wei and P. R. Reid. Quantitative determination of trinitroglycerin in human plasma. *Circulation* **59**:588 (1979).

10. V. F. Smolen, E. J. Williams, and P. B. Kuehn. Bioavailability and pharmacokinetic analysis of chlorpromazine in humans and animals using pharmacological data. *Can. J. Pharm. Sci.* **10**:95 (1975).

11. V. F. Smolen, H. R. Murdock, and E. J. Williams. Bioavailability analysis of chlorpromazine in humans from pupilometric data. *J. Pharmacol. and Exp. Therap.* **195**:404 (1975).

12. V. F. Smolen, H. R. Murdock, Jr. W. P. Stoltman, J. W. Clevenger, L. W. Combs, and E. J. Williams. Pharmacological response data from comparative bioavailability studies of chlorpromazine oral dosage forms in humans: I. Pupilometry. *J. Clin. Pharmacol.* **15**:734 (1975).

13. V. F. Smolen, R. D. Barile, and T. G. Theophanus. Relationship between dose, effect, time, and biophasic drug levels. *J. Pharm. Sci.* **61**:467 (1972).

14. V. F. Smolen. Theoretical and computational basis for drug bioavailability determinations using pharmacological data. I: General considerations and procedures. *J. Pharmacokin. Biopharm.* **4**:337 (1976).

15. V. F. Smolen, P. B. Kuehn, and E. J. Williams. Idealized approach to the optimal design, development, and evaluation of drug delivery systems: I. Drug bioavailability input$\rightleftharpoons$ pharmacological response output relationships. *Drug Dev. Comm.* **1**:143 (1974–75).

16. V. F. Smolen. Bioavailability and pharmacokinetic analysis of drug responding systems. *Ann. Rev. Pharmacol. Toxicol.* **18**:495 (1978).

17. W. S. Aronow. Use of Nitrates as Antianginal Agents. In P. Needleman (ed.), *Organic Nitrates*, Springer-Verlag, New York, 1975, p. 163.

18. H. I. Russek. The therapeutic role of coronary vasodilators: Glyceryl trinitrate, isosorbide dinitrate, and pentaerythritol tetranitrate. *Am. J. Med. Sci.* **252**:9 (1966).

19. S. F. Vatner and X. Hendrick. Mechanism of Action of Nitroglycerin, Coronary, Cardiac, and Systemic Effects. In P. Needleman (ed.), *Organic Nitrates*, Springer-Verlag, New York, 1975, p. 131.

20. V. F. Smolen. Pharmacokinetic Engineering Approach to Drug Delivery System Design and the Optimization of Drug Effects. *IEEE Proc. Int. Conf. Cybern. Soc.*, Washington, D.C., November 1–3, 1976, p. 340.

21. T. Winsor. Effects of Nitrates on the Peripheral Circulation. In G. C. Gensini (ed.), *The Study of Systemic Coronary and Myocardial Effects of Nitrates*, Charles C. Thomas, Springfield, Illinois, 1972, p. 267.

22. D. T. Mason, R. Zelis, and E. A. Amsterdam. Nitroglycerin and the Peripheral Circulation. In G. C. Gensini (ed.), *The Study of Systemic Coronary and Myocardial Effects of Nitrates*, Charles C. Thomas, Springfield, Illinois, 1972, p. 274.

23. C. Cowan, P. Duran, G. Corsini, N. Goldsclager, and R. Bing. The effects of nitroglycerin on myocardial blood flow in man. *Am. J. Cardiol.* **24**:154 (1960).

24. A. Klaus, B. L. Zaret, B. L. Pitt, and R. S. Ross, Comparative evaluation of sublingual long acting nitrates. *Circulation* **48**:519 (1973).

25. T. Winsor. Uber Methoden Zum Studium Antianginoser Wirkstoffe. *Muenchenek Med. Wochenschr. (Munich)* **114**:463 (1972).

26. T. Winsor, H. Kaye, and B. Mills. Hemodynamic response of oral long-acting nitrates: Evidence of gastrointestinal absorption. *Chest* **62**:407 (1972).

27. I. Hirshliefler. Peripheral hemodynamic effects of oral controlled-release nitroglycerin (Nitrong) in man. *Curr. Ther. Res.* **15**:158 (1973).

28. D. T. Mason and E. Braunwald. The effects of nitroglycerin and amyl nitrate on arteriolar and venous tone in the human forearm. *Circulation* **32**:755 (1965).

29. R. D. Allison. Clinical applications of impedance plethysmography. *Clin. Med.* **74**:33 (1967).

30. D. T. Danahy, D. T. Burwell, W. S. Aronow, and R. Prakash. Sustained hemodynamic and antianginal effect of high dose oral isosorbide dinitrate. *Circulation* **55**:381 (1977).

31. M. T. Rosseel and M. G. Bogaert. GLC determination of nitroglycerin and isosorbide in human plasma. *J. Pharm. Sci.* **62**:754 (1973).

32. J. O. Malbica, K. Monson, K. Neilson, and R. Sprissler. Electron-capture GLC determination of nanogram to picogram amounts of isosorbide dinitrate. *J. Pharm. Sci.* **66**:384 (1977).

33. D. F. Assinder, L. F. Chasseaud, and T. Taylor. Plasma isosorbide dinitrate concentrations in human subjects after administration of standard and sustained-release formulations. *J. Pharm. Sci.* **66**:775 (1977).

34. P. Needleman. Biotransformation of organic Nitrates. In P. Needleman (ed.), *Organic Nitrates*, Springer-Verlag, New York, 1975, p. 57.

35. R. E. Goldstein, M. D. Douglas, M. D. Rosine, D. R. Redwood, G. D. Beiser, and S. E. Epstein. Clinical and circulatory effects of isosorbide dinitrate: comparison with nitroglycerin. *Circulation* **43**:629 (1971).

36. V. F. Smolen, and E. J. Williams. Recommended Guidelines and Methodology for the Evaluation of Pharmacological Effectiveness and Comparative Bioavailability of Organic Nitrate Antianginal Drug Products, V. F. Smolen, Project Director Rep. Res. Prog., FDA Contract No. 223-73-3023, *Drug Bioavailability as Related to Physiological Response*, Vol. 1. Submitted to Bureau of Drugs, March 22, 1977.

37. N. Reichek. Long acting nitrates in the treatment of angina pectoris. *J.A.M.A.* **236**:1399 (1976).

38. Drug Efficacy Study: Final Report to the Commissioner of Food and Drugs. National Academy of Sciences, Washington, D.C., 1969, p. 161.

39. J. Abrams. Usefulness of long-acting nitrates in cardiovascular disease (Editorial). *Am. J. Med.* **64**:183 (1978).

40. T. Winsor and H. Berger. Oral nitroglycerin as a prophylactic antianginal drug: Clinical, physiologic evidence of efficacy based on a three-phase experimental design. *Am. Heart J.* **90**:611 (1975).

41. D. A. Chin, D. G. Prue, J. Michelucci, B. T. Kho, and C. R. Warner. Quantitative determination of isosorbide dinitrate and two metabolites in plasma. *J. Pharm. Sci.* **66**:1143 (1977).

42. S. J. Shane, J. J. Iazzetta, A. W. Chisholm, J. F. Berka, and D. Leung. Plasma concentrations of isosorbide dinitrate and its metabolites after chronic high oral dosing. *Br. J. Clin. Pharmacol.* **6**:37 (1978).

43. Food and Drug Administration. Guidelines for Conducting In Vivo Bioavailability Studies on Conventional Release, Chewable, and Controlled Release Coronary Vasodilator Drug Products, July 28, 1977. (Available from Dr. Jerome Skelly, FDA, Pharmacokinetics Branch, HFD-525, 5600 Fishers Lane, Rockville, Maryland 20852).

44. V. F. Smolen. Practical Pharmacodynamic Engineering in the Design–Development and Evaluation of Optimal Drug Products. In A. H. Beckett, H. S. Bean, and J. E. Canless (eds.), *Advances in Pharmaceutical Sciences*, Vol. 5 Academic Press, 1981.

45. I. W. F. Davidson, H. S. Miller, and F. S. Dicarlo. Absorption, excretion and metabolism of pentaerythrytol tetranitrate by humans. *J. Pharm. Sci.* **60**:274 (1971).

46. F. J. Dicarlo, M. C. Crew, L. S. Brusco, and I. W. F. Davidson. Methodology of pentaerythrytol tetranitrate. *Pharmacol. Therap.* **22**:309 (1977).

47. V. F. Smolen and R. E. Hannemann. Bioavailability and pharmacologic activity of oral and topical long-acting nitroglycerin: noninvasive assessment by computerized digital plethysmography. *Clin. Res.* **27**:2 (1979).

48. Department of Health, Educational, and Welfare, FDA. Drug products: Bioequivalence requirements and in-vivo bioavailability procedures. *Fed. Regist.* (Part III) **42**:1624 (1977).

49. M. G. Bogaert, M. T. Roseel, and A. F. de Schaepdryerk. The metabolic rate of nitroglycerin (Trinitrin) in relation to its vascular effects. *Eur. J. Pharmacol.* **12**:224 (1970).

50. P. Needleman. Organic nitrate metabolism. *Ann. Rev. Pharmacol.* **16**:81,(1976).

51. J. C. Parker, F. J. DiCarlo, and I. W. F. Davidson. Comparative vasodilator effects of nitroglycerin pentaerythritol trinitrate and biometabolites and other organic nitrates. *Eur. J. Pharmacol.* **31**:29 (1975).

52. R. L. Wendt. Systemic and coronary vascular effects of the 2- and 5-mononitrate esters of isosorbide dinitrate. *J. Pharmacol Exp. Ther.* **180**:732 (1972).

53. M. G. Bogaert. Organic nitrates in angina pectoris. *Arch. Int. Pharmacodyn. Ther.* **196**:25 (1972).

54. J. C. Krantz, Jr. and C. D. Leake. The gastrointestinal absorption of organic nitrates (Editorial). *Am. J. Cardiol.* **36**:407 (1975).

INDEX